Statistics for Social Science and Public Policy

Statistics for Social Science and Public Policy

Brennan: Generalizability Theory.

Devlin/Fienberg/Resnick/Roeder (Eds.): Intelligence, Genes, and Success: Scientists Respond to *The Bell Curve.*

Finkelstein/Levin: Statistics for Lawyers, Second Edition.

Gastwirth (Ed.): Statistical Science in the Courtroom.

Handcock/Morris: Relative Distribution Methods in the Social Sciences.

Johnson/Albert: Ordinal Data Modeling.

Kolen/Brennan: Test Equating, Scaling, and Linking: Methods and Practices, Second Edition.

Morton/Rolph: Public Policy and Statistics: Case Studies from RAND.

von Davier/Holland/Thayer: The Kernel Method of Test Equating.

van der Linden: Linear Models of Optimal Test Design.

Zeisel/Kaye: Prove It with Figures: Empirical Methods in Law and Litigation.

DeBoeck/Wilson: Explanatory Item Response Models: A Generalized Linear and Nonlinear Approach

Longford: Missing Data and Small-Area Estimation: Modern Analytical Equipment for the Survey Statistician

Nicholas T. Longford

Missing Data and Small-Area Estimation

Modern Analytical Equipment for the Survey Statistician

With 45 Figures

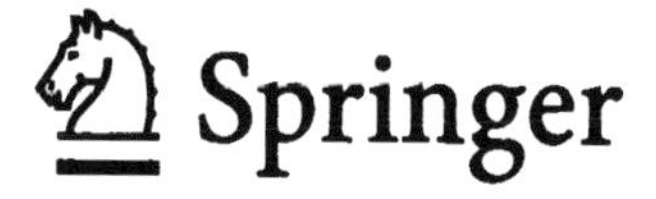

Nicholas T. Longford
SNTL
Oadby, Leicester LE2 5RL
England
NTL@SNTL.co.uk

Library of Congress Cataloging-in-Publication Data
Longford, Nicholas T., 1955–
Modern analytical equipment for the survey statistician : incomplete data and small-area estimation / Nicholas T. Longford.
p. cm. — (Statistics for social science and public policy)
Includes bibliographical references and index.

1. Surveys—Methodology. 2. Social surveys—Methodology. 3. Missing observations (Statistics) 4. Estimation theory. 5. Social sciences—Research—Statistical methods. I. Title. II. Series.
HA31.2.L66 2005
001.4′33—dc22 2005043229

Printed on acid-free paper.

ISBN-13: 978-1-84996-907-9

9 8 7 6 5 4 3 2 1

springeronline.com

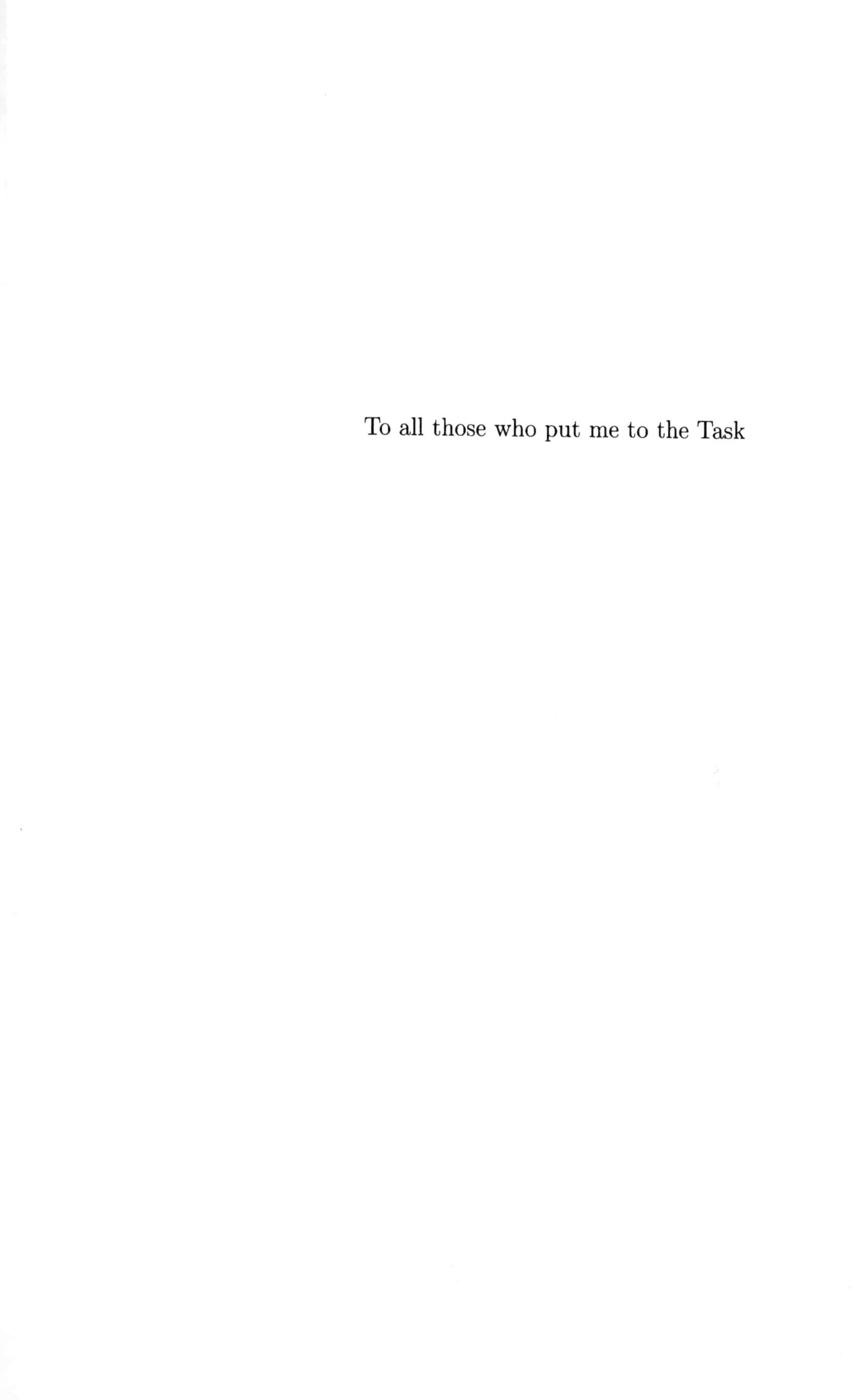

To all those who put me to the Task

Preface

This book evolved from lectures, courses and workshops on missing data and small-area estimation that I presented during my tenure as the first Campion Fellow (2000–2002). For the Fellowship I proposed these two topics as areas in which the academic statistics could contribute to the development of government statistics, in exchange for access to the operational details and background that would inform the direction and sharpen the focus of academic research. After a few years of involvement, I have come to realise that the separation of 'academic' and 'industrial' statistics is not well suited to either party, and their integration is the key to progress in both branches.

Most of the work on this monograph was done while I was a visiting lecturer at Massey University, Palmerston North, New Zealand. The hospitality and stimulating academic environment of their Institute of Information Science and Technology is gratefully acknowledged. I could not name all those who commented on my lecture notes and on the presentations themselves; apart from them, I want to thank the organisers and silent attendees of all the events, and, with a modicum of reluctance, the 'grey figures' who kept inquiring whether I was any nearer the completion of whatever stage I had been foolish enough to attach a date.

The first part of the book deals with analysis of incomplete data. The subject is a must for every survey analyst because large scale surveys without any missing data exist only in textbooks and superficial plans. Although [146] and [233] have exposed the deficiencies of trivial methods for handling incomplete data, they have influenced the practice in official statistics and epidemiology outside U.S.A. only at the margins. I have aimed the presentation at practicing and future survey analysts, setting aside much of the theory, and focussing on the general principles of letting all the substantial sources of uncertainty permeate through the entire estimation process, exploiting all the relevant information about the missing data and challenging the adopted untestable assumptions by sensitivity analysis that plays, within reason, the role of the devil's advocate. The solution, the method of multiple imputation, is respectful of the analyst's work and is built around the methods, tools and software that are well suited, and may have been prepared at some cost, for the ideal complete-data setting.

The subject of the second part is small-area estimation. Although not a concern in every survey, it is becoming a prominent problem in government statistics as clients of established national surveys demand more and more detail about geographical and other divisions of the country, while the survey management is reluctant to conduct more extensive surveys because of escalating costs and increasing rates of nonresponse. Empirical Bayes models are the principal methodological tool at present. I review these methods and develop an approach that relies on a 'good' model much less than model-based methods do, pursuing the creed of making the best of the available information, irrespective of its format or source.

The third part, a single chapter, is a diversion from the focus on survey analysis. It addresses the problem of model uncertainty by drawing on the solution from small-area estimation. In brief, selection (of models, estimators, and the like) is replaced by synthesis, linearly combining estimators or predictors based on alternative models. In the process, I question some of the established wisdoms, such as the finite-sample efficiency of the maximum likelihood estimator and the imperative of basing all inferences on a model judged to be valid by error-prone criteria.

Chapters 5, 10 and 11 directly, and the other chapters indirectly, draw on several publications, some of them written with coauthors. The numerous anonymous referees and journal editors not only helped us to improve the manuscripts but also pointed to aspects and areas in which more rigour and further research was (and in some cases still is) required. I have been tested hardest of all by reactions to the material in Chapter 11. The encouraging comments prevailed, although I may have been a bit too harsh on some of the existing conventions. I want to thank the Editors of the *Journal of the Royal Statistical Society*, *Journal of Official Statistics* and *Statistics in Transition* for their permissions to use material from my publications in their journals.

All the computing described in this book was carried out in `Splus` and `R`. The data analysed in Sections 5 and 10 can be obtained from their original sources; I am not allowed to distribute them, but the code for their analysis as well as for the various illustrations is available from me on request (`NTL@sntl.co.uk`). I hope that the reader will realise early on that a computational and graphical environment in which all the statistical computations can be done and high-quality illustrations drawn as a matter of routine is an essential part of an effective statistician's toolkit. I want to convey my apologies to Grazia Pittau for treating her like a guinea pig in this regard.

Research, on small-area estimation in particular, involved some travel overseas, to NSD, Bergen, Norway; ZA, Cologne, Germany; ZUMA, Mannheim, Germany; and CEPS/INSTEAD, Differdange, Luxembourg. I want to acknowledge the support of the Travel and Mobility of Researchers, a EUROSTAT programme that funded some of this travel and the assistance of the hosts with my research and general well-being. My former employer, De Montfort University, was generous in releasing me, up to a point, on these and other occasions.

I have greatly benefited from consulting engagements with Communities Scotland (formerly Scottish Homes), Edinburgh, and a three-year secondment at the Office for National Statistics, London. Ludi Simpson, by introducing me to a particular problem, and the U.S. National Center for Educational Statistics, by generous research grants, provided impetus that turned my attention to small-area estimation about a decade ago. Don Rubin has been an inexhaustible source of experience and wise advice on anything to do with missing data, and I have caught his incurable virus of multiple imputation.

Jim Ramsay gave me invaluable advice on manuscript preparation; I will not elaborate on the details of which elements I adhered to and which I have failed. Interactions with Albert Satorra have stimulated my interest in some 'missionary' aspects of the statistics profession, which probably come through in the text. Rolling the time back by a decade or two, Murray Aitkin helped to shape my ideas of how and why I want to work as a research statistician, and how this can be enjoyed, by myself and others.

I owe Nathan Jeffery for his competent IT support, on occasions beyond the call of duty. The best testament to the Springer-Verlag team is that this is not my first project with them ([152]).

Leicester, England
February 2005

Nick Longford

Contents

Preface ... VII

Part I Missing data

1 **Prologue** ... 3
1.1 Terminology. Some basics ... 3
1.1.1 Efficiency ... 8
1.1.2 Classes and types of estimators ... 10
1.2 Populations and variables ... 11
1.3 Missing data ... 13
1.4 Suggested reading ... 15
1.5 Exercises ... 16

2 **Describing incompleteness** ... 19
2.1 The problem of incompleteness ... 19
2.2 The extent of missing data and the response pattern ... 22
2.2.1 Monotone response patterns ... 26
2.3 Sampling and nonresponse processes ... 28
2.3.1 The nature of the nonresponse process ... 30
2.3.2 The importance of MAR ... 33
2.4 Exercises ... 34

3 **Single imputation and related methods** ... 37
3.1 Data reduction ... 39
3.2 Data completion ... 40
3.2.1 Mean imputation ... 40
3.2.2 Imputation from another variable ... 41
3.2.3 Nearest-neighbour imputation ... 42
3.2.4 Hot deck ... 43
3.2.5 Weight adjustment ... 44

3.2.6 Regression imputation ... 45
3.2.7 Using experts' judgements ... 47
3.2.8 Data editing ... 48
3.2.9 Single imputation. Summary ... 48
3.3 Models for imputation ... 49
3.3.1 Operating with uncertainty ... 50
3.3.2 Models for the nonresponse process ... 52
3.4 EM algorithm ... 53
3.5 Suggested reading ... 56
3.6 Exercises ... 57

4 Multiple imputation ... 59
4.1 The consequences of imperfect imputation ... 60
4.2 The method ... 61
4.2.1 Fitting a model for missing values ... 61
4.2.2 Generating plausible values ... 62
4.2.3 Analysis of each completed dataset ... 64
4.2.4 The MI estimator ... 64
4.2.5 The lost information ... 64
4.2.6 Assumptions and properties ... 66
4.3 Conditional distributions ... 66
4.3.1 Normally distributed data ... 66
4.3.2 Categorical variables ... 67
4.3.3 Categorical and continuous variables ... 68
4.3.4 Multivariate and multi-stage imputation ... 69
4.3.5 Imputation with monotone response patterns ... 70
4.3.6 The method of chained equations ... 71
4.3.7 From MAR to NMAR models ... 72
4.4 From theory to practice ... 72
4.4.1 Organising MI ... 72
4.4.2 Validity of the assumptions ... 73
4.4.3 MI adaptation of LOCF ... 74
4.4.4 MI-proper hot deck ... 75
4.4.5 Propensity scoring ... 77
4.5 NMAR and sensitivity analysis ... 78
4.6 Other applications of MI ... 79
4.6.1 Measurement error ... 80
4.6.2 Misclassification ... 83
4.6.3 Coarse data and rounding ... 84
4.6.4 Summary ... 92
4.7 Suggested reading ... 93
4.8 Exercises ... 93

5 **Case studies** ... 97
5.1 The UK Labour Force Survey ... 97
5.1.1 From LOCF to hot deck ... 101
5.1.2 Results and discussion ... 104
5.1.3 Imputation for absentees ... 108
5.2 The National Survey of Health and Development ... 110
5.2.1 Eliciting information about alcohol consumption ... 112
5.2.2 Excessive alcohol consumption ... 115
5.2.3 Sensitivity analysis ... 117
5.3 The International Social Survey Programme ... 119
5.3.1 Imputation for 'national identity' items ... 121
5.3.2 Attitudes to immigration ... 124
5.3.3 Sensitivity analysis ... 127
5.4 The Scottish House Condition Survey ... 130
5.4.1 Missing information ... 133
5.4.2 Estimating the misclassification probabilities ... 135
5.4.3 Generating plausible scores ... 137
5.5 Suggested reading. Software ... 138

Part II Small-area estimation

6 **Introduction** ... 143
6.1 Preliminaries ... 146
6.2 Choosing the estimator ... 149
6.2.1 Uniform choice ... 149
6.2.2 Tailored choice ... 150
6.3 Composition ... 151
6.3.1 Combining the district-level means ... 157
6.3.2 Suboptimal composition ... 159
6.4 Estimating the district-level variance ... 160
6.4.1 The sampling variance of $\hat{\theta}_d$ ... 161
6.4.2 The impact of uncertainty about σ_{B}^2 ... 164
6.5 Spatial similarity ... 167
6.6 Suggested reading ... 169
6.7 Exercises ... 170

7 **Models for small areas** ... 173
7.1 Analysis of variance ... 173
7.2 Auxiliary information ... 176
7.2.1 Several covariates ... 178
7.2.2 Two-level models and small-area estimation ... 181
7.3 Computational procedures ... 182
7.3.1 Restricted maximum likelihood ... 186
7.3.2 Implementing ML and REML ... 188

7.3.3 Computational issues ... 189
7.4 Model selection issues ... 192
7.4.1 Residuals and model diagnostics ... 195
7.5 District-level models ... 197
7.6 Generalised linear models ... 200
7.6.1 Two-level GLMs ... 202
Appendix. The REML adjustment of the Hessian ... 203
7.7 Suggested reading ... 204
7.8 Exercises ... 205

8 Using auxiliary information ... 207
8.1 From models to small-area estimates ... 208
8.1.1 Synthetic estimation ... 208
8.2 Composite estimation ... 212
8.2.1 Shrinkage and borrowing strength ... 214
8.3 Multivariate composition ... 215
8.3.1 How to choose $\mathbf{x}$? ... 217
8.3.2 Estimating $\boldsymbol{\Sigma}_{\mathrm{B}}$ ... 219
8.4 Applications ... 220
8.4.1 Related variables in a survey ... 220
8.4.2 Estimation for several subpopulations ... 221
8.4.3 Estimating compositions ... 223
8.4.4 Survey and register ... 224
8.4.5 Historical data as auxiliary information ... 226
8.4.6 Summary. Using all the relevant information ... 228
8.5 Planning and design for small-area estimation ... 229
8.5.1 Optimal design for the composite estimator ... 231
8.5.2 Variable subsample sizes and several divisions ... 234
8.6 Suggested reading ... 235
8.7 Exercises ... 236

9 Using small-area estimators ... 239
9.1 Non-linear transformations of the estimates ... 239
9.1.1 How important is bias? ... 241
9.2 Ranking and ordering ... 241
9.2.1 Inference about selected districts ... 244
9.3 Estimating many variances and precisions ... 246
9.3.1 Estimated or guessed variance ratio ... 248
9.3.2 Estimating precisions ... 252
9.4 Suggested reading ... 254
9.5 Exercises ... 254

10 Case studies 257
10.1 The UK Labour Force Survey 257
10.1.1 Multivariate shrinkage 262
10.1.2 Distribution of district-level rates 268
10.1.3 Estimation for age-by-sex subpopulations 271
10.1.4 Pooling information across time 274
10.2 Samples of Anonymised Records 276
10.3 Norwegian municipalities 282
10.3.1 Composition of the labour force by industrial sectors 289
10.4 The Scottish House Condition Survey 291
10.4.1 Estimation for subpopulations 296
10.5 Suggested reading 297

Part III Combining estimators

11 Model selection 303
11.1 The problem 303
11.1.1 EM algorithm 307
11.1.2 Example 308
11.2 Why model selection fails 310
11.2.1 Limitations of model selection 311
11.3 Synthetic estimation 313
11.3.1 One submodel 314
11.4 Analysis of variance 316
11.4.1 Minimax estimation 318
11.4.2 Estimating σ_{W}^2 319
11.4.3 Estimated coefficient $\hat{b}^*$ 321
11.4.4 Simulations 322
11.4.5 ANOVA with random effects 323
11.5 Ordinary regression 325
11.5.1 Estimating σ^2 326
11.5.2 Several covariates 327
11.6 Discussion 329
11.7 Other applications of synthesis 331
11.7.1 Meta-analysis 331
11.7.2 Multiple sources and prior information 332
11.7.3 Secondary outcomes and auxiliary information 333
11.8 Suggested reading 334
11.9 Exercises 334

References 337

Index 353

Part I

Missing data

1

Prologue

I hope it's not gone missing completely.

This chapter introduces the basic terminology related to survey sampling and estimation. It is used in all three parts of the book, but it is not the universally adopted terminology in the statistical literature.

1.1 Terminology. Some basics

The purpose of a survey is to enable making inferences about a domain or *population.* A population is a well-defined collection of units; any entity can be classified without ambiguity as to whether it belongs to (is a *member* of) a specified population or not. A *variable*, defined for a population, is specified by its value for each member of the population. A standard task is to estimate the mean of a variable in a population. This *population quantity* could be established with precision if the exact value of the variable were elicited from each member of the population. A more practical alternative, requiring much more modest resources (time, manpower, funds, good will of the respondents, and the like), is to *estimate* this value. The population quantity is estimated from a *sample* of subjects drawn from the population. The sample is drawn by a *sampling design*, denoted by π. It is a probabilistic prescription for how to obtain a sample. Formally, the sampling design is defined as a function that assigns to each subset of the population the probability that it would form the sample. For a large population, comprising millions of subjects, listing each subset and the corresponding probability is not feasible. Although most subsets have zero probability of forming a sample, the number of possible samples is usually still very large. In most settings, it is practical to describe the sampling design by a mechanism for drawing the sample; listing each possible sample and the associated probability is not a practical proposition.

For example, the simple random sampling design without replacement is aptly described by its name or by the following mechanism: draw a member of the population, and then keep drawing one member at a time from the pool of members who have not been drawn before. The draws are mutually independent and in each draw every candidate member of the population has the same probability of being included. Let N be the *population size* (the number of members of the population). In draw k, the probability of drawing a member of the population who has not yet been included in the sample is $1/(N-k+1)$. The number of subjects in the sample is called the *sample size* and is denoted by n. The sample size may be fixed — all the subsets that have positive probabilities have the same size n. Otherwise the sample size is said to be random and is described by the *distribution* of sample size.

The members of a population are usually related and the relationships define a structure. For instance, the members may be organised in clusters, and the clusters may be further clustered, so that there are clusters at several levels. A familiar example of such a structure are (human) subjects within households, households within postcodes (such as LE2 5YL in the UK), postcodes within postal sectors (LE2), and so on. It is meaningful to define the population size for each level of clustering, denoted by $N^{(1)} = N$ for the members (units at the elementary level, or elements), $N^{(2)}$ for clusters at level 2, $\ldots$, $N^{(L)}$ for clusters at level L. Sample sizes at the various levels of clustering are defined similarly; a cluster is counted if it is represented in the sample by at least one member.

The sample is a set of subjects. The order in which the subjects are drawn is unimportant. A subject may be included in the sample several times. The number of inclusions (*multiplicity*) distinguishes samples. Thus, for distinct elements a_1, a_2 and a_3, (a_1, a_2, a_3) and (a_1, a_3, a_2) are identical samples, whereas (a_1, a_2, a_2) and (a_1, a_1, a_2) are not. A sampling mechanism that describes the formation of a sample by including one element at a time is said to be without replacement if no member can be included in the sample more than once; the multiplicity of each member is either zero or one. Otherwise the mechanism is called with replacement. For example, in simple random sampling without replacement there are $C_n^N = \frac{N!}{(N-n)!n!}$ possible samples, each with the same probability $1/C_n^N$, whereas in simple random sampling without replacement there are $(N+n)!/n!$ distinct possible samples, but their probabilities are not equal.

We distinguish *population quantities* — values that could be established if the entire population were enumerated (if the requisite values were available for each member of the population), and *sample quantities* — values that depend only on the units included in the sample. Sample quantities are also referred to as *statistics*. A population quantity μ is estimated by a sample quantity $\hat{\mu}$. A good choice of $\hat{\mu}$ is such that $|\hat{\mu} - \mu|$ is small, in the sense to be defined. The quantity μ is referred to as the *target*, and $\hat{\mu}$ as estimate or estimator; we draw a distinction between the latter two terms below.

We assume that the studied population is *frozen*, undergoing no changes while being studied. Therefore, the target μ is fixed. In contrast, the value of $\hat{\mu}$ depends on the sample drawn (the *realised* sample). Therefore, we cannot measure the proximity of $\hat{\mu}$ to μ simply by the difference $\hat{\mu} - \mu$, its absolute value, ratio, or the like. In most settings, μ is not known; otherwise there is no rationale for conducting a survey to estimate it.

A sample quantity has two forms. Prior to drawing a sample, it is a random variable, as its value depends on the vagaries of the sampling process. Once a sample is drawn, it is a constant. We draw a similar distinction between estimators and estimates. An estimator is a random variable, usually given as a formula, a computational procedure, or a software programme that assigns a value for every conceivable sample. An estimate is the value of the estimator applied to the realised sample. Prior to drawing a sample, we consider estimators — we plan and implement procedures for processing the data to be collected. When the sample is available we submit the collected data to these procedures (estimators) and obtain their values, estimates.

Being objects of different types, estimators and estimates have very different attributes. The attributes of an estimate are, for example, its sign, being a rational number and whether it exceeds a particular constant. The attributes (properties) of an estimator require much more careful definitions.

The principal conceptual device for assessing the properties of an estimator is *replication*, defined as the act of repeating a process independently from its previous applications. The results of replications are called *replicates.* A replication of the sampling design yields, in general, a different sample, because the outcome of drawing a sample is subject to chance. In most contexts, replication is a theoretical concept, because there is no intention to conduct it in practice, even when it is physically possible. Usually, resources, or other circumstances, do not allow any replication, and the sampling design is applied only once, to obtain the realised sample.

Suppose a large number H of replications is conducted for a particular sampling (data-generating) process followed by evaluation of an estimator $\hat{\mu}$, that is, by applying an estimation process. The result of this exercise is a set of H estimates $\hat{\mu}_h$, $h = 1, \ldots, H$, values of the estimator $\hat{\mu}$. Loosely speaking, an estimator of a given target μ is regarded as good if the values $\hat{\mu}_h$ are tightly clustered around the target. As a standard, the *mean squared error* (MSE) is used for assessing the quality of $\hat{\mu}$ as an estimator of μ; it is defined as

$$\frac{1}{H} \sum_{h=1}^{H} \left(\hat{\mu}_h - \mu \right)^2$$

or, more precisely, as the limit of this expression when H grows over all bounds, that is, as $H \rightarrow \infty$. This limit is denoted by $\mathrm{MSE}(\hat{\mu};\, \mu)$. The second argument of MSE, the target μ, is usually dropped, but this is appropriate only when the target is obvious from the context. An estimator may be quite good for one target and poor for another. A more rigorous notation for MSE includes the sampling design as another argument, that is, $\mathrm{MSE}(\hat{\theta};\, \theta, \pi)$.

The *bias* of an estimator, denoted by $\mathrm{B}(\hat{\mu};\, \mu)$, is defined as the limit of the difference

$$\frac{1}{H}\sum_{h=1}^{H}\hat{\mu}_h - \mu\,.$$

It is a measure of the tendency to exceed or fall short of the target. Just like MSE, the bias also depends on the sampling design. The expectation of an estimator is defined as the average of its values in an (infinite) sequence of replications,

$$\frac{1}{H}\sum_{h=1}^{H}\hat{\mu}_h\,;$$

note its relation to the bias. The expectation of $\hat{\mu}$ is denoted by $\mathrm{E}(\hat{\mu})$, so $\mathrm{B}(\hat{\mu};\,\mu) = \mathrm{E}(\hat{\mu}) - \mu$ and

$$\mathrm{MSE}(\hat{\mu};\,\mu) \;=\; \mathrm{E}\left\{(\hat{\mu}-\mu)^2\right\}\,.$$

The variance of an estimator or, more generally, of a statistic $\hat{\mu}$ is defined as

$$\mathrm{var}(\hat{\mu}) \;=\; \mathrm{E}\left[\{\hat{\mu}-\mathrm{E}(\hat{\mu})\}^2\right]\,.$$

It is a measure of the dispersion of $\hat{\mu}$, without a reference to a target. It is easy to derive the identity

$$\mathrm{MSE}(\hat{\mu};\,\mu) \;=\; \mathrm{var}(\hat{\mu}) + \{\mathrm{B}(\hat{\mu};\,\mu)\}^2\,, \qquad (1.1)$$

for example, by using the finite-replication expressions for the variance and bias. The two components of MSE in (1.1), the dispersion and bias (squared), represent the respective haphazard (non-systematic) and systematic components of the estimation error $\hat{\mu}-\mu$. We should strive to reduce both of them, but reducing one at the expense of the other is not always useful. For illustration, suppose the target, unknown to the analyst, is $\mu = 7$. One estimator is unbiased, taking on values around 0 and 14, with equal probabilities (frequencies), whereas the other estimator yields values between 6.25 and 6.75, and so is biased. In this case, the biased estimator is far superior, because any of its realisations is much closer to the target than any realisation of the unbiased but large-variance estimator. Figure 1.1 illustrates the two estimators by their histograms. The estimators are represented by 2000 values each. The widths of the bars in the histograms are 0.25.

The *standard error* is defined as the square root of the MSE. (It is also called the root-mean squared error, or rMSE.) Its value is easier to interpret because it is on the same scale and is expressed in the same units as the estimate and the target.

A more detailed description of an estimator is by its *distribution*. The distribution characterises the frequency of the possible values in replications. The distribution function of an estimator is defined as the probability that the estimator's value is not greater than a given threshold:

Figure 1.1. A large-variance unbiased and a small-variance biased estimator of the same target T, marked by vertical dashes.

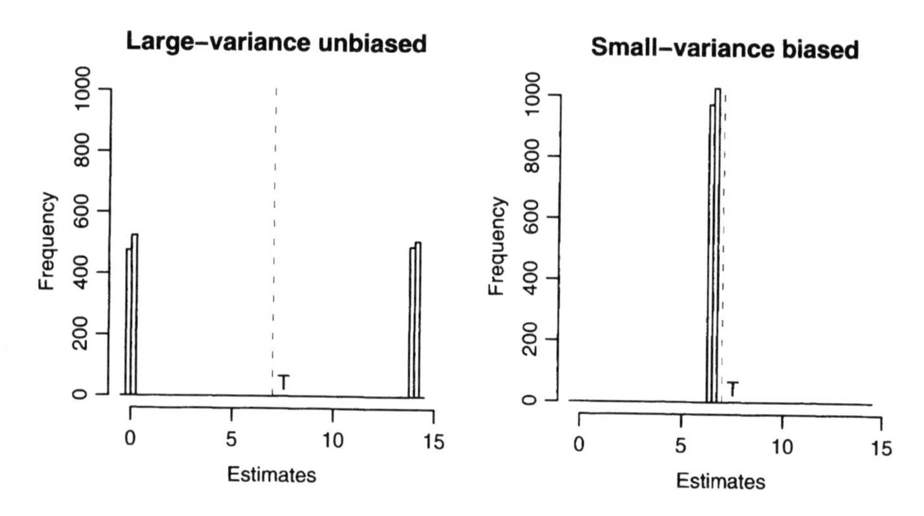

$$F_{\hat{\mu}}(x) = \mathrm{P}(\hat{\mu} \le x)\,,$$

for $-\infty < x < +\infty$. The probability is interpreted as the frequency of the event that $\hat{\mu} \le x$ in a large number of replications. When this function is differentiable (absolutely continuous), its derivative, $f_{\hat{\mu}}(x) = \partial F_{\hat{\mu}}(x)/\partial x$, is called the *density*. The histograms in Figure 1.1, after a suitable rescaling, approximate the densities of the corresponding distributions.

MSE and standard error are examples of *sampling-process quantities*. They refer to the sample as a random object (prior to its realisation) and can be established by replications of the sampling process. The distribution of any estimator or its summary are sampling-process quantities. Such a summary usually has to be estimated from a single sample.

Many commonly encountered estimators are unbiased and have (approximately) normal distributions; in notation,

$$\hat{\mu} \sim \mathcal{N}(\mu, \sigma^2_{\hat{\mu}})\,. \tag{1.2}$$

A normal distribution is given by its mean μ and variance σ^2. Subscripts of μ and σ^2 may indicate the relevant statistic, although $\mu_{\hat{\mu}}$ may appear too pedantic. The density of the normal distribution is

$$\phi_{\hat{\mu}}(x) = \frac{1}{\sigma_{\hat{\mu}}\sqrt{2\pi}} \exp\left\{ -\frac{(x-\mu)^2}{2\sigma^2_{\hat{\mu}}} \right\},$$

and its distribution function is given by the integral

$$\Phi_{\hat{\mu}}(x) = \int_{-\infty}^{x} \phi_{\hat{\mu}}(x) \mathrm{d}x \,.$$

The normal distribution with zero mean and unit variance, $\mathcal{N}(0,1)$, is called the *standard normal*, and its distribution function and density are denoted by Φ and ϕ, respectively. If $\hat{\mu} \sim \mathcal{N}(\mu, \sigma^2)$, then $(\hat{\mu} - \mu)/\sigma \sim \mathcal{N}(0,1)$. Their distribution functions and densities are related by the respective identities

$$\Phi_{\hat{\mu}}(x) = \Phi\left(\frac{\hat{\mu} - \mu}{\sigma}\right)$$

$$\phi_{\hat{\mu}}(x) = \frac{1}{\sigma}\phi\left(\frac{\hat{\mu} - \mu}{\sigma}\right) .$$

A *confidence interval* for a population quantity μ is defined as an interval delimited by sample quantities, $\hat{\mu}_{\mathrm{L}}$ and $\hat{\mu}_{\mathrm{U}}$, such that it contains the target μ with a probability equal to or exceeding a prescribed value:

$$\mathrm{P}(\hat{\mu}_{\mathrm{L}} < \mu < \hat{\mu}_{\mathrm{U}}) \geq 1 - \alpha \,, \tag{1.3}$$

where α is a small number. A conventional choice for α is 0.05. The (sample) quantities $\hat{\mu}_{\mathrm{L}}$ and $\hat{\mu}_{\mathrm{U}}$ are called the *lower* and *upper confidence limits*, respectively. Narrower confidence intervals are in general preferred, so long as the coverage rate, the probability in (1.3), is at least $1 - \alpha$. The probability may exceed $1 - \alpha$. In that case, we *could have* claimed that the confidence interval $(\hat{\mu}_{\mathrm{L}}\,;\, \hat{\mu}_{\mathrm{U}})$ has a greater coverage, but by failing to do so we merely under-rate the quality of our 'product'. Over-rating it, when the claimed coverage rate is not achieved, is not regarded as a good practice and could be viewed as a form of statistical 'dishonesty'.

A confidence interval for μ in (1.3) is obtained by inverting (1.2), that is, by solving it for μ. The solution is not unique, but the solution

$$\hat{\mu}_{\mathrm{L}} = \hat{\mu} + \hat{\sigma}_{\hat{\mu}}\Phi^{-1}(\alpha/2) \qquad \hat{\mu}_{\mathrm{U}} = \hat{\mu} + \hat{\sigma}_{\hat{\mu}}\Phi^{-1}(1 - \alpha/2)$$

is often preferred because it is symmetric around the estimator $\hat{\mu}$. Another solution is

$$\hat{\mu}_{\mathrm{L}} = -\infty \qquad \hat{\mu}_{\mathrm{U}} = \hat{\mu} + \hat{\sigma}_{\hat{\mu}}\Phi^{-1}(1 - \alpha) \,.$$

These confidence intervals involve approximations because an estimator $\hat{\sigma}_{\hat{\mu}}$ is used instead of the underlying standard deviation $\sigma_{\hat{\mu}}$. The approximation is usually close whenever $\hat{\mu}$ is based on many observations. Otherwise the t-distribution is applicable.

1.1.1 Efficiency

The principal difficulty faced by an analyst is not the implementation (evaluation) of estimators, but their choice — identifying the estimator best suited for a given target. The circumstances that make this choice difficult are that the properties of the estimators are not known (recall that we cannot afford any replications that would establish them), or are known only partially, subject to assumptions, some of which cannot be verified or about which we are not certain whether they apply. In practice, the properties themselves are estimated, so they may not be established with perfect precision. Then the choice of the estimator is also subject to uncertainty. Most properties of a typical estimator also depend on the sampling design.

In a typical report of an analysis, the estimate (the value of the estimator selected for an a priori specified target) is usually accompanied by its *estimated* standard error. The qualifier 'estimated' is usually omitted; this is not a good practice if the reported quantity is thereafter treated as a known sampling-process quantity.

An estimator $\hat{\mu}_1$ is said to be *more efficient* than estimator $\hat{\mu}_2$ for estimating a target μ if

$$\mathrm{MSE}(\hat{\mu}_1\,;\,\mu) \;<\; \mathrm{MSE}(\hat{\mu}_2\,;\,\mu)\,.$$

The MSE may depend on some unknown (population) quantities, so one estimator may be more efficient than another for certain values of these quantities. One estimator is said to be *uniformly more efficient* than another if it is more efficient for any set of these quantities. We prefer more efficient estimators because, *on average*, they are closer to the target than less efficient estimators. Two estimators based on a single sample are difficult to compare when their MSEs can only be estimated. An estimator that is more efficient than any other estimator for the same target is said to be efficient for that target (without any qualification). Such efficiency may be qualified as applicable within a class of estimators or for a specific single or a class of sampling designs.

An estimator may be efficient for one target and less efficient for another. For example, the sample mean of a variable recorded by a survey may be an efficient estimator of the national mean of that variable, but may be less efficient for estimating the mean of the variable for a given region, or for the mean of a related variable that has not been recorded by the survey.

It is meaningful to compare the MSEs of two estimators only when they refer to the same target. Properties of estimators depend on the sampling design. For a given sampling design, we may wish to identify the efficient estimator of a particular target. At the planning stage, we may be looking for a sampling design that enables the most efficient estimation of a target. For each candidate design we may identify the efficient estimator. In this setting, it is meaningful to compare estimators under different designs, but they have to be aiming at the same target.

Suppose estimator $\hat{\mu}$ is efficient for μ. Then a linear transformation of μ, namely $a + b\mu$, is efficiently estimated by the same linear transformation of $\hat{\mu}$, $a + b\hat{\mu}$, and $\mathrm{MSE}(a + b\hat{\mu};\, a + b\mu) = b^2\mathrm{MSE}(\hat{\mu};\, \mu)$. However, a non-linear transformation of an efficient estimator is usually not an efficient estimator of the same transformation of the target. A linear transformation of an unbiased estimator, say $a + b\hat{\mu}$, is unbiased for the same transformation of the target, $a + b\mu$; $\mathrm{E}(a + b\hat{\mu}) = a + b\mu$ if $\mathrm{E}(\hat{\mu}) = \mu$. But a non-linear transformation, say $g(\hat{\mu})$, may be biased for the same transformation of the target, $g(\mu)$. A simple example can be constructed using the inequality

$$\mathrm{E}(\hat{\mu}^2) > \{\mathrm{E}(\hat{\mu})\}^2 .$$

In fact, μ^2 is estimated without bias by $\hat{\mu}^2 - \hat{\sigma}^2_{\hat{\mu}}$, where $\hat{\mu}$ and $\hat{\sigma}^2_{\hat{\mu}}$ are unbiased estimators of μ and $\sigma^2_{\hat{\mu}}$, respectively. Suppose that the population mean μ is close to zero. Then $\hat{\mu}^2$ is less efficient for μ^2 than $\hat{\mu}^2 - \hat{\sigma}^2_{\hat{\mu}}$ or $\left(\hat{\mu}^2 - \hat{\sigma}^2_{\hat{\mu}}\right)_+$, its value truncated to be non-negative.

1.1.2 Classes and types of estimators

Suppose the surveyed country comprises a number of regions denoted by $k = 1, \ldots, K$, and the mean of a variable X is to be estimated for each region. An estimator, such as the sample mean, is applied to every region. The properties of the estimator, denoted by $\hat{\mu}_k$, usually differ from region to region. In this context, we refer to the pair $(\hat{\mu}_k, k)$ for a given region k as an estimator, and to the collection of these region-specific estimators as an *estimator type*. More generally, when considering the analysis of a collection of datasets using the same method or approach, each dataset is associated with an estimator (its distribution, and the like) and the term estimator type refers to what these estimators have in common; for instance, that they are derived by ordinary regression with a given set of covariates.

Since an estimator type involves several estimators, comparing estimator types is not straightforward. Two estimator types are said to be *compatible* if they have the same sets of targets. One estimator type is uniformly more efficient than another if the two types are compatible and the estimator of the former type is more efficient than the corresponding estimator of the latter type for each target.

Uniform efficiency of an estimator type is a rather rare property. Usually an estimator type is more efficient for some and less efficient for other targets than a compatible estimator type. In such a setting, we have to define a criterion for regarding an estimator type as superior (more efficient on average). An obvious proposal is to compare the totals of the MSEs, and give preference to the type with the lower total. More appropriate criteria take into account our (our clients') preferences. For example, if a certain precision is imperative for estimating each target, then the estimator type with the higher number of sufficiently precise estimators is preferred. Satisfying the precision threshold may be more important for some targets than for others; then each target can be associated with a weight. The total of the MSEs may also involve these weights. Further flexibility is afforded by considering (weighted) totals of a monotone transformation of the MSEs.

An estimator type may be related to several variables by a model. The details of the specification of this model define different estimators. The collection of such estimators is called an *estimator class*. For example, without specifying the covariates and other details, estimators based on a linear regression model that use the regression parameter estimates in a particular way form a class of estimators. Maximum likelihood estimators are another general class of estimators.

1.2 Populations and variables

Statistics as a scientific discipline and a profession encompasses a wide range of activities that defy a simple delineating description or definition. In any case, there is no consensus on what constitutes a statistical activity. For the setting of this monograph, we propose the following characterisation. Statistics is the scientific discipline concerned with making statements about populations based on their incomplete observations. The term *population* stands for a collection of units (subjects) that are of interest. A variable is a function, an assignment of a value to each member of the population. The population of interest is characterised by one or several summaries of the values of a variable in a population. Examples of such (univariate) summaries are the mean, median, mode (the most frequently occuring value), a percentile and the variance. If the value of the variable were recorded for every subject in the population, evaluation of any summary would be straightforward. Statistical methods address the problem of *making inferences* about such summaries when the variable in the population is observed *incompletely*. Complete (and perfect) observation of the entire population is referred to as *enumeration*. Examples of incompleteness are observations on only some members of the population and observations that are affected by imperfections in the process of recording (measuring, eliciting, or transcribing) the values of the variable. This makes sampling on the one hand, and measurement error and misclassification on the other, key themes in statistics.

As an alternative, a population can be defined by a rule that arbitrates about any conceivable entity whether it is a member of the population or not. We emphasize that two populations are regarded as distinct even when they have a substantial overlap. The rules specifying their membership differ. Similarly, two variables coincide only if they are defined for the same population and their respective values coincide for each member of the population. In particular, a variable may have several versions, such as an ideal (*latent*) version, defined conceptually, and a recorded (*manifest*) version obtained by the application of a specific instrument. For example, the ability of students in a particular population and a particular subject area is a latent variable and the results of a test or examination are its manifest version. A latent variable may have numerous manifest versions.

Making inferences means making guesses about the unknown value of the summary, based on the available values (data) and the processes applied in their collection. The guesses may be in the form of a value (estimate), a range of plausible values (confidence regions) or any other interpretable format. Such statements are, however, only intermediate to making decisions that would have been relatively easy to make had the population been enumerated. Inferences can be regarded as attempts at undoing the inadequacies of the observations: not collecting the information from every member of the population and, when collecting it, not doing so accurately.

The principal reasons for these inadequacies are limited resources and unavailability of the members of the population or their unwillingness to cooperate with the data collection effort. Given its inevitability, the statistician's task is to limit its impact. The main principle in this is to exercise control, or at least have an understanding of the processes involved: sampling and imperfect measurement. For sampling, a sampling design is specified, and so the process, if perfectly implemented, is known and under our control. The imperfection of the measurement can be studied outside the confines of collecting the survey data, although it is essential to set the measurement or observation in the same context, and apply it in the same population. If the 'ideal' value of a variable on a subject can be established, then the measurement by the adopted method can be compared with it in a straightforward manner to assess the extent of the deviation. When the 'ideal' value cannot be established, replications of the measurement on subjects inform us about the level of (within-subject) variation. This is one component of the imperfection in measurement; the other, systematic deviations (biases), cannot be estimated without collecting some additional information, perhaps using more sensitive (and expensive) instruments or procedures.

The measurement process is described by the conditional distribution of the observed value X given the ideal value X^*. Of interest is the conditional distribution with the roles of the two variables interchanged: X^* given X. The two probabilities are related by the Bayes theorem

$$\mathrm{P}(X^* = k \,|\, X = h) = \frac{\mathrm{P}(X = h \,|\, X^* = k)\mathrm{P}(X^* = k)}{\mathrm{P}(X = h)}, \qquad (1.4)$$

for discrete variables, and a similar expression, with probability P replaced by density f, for absolutely continuous variables. Note that the marginal probabilities for X and X^* are factors in (1.4), so care has to be exercised in extrapolating inferences about the distribution $(X^* \,|\, X)$ from one population to another.

1.3 Missing data

In plain language, missing data refers to the difference between the data we planned to collect and what we have managed to collect. The plan may be a genuine or a fictional one. An example of a genuine plan is the intention of a typical survey to collect the precise values of a list of variables from each subject in a sample drawn from a specified population by a specified sampling design, such as simple random sampling. Some subjects in the sample refuse any cooperation outright; they are total non-respondents. Others may fail to respond to some of the questions, for a variety of reasons and motives. The subjects may find the experience of responding burdensome, may be unwilling or unable to recover the requested information from their records (or recall or reconstruct it from memory), may not know the answer, may find the question embarrassing, or may be unwilling to carry on with the interview any longer for a multitude of reasons — obvious, inexplicable, disclosed to the interviewer, or neither. Further losses of data may occur in its transfer and transcription to the electronic medium, and in its further processing.

An example of a fictional plan is to collect information about subjects' long-term diet. The unattainable ideal is to record with precision the quantities of all components of food (nutrients, such as protein, cholesterol, carbohydrates, starch, and vitamins) for a random sample of subjects over a period of several years. These quantities are required for studying how the incidence of certain medical conditions is related to the long-term diet. The best that can be expected of the selected subjects is that they keep diaries of all the food and drink they consume over a week, with some indication of quantity of each item. For a diligently completed diary, the missing data in this context would be the diary for all the other weeks of the subject's (adult) life. So, most of the data is missing. However, the diary for a week informs us quite well about certain targets, because subjects do not alter their diets radically from one week to the next in any systematic way, perhaps with the exception of major holidays. In a completed diary for one of the 2600 weeks of a 50-year-old subject, we have collected much more than one 2600th part of the desired information. Information cannot be 'weighed' by the number of digits, kilobytes of data or quantity of ink used. A more subtle scale, tailored to our needs, is defined by the quality of the resulting inferences, assuming that we do our best with the data in our possession.

Resources (funding, available staff, time in which the survey has to be completed), are usually insufficient to locate and interview every member of the surveyed population. We may regard as missing data all the information that would have been collected if the survey interview had been conducted with every member of the population and if all of them had disclosed every detail relevant to the studied subject matter, and if all the collected details were recorded in the database used in the subsequent analyses. This indicates that we have a considerable freedom in what we declare as missing data. We should handle this self-granted responsibility with care. Less missing data is better than more, but pretending that we have none, ignoring the imperfections in the data collection and processing, is not appropriate either.

Possession of expertise and ability to deal with missing data is by no means a licence to neglect efforts aimed at reducing the extent of missing data. The best methods, even with the anticipation of new developments in statistical analysis, will never make up for the losses due to nonresponse and reasons for failure to collect all the planned data. All such methods should be regarded as a form of statistical damage control, or as statistical 'fire-fighting' equipment. Apart from attending to all emergencies, promptly and well equipped, a responsible fire-fighter studies and implements preventive measures. In that respect, less work at the frontline is better business. Other professions adhere to a similar creed. Avoiding emergency surgery by encouraging safer everyday conduct and healthier lifestyle is an integral part of a good health care system. The quality of legal advice is measured not by the number or rate of legal suits and trials won, but by the quantity and extent of adversarial confrontation that is avoided.

In summary, we should not look for missing data where there is none, but have our equipment for dealing with it in good working order when its use can reasonably be expected to be constructive, and appreciate, encourage and contribute to the effort of reducing the extent of missing data and its impact on the quality of the inferences made. Similar standards are difficult to formulate for statistics in general. Much of the output of academic statisticians focusses on illustrating novel methods, new uses of established methods, and deriving optimal solutions. Often the questions are grafted onto the solution, to appeal to artificial scenarios. In this monograph, we attempt to distance ourselves from this mode of operation by considering examples with inflexibly stated questions, by clients who have firmly set agendas. These are the principal motives for conducting the surveys analysed in the examples in Chapters 5 and 10.

Other things being equal, simpler solutions are preferred because they are easier to understand, adapt to changed circumstances, and are often laden with fewer caveats. Complexity is unavoidable when simple solutions are far from optimal. We should have a comprehensive tool kit, with all the tricks and intricate equipment, but pick the simplest tools that do the job.

Most analytical tools, for estimation and other forms of statistical inference, assume that the data are in a prescribed format and have no imperfections. Some forms of missing data are a kind of imperfection that either disable the routine application of a method, or bring the assumptions underlying the implemented method into question. The responses to and resolutions of such problems can range from a quick fix that disregards its consequences to a complete turnabout in the goals of the analysis — from the substance (the original purpose of the survey) to the study of a *nuisance* (missing values, an undesirable phenomenon) that has a parasitic existence in all large-scale data collection exercises. And, insufficient quality of the data may be regarded as a respectable excuse for abandoning the analysis altogether.

The attitude promoted in this monograph is that missing data or, more generally, *messy* data, is a respectable subject in statistics, and essential in a wide range of contexts. The respect is derived from its potential to contribute to the general goals of statistics — promoting scientific endeavour in all fields where incomplete data (information) is encountered. The subject is essential because it addresses a ubiquitous feature of large-scale survey databases and other data collections and contributes to the quality and credibility of the inferences. Statistical research and practice provide numerous theoretical and empirical examples of inferences that are misleading and deceptive because of a superficial treatment of missing data.

The main themes in studying messy data are: understanding the processes that generate the 'mess' (nonresponse, measurement error, misclassification, rounding, and the like) and collecting information about them, making provisions to do the best that can be done with the data at hand, without compromising the general goals of efficient inference and unbiased (honest) assessment of its quality, and contributing to the design of studies in which mess can be expected. With messy data, the confidence should be reduced as compared to the hypothetical data that would have contained no mess. Such a reduction in the assessed confidence should be indicated in the conclusions of the analysis. Otherwise, the analyst achieves a temporary kudos because greater confidence is always desired. However, if the confidence is not justified the kudos may soon be deflated and the purpose of the whole analytical enterprise compromised because a different decision might have been made if the confidence were assessed with greater 'honesty'.

In this respect, the subject of missing data is not for the researcher who has to deal with a single problem in which missing data has occurred or some other form of data-mess has been identified. Our target is the professional who anticipates being involved in handling incomplete data, as a survey designer, data manager, statistical analyst, or a user of the analyst's output (a client), for many years to come, so that the investment in acquiring expertise would have rewards beyond the intellectual.

1.4 Suggested reading

This chapter is intended merely as a 'refresher' on the basics of survey sampling and as a reference for the terms used in the rest of the monograph. The foundations of survey sampling are essential for the following chapters. There are a number of very good texts on survey sampling; [124] and [30] are undisputed classics that have withstood the test of time. [242] is a popular text with a more modern approach. Reference [274] may have a greater appeal for the reader with a stronger mathematical background.

A comprehensive computing and graphical environment is essential for both practicing and theoretical academic statisticians. My strong preference is for `Splus`, [14] and [279], or its freely available version `R`, [114], [41] and

[215]. `Gauss` and `matlab` are suitable alternatives. If you are about to make a commitment, ask your colleagues what environments they work in and why. There is some advantage in conforming to the majority, but not if their practice is restricted by the capacity and range of the software. In particular, the analyst's control over every detail of the analysis, the graphical or tabular presentation of its results and no limits to how the data can be manipulated is essential.

Linear models and the linear algebra that supports their analysis are an indispensible part of the statistician's analytical equipment; [253], [177], [51], [250] and [251] (any one of them) provide ample background. Although the monograph adheres to the frequentist paradigm, most of the presented material can be easily reformulated for the Bayesian. [77] gives a lucid and engaging introduction to and is an effective advertisement for Bayesian analysis. Although the Bayesian paradigm has taken firm hold in computational statistics in the recent years, much of the survey sampling practice is affected by it only on its periphery.

Matrices appear in statistics in two key roles. They represent datasets (as subjects by variables) and variance, covariance and correlation matrices describe the associations among variables. Many statistical concepts are neatly presented by matrix algebra. Without matrices, our equations would be full of summations and indices; by using matrices, they are much more compact and easier to comprehend and manipulate. Although matrices are introduced and their properties discussed in most texts on linear regression, [96] goes beyond the minimum required without losing the focus on applications in statistics. Modern statistics requires not only computers but also expertise in computing and numerical methods. References [270] and [128] are excellent resources for them.

Statistical operations, including estimation, are easier to conduct with continuous (normally distributed) data and random variables. In contrast, lay people, such as survey subjects, are often more comfortable with categories, and many variables collected by surveys are discrete. Reference [1] provides a well-rounded background to analysis of discrete data.

1.5 Exercises

1. In a textbook example, but preferably with a survey that you are familiar with, consider how additional resources could be wisely spent: to reduce the sampling error by increasing the sample size, improve the measurement process, reduce the nonresponse, construct a better sampling frame (to combat non-sampling errors), collect more information by a more extensive questionnaire, use more advanced data management, or use different methods of analysis.

2. Review common sampling designs and estimation of population means, proportions and totals in a standard textbook on survey sampling (e.g., [242]).
3. Review the advantages and drawbacks of the common sampling designs. In particular, why is simple random sampling not applied universally? What is the purpose of stratification, clustering and using unequal probabilities of selection?
4. Prove the identity in (1.1). Construct other measures of dispersion and bias and combine them into alternative measures of the quality of an estimator. Describe the difficulties in defining these and other measures of the quality. Consider, for example, the mean absolute deviation $\mathrm{E}(|\,\hat{\mu}-\mu\,|)$, $\mathrm{E}\left\{(\hat{\mu}/\mu - 1)^2\right\}$ or $\mathrm{P}(|\,\hat{\mu}-\mu\,| > \Delta)$ for a given positive constant Δ.
5. Implement a simple sampling design in your preferred computing environment. Either use a population (that is, a sampling frame) from another source, or define the values of a single variable for a large number of units (tens of thousands at least). Use a random sample from the uniform distribution for drawing the sample. (For example, a 1% simple random sample is drawn by including all members whose value of the draw from the uniform distribution on $(0, 1)$ falls below 0.01.)
6. Apply an estimator of the population mean to the sample obtained in the previous example and estimate the sampling variance of the estimator. Replicate the process a large number of times (at least 100 times), and compare the distribution of the estimates with the population quantity and the (theoretical) sampling variance.
7. On a smaller example, simulate a misclassification process. Simulate the values of X^* from a discrete distribution on small integers (say, from 1 to 6), and apply misclassification by increasing or reducing each value with a small probability p. If the result is a value outside the range (1–6), truncate it. Compare the estimates of the population mean for the original and 'misclassified' variable.
8. Collect a few examples of (definitions of) a latent variable and several of its manifest versions, and discuss how the difference between latent and each manifest variable, and among the manifest variables, could be described. In particular, consider so-called *parallel* manifest variables that have the same association with the latent variable. Define meaningful ways of (partial) ordering of the manifest variables, e.g., by their proximity to the latent variable and by the effort (cost) required to obtain their values.
9. Draw a random sample from $\mathcal{N}(0, 1)$ and use it to estimate the mean $\mu = 0$. Apply quadratic and exponential transformations to the data and show that μ^2 and $\exp(\mu)$ are estimated very poorly by $\hat{\mu}^2$ and $\exp(\hat{\mu})$, respectively. Propose more efficient estimators. Construct the symmetric (two-sided) confidence interval for μ with coverage probability 0.95, and use it to construct confidence intervals for μ^2 and $\exp(\mu)$.

2

Describing incompleteness

This chapter is concerned with describing the extent and patterns of missing values in a dataset. The nonresponse process is introduced as a nuisance accompaniment of the sampling process and the ground is prepared for a discussion of the several common schemes for addressing data incompleteness in Chapter 3.

2.1 The problem of incompleteness

Most surveys rely on subjects' cooperation. We should therefore consider their perspective. As survey designers, interviewers or analysts, we may also be survey subjects. We can easily point to settings or circumstances in which we might respond negatively to an invitation to complete a questionnaire by an unsolicited phone call, or to a request for a face-to-face interview. There are dozens of activities more inspiring, entertaining, stimulating and rewarding than responding to a survey. So, the spectrum of our responses ranges from pretending total incomprehension, through polite or rude refusal, with or without a credible excuse, to reluctant cooperation that may be terminated as soon as we experience some further inconvenience, discomfort or some other perceived unpleasantry. We bear any intrusion with reluctance and jealously protect our privacy.

As a commodity, information is expensive but perishable — what is valuable today is discarded tomorrow or, at best, next week. Although the extent of missing data may be reduced by repeated calls and other time-consuming measures, a survey and its analysts and clients cannot always afford to wait until these measures have run their course.

However carefully a survey may be designed, the best plan is merely an ideal because complete cooperation of all the subjects, an assumption implied by the plan, is but an unattainable ideal. A simplified stereotype of a plan may be to collect the values of K variables from a random sample of n subjects drawn from a specified population. We may fail to identify the population precisely because of migration, changes of status, errors in the sampling frame, and the like. Further, we may fail to contact some of the selected subjects or fail to enlist their cooperation. The cooperation may be interrupted during the interview or completion of the questionnaire, some questionnaire items may remain not responded because of oversight, deliberate omission, inability to respond, nonexistence of an appropriate response, and the like. Further losses can occur in the process of transcribing the collected responses to the computer (due to illegible hand-writing and clerical errors).

Such missing data is visible, easy to detect by inspecting the constructed database, if it is constructed appropriately. The data field reserved for a particular value (of a variable for a subject) is either empty or contains a symbol that indicates that the value has not been recorded. There may be several such symbols, one for each kind of missing value: for 'do not know', 'not willing to tell', for an apparently inadvertent omission, and the like.

What about subjects from whom we elicited no information? Why should the database be burdened by their records, full of missing values? The implied viewpoint tends to prevail at present. We will argue against it, and against the practice it encourages, on the grounds illustrated by the following comparison. Suppose two surveys, A and B, are conducted in the same population using the same sampling design, instruments and methods of data collection. Survey A has sample size 7650 and complete information is elicited from each selected subject, so that no data is missing. Survey B has sample size 10 000, but only 76.5% of the selected subjects cooperate with the survey completely, and no information is elicited from the remainder. In survey A, the planned and realised designs coincide, whereas in survey B they differ. If the analysis does not reflect the difference between the two surveys, or between the planned and realised sampling designs, we should seek fault with the method applied, not our intuition.

The sampling design is important because the claimed properties of the estimators used are contingent on the sampling design, assuming that it is implemented perfectly. One element of such perfection is that there is no missing data. The purpose of the sampling design is to extract the maximum information with the resources available for the survey. In practice, this is interpreted as ensuring good representation of the population — that the sample is a faithful image, in the miniature, of the population or, more formally, that the sample (empirical) distribution function of the values of any variable is an unbiased estimator of its population counterpart.

The sampling design might ensure this, but not if it is infiltrated with nonresponse. If the sample drawn is representative, and is then reduced by nonresponse, the remainder of the original sample (the respondents) may no longer be representative. For example, if non-responding subjects tend to be wealthier than the respondents, our conclusion about the wealth of the population is distorted. If we regard the complete respondents as the (original) sample, we have no means of detecting such a distortion. Non-respondents are the subjects who tell us nothing, so we have no means of knowing that their absence from the database spoils the good representation that was arranged by the sampling design. We should strive to overcome this problem, even if in some circumstances it may appear prudent to defuse it by focussing on the population of respondents. Although with apparently greater competence, we would then solve a less relevant problem, because the original inferential task relates to the complete population, not to any of its opportunistically defined subpopulations.

The lack of any evidence that nonresponse causes a problem does not justify ignoring it, because the appropriate interpretation of no evidence is 'do not know'. For instance, no evidence may arise as a result of no inquiry. To justify ignoring nonresponse, evidence is required that it causes no problem.

The first step in dealing with nonresponse, or controlling its impact, is a survey of the damage. For missing data, this amounts to describing the extent of missing values, classified according to a suitable nomenclature. Although the party in charge of data collection has incentives to present the problem with as little fanfare as possible, there are ample long-term rewards for honesty and integrity. Suppose a survey has 20% of total nonresponse (non-contacts and outright refusals), and it is much lower than in surveys of similar populations and with similar content and protocol. The relatively high response rate does not justify ignoring the problem of nonresponse altogether. We should, at least informally, play the devil's advocate and contemplate what impact the 20% of the subjects might have had on the planned or intended inferences, had they all responded. It is easy to construct scenarios in which as little as 5% nonresponse results in a substantial distortion of the inferences. For instance, if in a country with low unemployment rate most of the unemployed do not respond to a survey that inquires about their employment status, and most employed and other subjects do, the estimate of the unemployment rate is bound to be problematic. The percentages (rates) of nonresponse (for each variable recorded in the survey), although easy to establish, are but one aspect of the problem. The impact on the planned inferences is what matters because the survey and its analysis have been undertaken specifically for the purpose of drawing the inferences.

The choice of the method for dealing with missing data is informed not only by the extent but also by the *pattern* of the missing data — whether subjects tend to omit responses to isolated questions or to whole sections (contiguous blocks) of questions, whether some questions are (almost) always or never responded when some other questions are responded or not, or whether nonresponse is associated with the values of one or a set of variables.

We conclude this section on a note of pedantry. Although the literature commonly refers to 'nonresponse', a more precise term for missing values is 'no record'. That is, a subject might have responded to a particular questionnaire item, but the processes that followed led to a missing code (blank) being entered, appropriately or not, in the corresponding location in the database. Although we prefer the phrase 'value not recorded', it is impossible to avoid the term nonresponse, as there is no alternative single word for the failure to record a value.

2.2 The extent of missing data and the response pattern

In this section, we define a terminology for missing data. We deal only with its *visible features* that can be summarised in one word as frequency of various combinations of missing and recorded values in the records. Section 2.3 discusses invisible features of missing data; they are properties of the process of nonresponse (missingness). We introduce first the general setting, some notation and related conventions.

We consider a fixed (frozen) population, so that there is no ambiguity about any entity whether it is a member of the population or not. The size of the population (number of its elements) is denoted by N. In general, we use capitals for population quantities and (the corresponding) lowercases for sample quantitites, although this notation is difficult to adhere to consistently. For example, boldface capitals are also used for matrices and boldface lowercases for their rows.

A population quantity can be derived with precision only if the relevant data items are available for the entire population or its a priori defined subset. Sampling has no impact on a population quantity. A sample quantity depends on the sample — it is a random variable prior to sampling, and a constant thereafter. Its value can be established when the sampling process is executed perfectly. A sampling-process quantity depends on the sampling process. That is, its value could be established with a specified precision if the sampling design were executed sufficiently many times. Most sample quantities are estimators; most sampling-process quantities describe estimators. For example, the population mean is a population quantity, it is estimated by the sample mean, a sample quantity, and the bias and sampling variance of the sample mean are sampling-process quantities. The sampling variance may be estimated; the estimator is a sample quantity.

Let n^* be the planned sample size of a survey; it may be a random variable. Suppose the survey collects the values of K variables. The *complete data* is the hypothetical dataset that was planned to be collected by the survey. Anticipating nonresponse, the planners may have resigned themselves to obtaining this dataset with some of its values missing, but they issued instructions and implemented measures aiming to collect every item of the complete dataset. In most instances, it is a $n^* \times K$ rectangular array. The collected data is referred to as the observed data, and it may be characterised as *incomplete*; the missing data is, in this context, defined as the difference between the complete and incomplete datasets.

We can define the terms 'complete', 'incomplete' and 'missing' for subsets of data. These subsets can be formed by keeping only some of the variables, only some of the subjects (reducing our attention to a subpopulation), and by the combination of these two ways of reducing the data. A variable is said to be recorded completely if its value is recorded for every subject; that is, if the dataset reduced to the single column is complete. Similarly, the record of a subject is complete if the value of each variable for the subject is recorded. Otherwise, the record is called incomplete. A record is called *empty* if all its values are missing. A record that is neither empty nor complete is called *partial*. We could use the term 'empty' also for a variable that has not been recorded for any subject.

The extent of missing data can be summarised by the numbers or percentages of empty and incomplete records. More detailed summary is provided by these numbers or percentages for various important subsets of variables, such as blocks of questionnaire items. Further, the number or percentage of missing values can be given for each variable.

A rather coarse classification of the nonresponse is to unit and item nonresponse. Unit nonresponse refers to an empty record, when the unit (subject) has provided no data. Item nonresponse refers to a missing item — the subject concerned cooperated with the survey, but only partially. More detail can be introduced by distinguishing parts, or sections, of the survey. Not cooperating with a section can be called section nonresponse. For example, the section may be the questionnaire administered at a given time point in a longitudinal study.

Example 1

In a survey with a planned sample size of 2000 (human) subjects, 174 were outright refusals and further 229 sampled subjects were not contacted (either not located or not found at home). Further, among the $2000-229-174 = 1597$ responding subjects, complete records on the twelve variables on which we focus are available for only 1088 subjects.

The summaries defined for this dataset are: the rate of total nonresponse, $(1-1597/2000)\times 100 \doteq 20\%$, and the rate of partial (incomplete) cooperation, $(1-1088/2000)\times 100 \doteq 46\%$. The complements of these rates, 80% and 54%, are the respective rates of at-least-partial and perfect cooperation. Table 2.1 gives the nonresponse rates for each of the twelve variables. Figure 2.1 presents these rates graphically.

These summaries indicate that variables A–F are responded by most of the 1597 cooperating subjects. For example, the response to A is not recorded for only $407 - 403 = 4$ of them. The nonresponse rates are much higher for variables G–L. The total number of missing values is $407 + 415 + \cdots + 761 = 7225$, out of $12 \times 2000 = 24\,000$, but $12 \times 403 = 4836$ of them are for unit nonresponse (total non-respondents). The remainder, 2389 values, are distributed among the 509 subjects who have partial records. These subjects have only 89 missing values on the variables A–F. On the other six variables, G–L, they have 2300 missing values, about four-and-a-half per subject. This implies that many of these subjects have five or all six values missing.

Table 2.1. The nonresponse rates for the twelve variables, A–L, in a dataset. A fictitious example.

Variable	A	B	C	D	E	F
Number of missing values	407	415	413	431	422	419
Nonresponse rate (%)	20.3	20.7	20.6	21.5	21.1	20.9
Variable	G	H	I	J	K	L
Number of missing values	912	844	717	728	756	761
Nonresponse rate (%)	45.6	42.2	35.8	36.4	37.8	38.0

Figure 2.1. A graphical display of the nonresponse rates for variables A–L, given in Table 2.1.

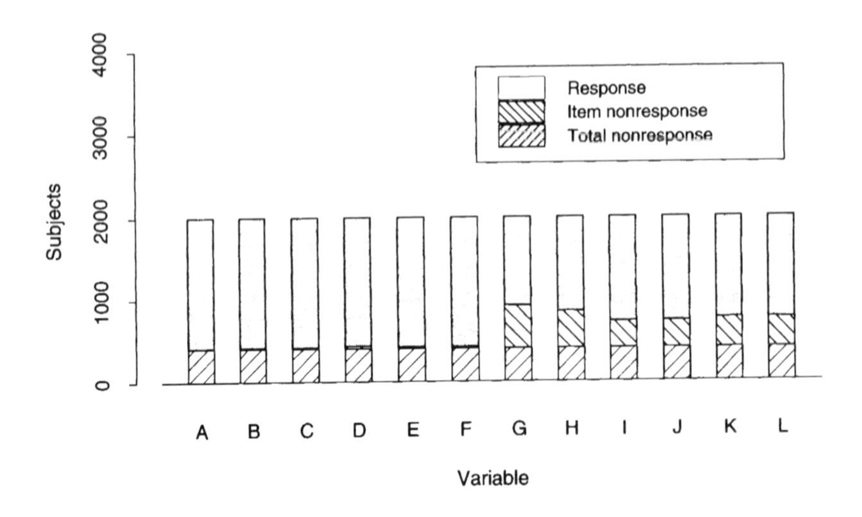

Although offering important insight, Table 2.1 does not contain all the information that might be useful to have. For example, we cannot establish how many subjects have empty records on the sets (segments) of variables A–F and G–L. For A–F, it may be only the 403 total non-respondents, and at most four others, whereas for G–L it could be as many as 314 in addition to the total non-respondents.

For a more detailed description of the nonresponse (or response), we define the *response pattern*. The *indicator of response* is an object of the same shape and size as the complete dataset, in our case a $n^* \times K$ matrix, in which

Table 2.2. Response patterns in an incomplete dataset. A fictitious example.

	Pattern						
	000000	100000	101000	111000	111001	1110111	111111
Subjects	407	6	2	4	3	9	1569
	Pattern						
	000000	001000	001100	001110	001111	011111	111111
Subjects	717	11	28	5	83	68	1088

one symbol is used to indicate that the corresponding value in the dataset is missing, and another that it is recorded. As a convention, 0 is used for a missing and 1 for an available (recorded) item. The indicator of response is denoted by **R**. (We can refer to **R** also as the *indicator of nonresponse.*) An obvious generalisation is to use different symbols for each kind of missing value. For example, -1 may be reserved for 'no contact', -2 for 'refusal', '-3' for 'do not know', and similar. For simplicity, we assume that such detail is not given and **R** comprises zeros and unities.

The response pattern for a subject (record) is defined as the corresponding row of **R**. It is a (binary) vector and, by 'gluing' its elements together, it can be represented as a sequence of zeros and ones. Thus, $\mathbf{1} = 11\ldots1$ represents a complete record, $\mathbf{0} = 00\ldots0$ an empty record, and so on. For a small number of variables, the patterns can be summarised by their tabulation. For K variables, there may be up to 2^K distinct patterns. It is useful to find out whether only a limited set of patterns occur in the data, or whether the vast majority of records have one or a small number of patterns. Table 2.2 gives an example, summarising the patterns of the same dataset as in Table 2.1. The patterns are summarised separately for the sets of variables A–F and G–L, both to conserve space and to get a better insight.

First we note that the number of distinct patterns, seven for both A–F and G–L, is much smaller than what we may have feared — $2^6 = 64$ for either set of variables. For variables A–F, there are, in addition to the 403 total non-respondents, four subjects with empty records. For variables G–L, there are $717 - 403 = 314$ such subjects; 195 subjects have one of the five partial response patterns. The most frequent partial patterns are 001111 and 011111. Subjects with this pattern appear to have started their cooperation on the block G–L with delay. (We explore their response pattern on the block A–F below.) A notable feature of the patterns for variables G–L is that the responses are concentrated in contiguous sets of variables, such as I–K for pattern 001110.

Table 2.2 still fails to inform about the pattern for the entire set of variables, A–L. Since the number of patterns does not exceed 49, we could list

Table 2.3. The cross-tabulation of the response patterns for the sets of variables A–F and G–L.

Pattern for A–F	Pattern for G–L						
	000000	001000	001100	001110	001111	011111	111111
000000	407	0	0	0	0	0	0
100000	6	0	0	0	0	0	0
101000	2	0	0	0	0	0	0
111000	4	0	0	0	0	0	0
111001	3	0	0	0	0	0	0
111011	9	0	0	0	0	0	0
111111	286	11	28	5	83	68	1088

them, although the two-way table of patterns for the variables A–F and G–L, displayed in Table 2.3, may be easier to digest. All the counts in this table are concentrated in the first column and last row. This indicates that no subjects have partial records on both segments A–F and G–L. The records are either empty (407 records), complete (1088 records), complete for A–F but empty for G–L (286 records), partial for A–F and complete for G–L (24 records), or complete for A–F and partial for G–L (195 records).

We can define a partial ordering according to the pattern of nonresponse. One variable is said to be recorded more than another if the only response patterns occuring for the two variables are 00, 11, 10; that is, when the first variable is not recorded, neither is the second. Records, or their patterns, can be compared similarly. For example, 111011 represents more response than 111000, although 110011 does not represent more response than 001000.

The patterns can be displayed graphically, by a $n^* \times K$ array of cells (symbols or squares) with different symbols, colours, shading, or the like, indicating whether the item has been recorded or not. A clearer impression of the distribution of the patterns is created if the subjects are permuted so that records with the same pattern form a contiguous segment. When the sample size n^* is large, it is practical not to draw the cells but represent a given number of records (rows) by a unit height in the rectangle representing the data. The variables can also be permuted to make the presentation clearer. An example is given in Figure 2.2.

2.2.1 Monotone response patterns

The variables in a dataset have a partial ordering according to the extent of their missing values. The response patterns of a dataset are said to be *monotone* if the variables can be permuted so that any variable is recorded

Figure 2.2. A graphical summary of the patterns of nonresponse.

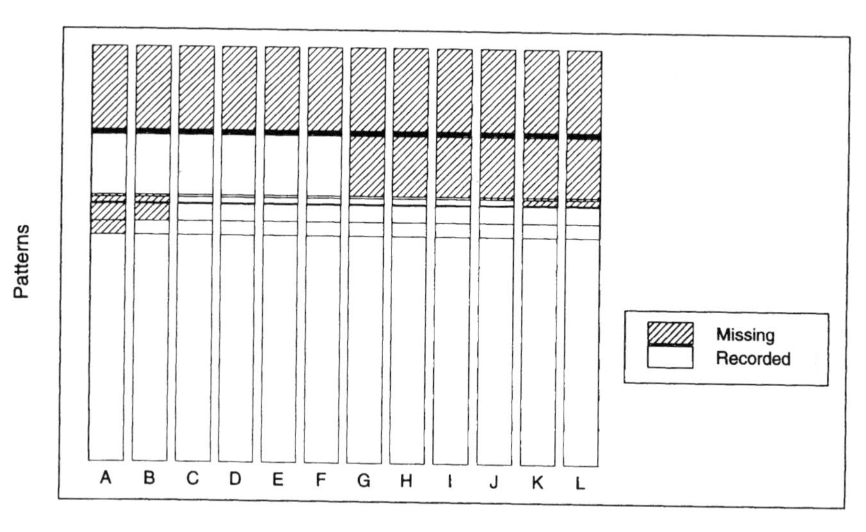

more than the following variable; nonresponse to a variable by a subject is followed by the subject's nonresponse to all the subsequent variables.

For vectors $\mathbf{X}_1$ and $\mathbf{X}_2$ of the same length, we introduce the notation

$$\mathbf{X}_1 \succeq \mathbf{X}_2$$

if $\mathbf{X}_1$ exceeds or is equal to the value of $\mathbf{X}_2$ for every subject. The symbols $\succ$, $\prec$ and $\preceq$ are defined similarly. For instance, $\mathbf{X}_1 \succ \mathbf{X}_2$ if $\mathbf{X}_1$ exceeds $\mathbf{X}_2$ for every subject. Variable $\mathbf{X}_1$ is recorded more than $\mathbf{X}_2$ if for the corresponding vectors of response indicators we have $\mathbf{R}_1 \succeq \mathbf{R}_2$.

For a dataset $\mathbf{X}$ with columns $\mathbf{X}_1, \ldots, \mathbf{X}_K$, and response indicator $\mathbf{R}$ with columns $\mathbf{R}_1, \ldots, \mathbf{R}_K$, monotone response patterns are defined by the string of ordering $\mathbf{R}_1 \succeq \cdots \succeq \mathbf{R}_K$. We can distinguish between 'recorded more than' and 'recorded at least as much as', but this will not be essential at any point.

In Section 2.3, we consider methods for completing the recorded (incomplete) data by substituting a value for each missing item. We assume that the value is well defined, even though it was not recorded. Since we do not know the value, we search for information on which to base our guess. For a subject, the available part of the record is an obvious candidate for this purpose. The more was recorded from the subject, the better our prospects of a good guess. Obviously, fewer missing items have to be filled in for (*imputed*) when more items are recorded. But we also possess more information on which to base the imputation. If we want to use all the information available about a subject we have to devise a different way for each pattern. So, the distribution of the patterns helps us draft a strategy for this task. In Chapter 4, and Section 4.2 in particular, we find that efficient methods for imputation are much easier to implement when the data has monotone response patterns.

2.3 Sampling and nonresponse processes

Why did we fail to collect a particular item of information? At first sight, this question is solely about nonresponse. On reflection, there are two classes of answers: because we did not intend to (as when the subject is not in the sample), and because we failed to elicit a response that, in principle, could have been recorded.

By a (random or stochastic) *process* we refer to one or a collection of random variables that describe a studied phenomenon or some of its ingredients. In a typical survey, we may consider a *data-generating* process describing how the members of the population acquire their values of a random variable or vector, the *sampling* process, describing how some members of the population end up being the subjects in the sample, and the *nonresponse* process, describing how we fail (or succeed) to elicit and record the elements of the planned (complete) dataset. In this chapter, we are not concerned with the data generating process (for instance, how certain members of the labour force end up being unemployed, at a certain time point), although the purpose of the survey may be to learn about this process. The nonresponse process is formally defined as the conditional distribution of the response indicator $\mathbf{R}$ given the complete data $\mathbf{X}^*$,

$$(\mathbf{R} \mid \mathbf{X}^*) \, .$$

In formulas, we refer to distributions of random variables or vectors by parentheses ( ), to conditioning by the vertical bar $|$, and to equality in distribution by the symbol $\sim$. For example,

$$(\mathbf{R} \mid \mathbf{X}^*) \;\sim\; (\mathbf{R})$$

denotes that the conditional distribution of the response indicator $\mathbf{R}$ given the complete data coincides with the (unconditional) distribution of $\mathbf{R}$. That is, $\mathbf{R}$ and $\mathbf{X}^*$ are independent. This distributional identity is not true in general. The missing data is denoted by $\mathbf{X}_{\mathrm{mis}}$.

A typical survey involves several other processes, such as questionnaire development (piloting) and interviewing. Although the interviewer is meant to be an inert instrument in eliciting responses, different interviewers might have elicited differing responses from the same subject, had such a replication been realised (a repeated interview, separated by a period in which the subject has forgotten the experience of having been interviewed for the first time, and would not recall the responses he or she gave earlier). For instance, the interviewer in a survey has to make an assessment of the need for repairs of the inspected dwelling; different interviewers (surveyors) may come to different conclusions when inspecting the same dwelling. The underlying *assessment* process has an impact on the quality of the collected data, and consequently on the quality of the inferences. We could consider an *ideal* assessment for each subject, and the assessment by the surveyor or interviewer as its *manifest* (error-prone) version. The ideal assessment is a completely missing variable, but the realised assessment contains a lot of information about it, especially when the assessors make 'mistakes' only rarely, and most of them are only minor. This is an example of planned 'nonresponse' and it indicates that methods for dealing with missing data may be applicable in some less conventional settings. They are explored in greater detail in Section 4.6.

The nonresponse process describes the momentary influences on the subject's response. If the subject were asked the same questions about a stable attribute, such as consumption of a food item, he or she may respond differently, depending on the momentary disposition, vagaries of the recall and formulation of the response. In this case, the ideal response is missing for every subject and the recorded response is its manifest version; it informs about the ideal value imperfectly.

The sampling process reduces the information from the population to the (complete) sample. The role of the sampling design is to minimise the loss of information given the resources available for the conduct of the survey. Given adequate resources and perfect implementation, the design ensures that we can make (sample-based) inferences about the population. An imperfect response process reduces the complete sample further, to the incomplete sample (information). The main qualitative difference between the sampling and nonresponse processes is that the former is under our control, by means of the sampling design prescribing the probabilities that a subset of the population forms the sample. The sampling process has a formal description as a function π on $\exp(\mathcal{P})$, the set of all subsets of the studied population $\mathcal{P}$; for $s \in \mathcal{P}$, $\pi(s)$ is the probability that s forms the sample.

In contrast, the nonresponse process is usually oblivious to the sampling design — the subject's reasons for not responding are unrelated to the sampling plan. Because it is outside our control, we should be concerned that the nonresponse process may spoil the representativeness of the sample. We can easily construct scenarios in which the representativeness is severely undermined. As an example, suppose in a survey aimed to estimate the unemployment rate, the unemployed tend to be much more difficult to contact or they are more reluctant to respond to the relevant questionnaire items. More subtle processes may be at play, such as when non-studying young men in urban areas have a lower response rate, or when the response rates among quite finely divided subpopulations do not differ a great deal, but in certain groups unemployed and in others employed subjects are less likely to respond.

This suggests two approaches. To ignore the issue, since the 'correct' answer is beyond the realm of possibilities, or to give up on the original goal of estimating the specified population quantities altogether because of a gross failure in the data collection process. Neither approach is very constructive. Instead, we will speculate about the possible nonresponse processes, draw inferences assuming these processes, and then explore how the inferences change as the assumed process is altered. In this way, we take a risk, but assess, informally, its magnitude. We will also look for means of reducing the risk by searching for insights about the nonresponse process. First we define a typology for the nonresponse processes, starting with the setting of a survey in which a single variable is recorded.

2.3.1 The nature of the nonresponse process

Since nonresponse is a process akin to sampling, we could describe it using the terminology from sampling theory. As nonresponse could in principle be described and motivated as a result of certain decisions or actions, it is also called the nonresponse *mechanism*. The ideal, usually not attainable, is to find a complete description of this mechanism, so that, for instance, we could simulate it on a computer.

In the simplest conceivable nonresponse mechanism, subjects who fail to respond are as if selected by simple random sampling (SRS) from all the subjects selected by the sampling process. The nonresponse mechanism is independent of the complete data:

$$(\mathbf{R} \mid \mathbf{X}^*) \sim (\mathbf{R}) . \tag{2.1}$$

With such a mechanism, the data are said to be *missing completely at random* (MCAR). As SRS is a very special sampling process, we cannot expect, without exercising any control over it, that the nonresponse would be MCAR. Usually we have no means of establishing that a nonresponse mechanism is MCAR. A more plausible assumption is that the mechanism belongs to a more general class.

A class of sampling designs more general than SRS is *stratified* simple random sampling (sSRS). In sSRS, the population is classified into strata (subpopulations), and simple random sampling (with stratum-specific probabilities of inclusion) is applied in each stratum. The stratification is given by a categorical variable defined in the surveyed population. Stratification based on a (categorical) variable A is said to be more detailed than stratification based on B, if B can be formed by aggregating (collapsing) some of the categories of A.

In a more general sampling design, the probability of inclusion is a function of one or several variables, and the inclusions are mutually independent. Such a design can be motivated by defining a sequence of designs with more and more detailed stratification. In the corresponding nonresponse mechanisms, data is said to be *missing at random* (MAR). A key characterisation of MAR is that the response indicator depends on the complete data only through its recorded part:

$$(\mathbf{R} \,|\, \mathbf{X}^*) \sim (\mathbf{R} \,|\, \mathbf{X}) \,. \tag{2.2}$$

That is, the missing data $\mathbf{X}_{\text{mis}}$ contains no information about $\mathbf{R}$. Note that missing data contains information about most population quantities. Although much more general than MCAR, it is easy to construct mechanisms that are not MAR. In all such mechanisms, data is said to be *not missing at random* (NMAR). In NMAR, the response indicator depends on the missing data. NMAR contains all manner of 'strange' mechanisms, as illustrated in Figure 2.3. In each panel, the histogram of the complete data is composed of the missing values, represented by the shaded bars, and the recorded values by the plain bars above them. In panel MCAR, the probability of missing, equal to 0.25, is the same within every interval (bar). Panel NMAR 1 depicts a mechanism with higher response rates for the smallest and largest values of X, NMAR 2 a mechanism with lower response rates for the extreme values, and NMAR 3 a mechanism with response rates decreasing with the value of X. These examples are in no way exhaustive. Any idiosyncratic mechanism is an example of NMAR. MAR mechanisms that are not MCAR are more difficult to represent graphically because they involve at least two variables.

On the one hand, we should be aware of NMAR mechanisms and contemplate how they might affect our inferences. On the other hand, we should be realistic and, while not subscribing to the assumption of a limited class of nonresponse mechanisms, such as MCAR, restrict our attention to the range of NMAR mechanisms that are plausible. Intelligence about the studied setting that reduces this range is particularly valuable.

Example 2

Suppose a survey collects the values of a single categorical variable X from a sample s, with a sampling design defined by π. If the nonresponse mechanism is MCAR the probability of response is the same for each value of X. If the nonresponse mechanism is MAR the probability of response does not depend on the subject's value of X, but may depend on the (known) inclusion probability π_i. An example of NMAR arises when the probabilities of response depend on X. For example, the subjects with a particular value of X are much more reluctant to respond, and those with other values of X are more forthcoming.

Several variables in $\mathbf{X}^*$

Although the definitions of MCAR, MAR and NMAR are easier to interpret for single variables, their definitions in terms of $(\mathbf{R} \,|\, \mathbf{X}^*)$ apply to sets of variables in $\mathbf{X}^*$. Simply, the joint distribution of the $n \times K$ elements of $\mathbf{R}$ is independent of the complete data $\mathbf{X}^*$ (MCAR), or depends on it only through the incomplete data $\mathbf{X}$ (MAR).

Figure 2.3. Examples of MCAR and NMAR mechanisms. Missing values are represented by the shaded sections of the bars.

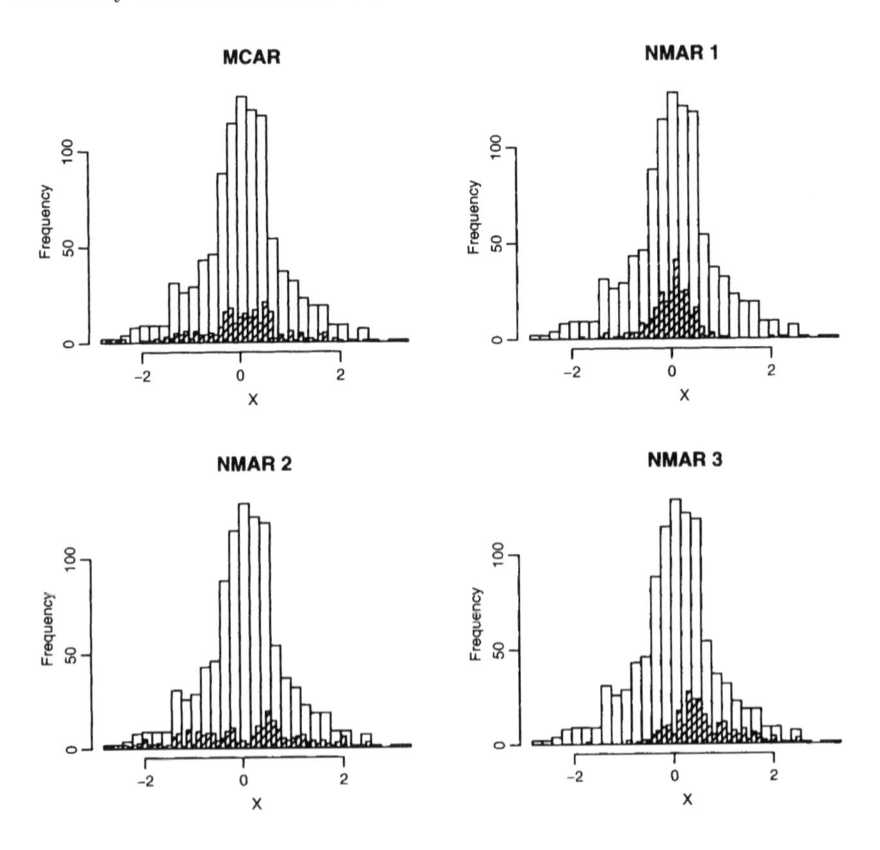

It is useful to separate the survey variables $\mathbf{X}$ into those that may be recorded incompletely, $\mathbf{Y}$, and those that never contain any missing values, $\mathbf{Z}$;

$$\mathbf{X} \sim (\mathbf{Y} \;\; \mathbf{Z})\,.$$

For example, the values of some of the variables in $\mathbf{Z}$ may be available prior to interviewing and those in $\mathbf{Y}$ are established by the interview. Variables that describe the circumstances of the interview (whether completed or not, whether conducted at the first appointment, and the like), usually belong to $\mathbf{Z}$. We can draw a distinction between completeness of a variable in the process of data collection and in the realised dataset. The former refers to hypothetical replications of the survey. When the sample size is large the distinction is unimportant.

2.3.2 The importance of MAR

The importance of MAR stems from a characterisation alternative to (2.2): when MAR applies the joint distribution of $\mathbf{X}$ for subjects with incomplete records is the same as for subjects with complete records:

$$(\mathbf{x} \mid \mathbf{r} = \mathbf{1}) \;=\; (\mathbf{x} \mid \mathbf{r} = \mathbf{r}^*)\,, \tag{2.3}$$

where $\mathbf{r}^*$ is any response pattern for $\mathbf{x}$ (a row of $\mathbf{X}$). The characterisation in (2.3) provides an important recipe for dealing with nonresponse. We establish, or estimate, the associations among the variables in $\mathbf{X}$ for subjects with complete records (pattern $\mathbf{1}$), and then assume that it applies also for the incomplete records. Before doing this, we have to be satisfied that the nonresponse mechanism is MAR. This we can rarely accomplish analytically, but that should not stop us from proceeding by assuming MAR. The best we can do is to reduce as much as possible the error incurred in the inferences that can be attributed to the assumption. Drawing inferences from $\mathbf{X}$ is much easier under MAR because NMAR includes a range of mechanisms in which some combinations of values of $\mathbf{X}$ that are infrequent among the complete records are quite frequent among the incomplete records. Whether MAR applies, as well as the departure from it, depends on the variables $\mathbf{X}$. If a nonresponse mechanism is MAR it will remain so when variables are added to $\mathbf{X}$. However, a NMAR mechanism need not become MAR when variables are added to $\mathbf{X}$. The variables considered, $\mathbf{X}$, are an important qualification of MAR and NMAR.

This suggests that when planning a survey we should think not only about recording the *outcome* variables directly connected with the desired inferences, but also variables that promote MAR. Although such *auxiliary* variables may also be recorded incompletely, they may be helpful nevertheless.

Example 3

One-week diaries of alcohol consumption in a survey of middle-aged people in the UK are analysed by [166]. Diaries are regarded as the most reliable way of collecting information about the consumption of food and drink, even though incomplete and empty (no-response) diaries are quite frequent. Keeping a diary for a whole week requires a lot of commitment from the subjects. In the survey, almost all subjects completed the diary for the first two days, but many dropped out thereafter. The subjects were also asked to recall how much alcohol they consumed during the previous week and were given a set of four brief questions about problems related to their past alcohol consumption (CAGE, [61]).

The response rate to the four recall questions (about drinking beer, wine, sherry and spirits) was much higher because the questions can be responded within a short time, after a cursory recall. The higher response rate comes at the price of lower reliability. The CAGE questions (response options Yes/No) also had very little nonresponse. Numerous other variables were collected, such as smoking habit, gender, body mass and height.

An obvious concern with diary data is that subjects may drop out from keeping it because of embarrassment over excessive consumption. Thus, the incomplete diaries would deceive the analyst by stopping at a day preceding excessive consumption. Such deception is an example of NMAR. From the recorded data we cannot infer whether it is present, and to what extent. However, the other variables related to alcohol consumption may provide some insights. Concerns about NMAR would be well supported if there were many subjects who declared substantial consumption in the recall and much lower consumption in their incomplete diaries, even after pro-rating for the number of completed diary days.

The recall variables play the role of auxiliary information that makes MAR more plausible. As an outcome they are not suitable, but as informants about the missing values that would have been derived from the diaries they are ideal. Details of the analysis are discussed in Section 5.2.

2.4 Exercises

1. Find or construct examples of nonresponse mechanisms that are MCAR, MAR and NMAR, and examples that are NMAR, without conditioning on a particular variable, but are MAR otherwise.
2. For a given incomplete dataset of at least 1000 subjects and several variables, write a programme (`Splus` function) to summarise the response patterns by a table and graphically. Look for ways of excluding as few subjects as possible to make the patterns monotone.
3. Unit nonresponse is encountered in a survey of a particular human population. The distribution of age within the sexes is known from a census or register. To assess whether the nonresponse presents a problem for the planned (complete-data) analyses, tests are carried out of the hypotheses that the proportions of the sexes and the sample distributions of age within the sexes are compatible with the population distribution. Provide a critique of this approach.
4. Simulate the values of a log-normally distributed variable in a population of at least 20 000 subjects. Regard the variable as the annual income. Define a small number of cut-points for 'income brackets' and devise methods for estimating the population mean income from the tabulation according to these income brackets. Draw a large number of samples from the population (according to the same sampling design, say, SRS without replacement with sample size 500), and compare the distributions of the sample means for the income and the income bracket.
5. Formulate the problem of estimating the population mean income from the income bracket data as a case of missing information.

6. In a national crime survey, interviews are conducted with a sample drawn from the country's population of households. An adult member of the household is asked to recall all instances of crime committed against any member of the household. Why does the survey not collect any information about the crimes committed *by* the interviewees and members of their households? What is the likely difference between the records of victimisation from the interviewees and records from the Police?
7. Data about total alcohol consumption in a year in the UK could be obtained from the records of payments of excise duty on alcohol. What information about alcohol consumption may be obtained by surveys of the (adult) population that could not be extracted from the excise duty enumeration?
8. Suppose a survey with sample size 8000 collects information about 30 variables, but item nonresponse occurs by MCAR with the same probability, 0.01, for every item and the event of nonresponse is independent across items. Calculate the expectation and variance of the number of incomplete records. Simulate this setting on a computer and verify the calculation. Alter the nonresponse process so that the events of nonresponse are dependent within subjects.
9. Describe the response patterns obtained in the previous example, by tables and graphs, and relate the within-subject dependence of response to the distribution of the patterns.

3

Single imputation and related methods

This chapter describes some commonly applied methods for incomplete data and points out their deficiencies. For the assessment of these methods, we adopt the standards of *efficiency* and not overstating the precision (*honesty*).

By efficiency we mean estimation with as small mean squared error (MSE) as possible, given the known or assumed details of the sampling process and associated information. Estimator $\hat{\theta}_1$ is said to be more efficient than estimator $\hat{\theta}_2$ if its MSE in estimating the same target θ is smaller; $\mathrm{MSE}(\hat{\theta}_1\,;\theta) < \mathrm{MSE}(\hat{\theta}_2\,;\theta)$. Estimator $\hat{\theta}$ of a population quantity θ is said to be efficient (without any qualification) if $\mathrm{MSE}(\hat{\theta};\theta)$ is smaller than the MSE of any other estimator of the same quantity θ. Properties of estimators depend on the (realised) sampling design, and so the design is an implied argument of MSE. Sampling designs can also be compared for efficiency. A sampling design π_1 is said to be more efficient for a given population quantity θ than another design π_2 if an efficient estimator of θ under π_1 has smaller MSE than an efficient estimator of θ under π_2. In most settings, MSE depends on unkown quantities (parameters), and so can only be estimated.

By honesty we mean estimation of MSE with non-negative bias. Of course, estimation of MSE without bias is preferred, but this is not always possible. Overestimation of $\mathrm{MSE}(\hat{\theta};\theta)$ can be regarded as 'under-selling' the estimator $\hat{\theta}$. In contrast, underestimation of MSE amounts to dishonesty — the precision implied by the estimator $\widehat{\mathrm{MSE}}(\hat{\theta};\theta)$, regarded as the underlying quantity $\mathrm{MSE}(\hat{\theta};\theta)$, is not justified. In this perspective, overestimation is less serious an error than underestimation by biases of the same order of magnitude.

We assume that an agenda for the analysis of the data collected by a survey has been set, by one or several parties (analysts), and they could cope with the analysis if the data were complete. The first step is therefore to alter the dataset so that it could be submitted to the planned (complete-data) analysis. The methods for accomplishing this can be classified as data *reduction* and data *imputation* (completion), according to the course of action taken with the incomplete records — discarding them or completing them. An obvious virtue of imputation is the aim, however unrealistic, to recover the complete dataset.

A typical imputation method draws on the recorded data, assuming that the patterns of values or associations observed among the complete records tend to occur also among the records that were not observed completely. In contrast, data reduction is straightforward, requiring no intelligence about the dataset or the nonresponse process. A feature common to these methods is that they refer to a complete-data analysis. Methods that do not involve a complete-data analysis tend to be complex because they have to combine descriptions of the processes that yield the complete data (sampling or data generation) and that introduce incompleteness or, more generally, imperfection (departure from the plan).

Insisting on complete-data methods is practical because these methods may have been implemented in preparation for the analysis, and the survey may have been designed so that a specific method would be suitable. The user's familiarity with the method is another factor. Most analysis tools are suitable only for complete data and the expertise in its analysis is available much more widely and with greater competence than for dealing with incomplete data. Modelling the nonresponse process entails added complexity, and is generally regarded as an undesirable distraction from the main goal of drawing inferences about the studied population. Although not impossible, it is much more difficult to plan an analysis with (unplanned) missing values than for a complete dataset.

We assume therefore that the available tools for analysis are limited to handling datasets that are complete, that were or could have been obtained if no deviation from the plan had taken place. A good plan calls for collecting a dataset that could be analysed, efficiently, by the available tools. A key feature of a dataset that enables its easy handling and analysis is *rectangularity.* A dataset is said to be rectangular if it comprises complete records, each with the values of the same set of variables. Such a dataset is usually represented as a matrix, with n^* subjects (units) as its rows and K variables as its columns. Rectangularity is spoilt when some of the Kn^* values are missing, in such a pattern that there are some partial records and partially recorded variables.

After discussing several approaches (classes of methods), we conclude that generating a completed dataset that is, item by item as close as possible to the complete dataset is not the appropriate goal. The purpose of the survey analysis is inference, in the form of a multitude of estimates or other statements about the studied population, and so the dataset should be edited with the purpose of enabling such inferences according to the commonly adopted or implied standards of efficiency and honesty.

3.1 Data reduction

In data reduction, we discard all the incomplete records and analyse the remainder. The reduced dataset has the (rectangular) structure amenable to the planned analysis, although the sample size has been reduced.

Data reduction has two drawbacks. An incomplete record is discarded even when only one of its less important items is missing, or when a good guess of the missing value(s) could be made. Thus, we may discard valuable information. This is an acute problem especially when there are a variety of response patterns. Further, the analysis of the reduced dataset relies on the assumption that the subjects with complete records (respondents) are just as a good a representation of the sampled population as the original sample (all the selected subjects). That is, data incompleteness (at least one item missing) is a process akin to MCAR.

Example 4

The UK Women's Cohort Study (WCS) is a survey of over 35 000 middle-aged women recruited from the UK participants of a larger survey conducted by the World Cancer Fund. The objective of WCS is to study the association of cancer (its occurence and death as its attributed cause) with diet. The subjects, contacted by mail in 1996, were requested to complete, without any supervision, a lengthy questionnaire about their diet, socio-economic background, anatomical measurements, medical and child-bearing history, and the like. The first section of the questionnaire comprises about 200 questions presented in the format

How often have you eaten these foods in the last 12 months?

with ten response options ranging from *Never* to *Six times a day*, coded as 0 and 9, respectively. The rates of nonresponse for these food-frequency questionnaire (FFQ) items are between 1% and 5%. The reported frequencies are converted to quantities of nutrients (protein, starch, carbohydrates, vitamins, and the like) to obtain a subject's dietary profile. The profile can be evaluated only when the responses are available for every item. Without a special provision, a single missing item can disrupt the calculation of the profile. Data reduction, applied to all the FFQ items, would reduce the sample size to around 10 000 (less than 30%), an unacceptable sacrifice to computational convenience.

The operationally implemented solution imputes 0 (*Never*) for each missing FFQ response. For most questions, this is the obvious category to impute because it is the most frequent response. Also, we may conjecture that many omissions are a result of the confusion between *Never* and no response. The instructions clearly state that one of the options should be selected for every question, but subjects may be distracted or lose concentration while responding to a long sequence of mundane questions. □

Data reduction is effective with a limited set of response patterns, when most of the values in the partial records are missing. But in most large-scale surveys, data reduction is poorly suited because the loss of information relative to the recorded dataset is unacceptable.

As an aside, data reduction is very ineffective when the complete-data analysis relies on some form of balance or orthogonality. An example of balance arises when equal numbers of subjects are planned to be in each cluster. In this case, either the number of subjects in each cluster has to be reduced, to restore the balance, or some incomplete clusters have to be discarded altogether. Many subjects with complete records may have to be discarded for the sake of an inflexible complete-data analysis.

3.2 Data completion

In the following sections, we discuss several common imputation schemes that generate a dataset that could be submitted to a complete-data analysis. The schemes can be classified as *deterministic* and *stochastic*. The completion by a deterministic scheme depends only on the recorded (incomplete) data. The replication of such a scheme on the same incomplete dataset yields the same completion. Stochastic schemes involve chance, typically in the form of random draws. A replication of such a scheme yields a different completion even with the same incomplete dataset — the imputed values are random, even after conditioning on the recorded data.

3.2.1 Mean imputation

In this scheme, the mean of the observed values of an incompletely recorded variable y is imputed for each missing value of y. This is very easy to implement for ordinal variables. The imputed values are as 'normal' as can be, given that a single value has to be chosen. The unattractive feature of the scheme is that the completed dataset has several values of y equal to the mean, even when all the observed values are unique or occur with small frequencies. The values of many ordinal variables are rounded; for them, the imputed values stand out like a sore thumb, unless they are also rounded. But such rounding introduces a consistent 'bias' for each completion. By no stretch of imagination can we claim to have recovered the complete dataset, even though we have restored its rectangularity and made it amenable to the complete-data analysis.

By imputing the mean (without rounding), we fix the values of the variable on average; the sample mean has not been altered by the imputations. In contrast, the sample dispersion of y is reduced, because 'model' values are imputed, not departing from the sample mean. It might be more appropriate to impute the population mean, but it is not known. By imputing the sample mean, we are committing a systematic error. However, imputing the population mean would not resolve the problem of reduced variation, and the constant imputed value is an obvious glitch in the completed dataset.

Imputing the mean is a univariate scheme, not informed by the values of the other variables. The scheme fails to maintain the associations among the variables. For example, imputing the average body mass of adult men (say, 70 kg) is appropriate for men of average height (say, 175 cm), but is not a plausible value for a man of height well above average, say, 200 cm. We could respond to known height by imputing a 'typical' body mass for *that* height. The values of other variables may similarly inform the choice of the imputed value. Methods for this are discussed in Section 3.2.6.

3.2.2 Imputation from another variable

Suppose some of the recorded variables are closely related, so that their values for a subject tend to be similar. If one value is missing, the value of another variable may be used instead. For each variable k, we may define a substitute variable h that would provide the replacement value. This arrangement may be reciprocal; variable k would provide a replacement value for variable h. Such a scheme does not impute for every missing value because the values of both variables k and h may be missing. This eventuality can be taken care of by defining 'second' substitutes; such a variable h_2 would provide the value for variable k when both variables k and h are missing. Further (third, fourth, and so on) substitutes can be defined, leading to a complex scheme that defines a replacement for every missing value, unless the record, or its relevant part, is empty. A transformed variable, or a variable constructed from several variables, may be used instead of an originally recorded variable.

A familiar example of this scheme is 'last observation carried forward' (LOCF) in longitudinal surveys.

Example 5

The UK Labour Force Survey (LFS) employs a rotating panel design in which each sampled residential address is planned to be contacted first when selected into the sample, and then 3, 6, 9 and 12 months later. The key outcome variable is the employment status of each adult resident at the address — whether the subject is employed, unemployed or economically inactive (not in the labour force) at the time of the scheduled interview. Within any three months, few subjects change their status, so imputing the status recorded three months ago (when available) for the current status is a fairly safe bet. It is difficult to devise an imputation scheme that would yield the correct status more frequently. However, as a consequence of this scheme, the transitions among the employment states are under-represented. This distortion is negligible for the middle-aged in certain socio-economic groups, who tend to be in secure employment, but far from trivial for the young who are developing their careers and exploring career options — some switch in quick succession between being students (economically inactive), working in short-term jobs, and having spells of unemployment and economic inactivity (e.g., caring for their small children). □

In the multivariate version of the LOCF scheme, a whole vector is brought forward, for example, for employment status, income, the strategy adopted in job search and perception of employment opportunities. A dilemma arises when the values of these variables are missing in various patterns. Should a partial record be overwritten by the values from the previous occasions, or should the imputations be restricted to the missing values? By overwriting, we discard some recorded values (the 'truth'); otherwise we may come across contradictions or implausible combinations of values, such as unemployment combined with high income.

When a trend is present, such as decreasing unemployment, there are more transitions from unemployment to employment than converse. This may be obvious from the recorded data, but it cannot be reflected in the imputations. Should the imputed status for all non-respondents who were unemployed three months ago be 'employed'? This is inappropriate if only 10% of those who responded on both occasions and who were unemployed on the previous occasion are now employed. As spells of unemployment tend to get shorter, bringing forward unemployment status from the previous wave becomes less appropriate.

Vertical and horizontal imputation

Mean imputation and imputation of an another variable are examples of *vertical* and *horizontal* imputation, respectively. In the former, imputation is based on the information in the same column as the missing item, and in the latter, information is used only from the same record (row). Vertical imputation can be based on a summary other than the mean. Median and mode are the obvious alternatives for deterministic imputations. For instance, the mode is imputed in Example 4 for most FFQ questions. In horizontal imputation, any rule for combining the recorded values of the other variables for the subject can be used.

Features of vertical and horizontal schemes can be combined, drawing on the advantages of both. For example, separate horizontal schemes may be defined for each category of a discrete variable or the details of a vertical scheme may depend on the (recorded) values of the other variables.

3.2.3 Nearest-neighbour imputation

In nearest-neighbour imputation, the incomplete record of a subject (called *recipient*) is completed by the values of the same variables of another subject (*donor*) whose record is complete. Let the variables with missing values for a particular recipient be $\mathbf{k} = (k_1, \ldots, k_m)$. For the recorded variables $\mathbf{k}^{(c)}$, the complement of **k**, a rule is defined that identifies a subject with a complete record on **k** that is closer to the recipient than any other. This is the nearest neighbour. When there are several equally well qualified nearest neighbours the donor is selected at random from among them and its values of the variables **k** are imputed for the corresponding values of the recipient. A simple rule for identifying a donor is by agreement (*match*) of the values of the variables in $\mathbf{k}^{(c)}$. The variables may be listed in the order of importance, so that a match of the values of the first variable is more important than a match of the values of the second variable, and so on. Matching of values as a criterion can be relaxed so that it suffices if the values do not differ by more than a set threshold. This is a practical arrangement especially for continuous variables. More generally, a distance can be defined between any two subjects with the requisite response patterns, and the donor is selected as the subject with the shortest distance from the recipient. Care has to be exercised in the definition of the distance, so that the relative importance of the contributing variables is appropriately reflected.

The donor need not have a complete record. Some variables may be ignored in matching or calculating the distance, or their contributions may be so small that the identified donor would be the nearest neighbour of the recipient for any completion of its record. Also, distances can formally be defined even for missing values. For example, the distance between score 4 and a missing value for the same variable, defined on the scale 0–10, can be defined as 6, the largest possible distance. In such a scheme, the distance for two missing values should be defined as 10 (as between 0 and 10), although there may be some rationale for a shorter distance, especially when the scores of 0 and 10 are very rare.

A drawback of this scheme is that the quality of the imputation is uneven. Some recipients have many close 'neighbours', while others are in relative isolation. Conversely, some donors may be very popular — their values are used for many recipients, whereas other subjects, even some with complete records, would not be donors for any recipients.

3.2.4 Hot deck

Hot-deck imputation is closely related to nearest-neighbour schemes. In hot deck, a pool of donors is defined for each recipient, and a donor is drawn from the pool at random. The pool is defined so that it contains the subjects who are similar to the recipient and have recorded values for the variables $\mathbf{k}^{(c)}$. The imputation can be organised so that the recipients are also grouped, into sets that share the same pool of donors.

The definition of hot deck can be generalised by assigning weights to each member of the pool and making the probabilities of their selection unequal. The weights can be based on a distance measure, as its decreasing function. With weights, each pool may comprise the whole sample, and each ineligible donor assigned zero weight.

Hot deck should be applied to all the missing values of a record simultaneously, so that the association of the imputed values is similar to the association of the recorded values. By way of an example, consider hot-deck imputation for the employment status in LFS for recipients with missing values at time points 4 and 5 (Example 5). If a recipient's status is imputed separately for the two time points, the imputed values will differ more frequently than might be expected. This would be the case even if the same pool of donors (subjects) were used on the two occasions. In contrast, if the status at both time points is imputed from the same (randomly selected) donor the imputed values will be identical about as frequently as among the potential donors — subjects similar to the recipient. In brief, plausibility of each imputed value is not sufficient for the plausibility of the set of imputed values of the record.

How large should a pool of donors be? Small pools offer too little variety of imputed values, whereas large pools may contain many potential donors that are very distant from the recipient. If estimation of the recipients' values is the goal, then small pools, defined by appropriate criteria, are better. Small pools may under-represent the variation of the values, and large pools may over-represent it. Setting aside ties, the nearest-neighbour method can be characterised as hot deck with pools comprising one subject each.

3.2.5 Weight adjustment

Records in a survey dataset are usually associated with sampling weights. The sampling weight for a member of the population is defined as the reciprocal of the probability that the member would have been included in the survey, as per plan, that is, in the complete dataset. The weights for the subjects (selected members) are factors in many common estimators of population quantities.

Weight adjustment is a device for reflecting the survey nonresponse in such estimators. It is motivated by the desire to maintain the good properties of the complete-data estimators without having to alter them substantially. The only change that takes place is in the sampling weights. The changes made can be related to estimation of the probabilities of selection in the *realised* design. For example, if a greater fraction of men than women fail to respond the weights associated with men are increased so that the fewer men in the subsample of respondents would represent well the men that were intended to be in the sample.

A common implementation of weight adjustment is based on a classification of the subjects into groups. The weights are then adjusted by multiplicative factors, specific to each group, so that the totals of the weights in the groups are proportional to the subpopulation sizes of the groups. When the groups are strata, or interpreted as such, weight adjustment is referred to as *poststratification*, since it amounts to an adjustment of the stratification (made *after* the data collection).

The weight-adjustment groups can be defined by cross-classifying several categorical variables, although the population size of each group (a combination of the values of the variables) has to be known. If there were no nonresponse, the total of the sampling weights for a group would differ from the population size by a random quantity. Forcing the match of the totals of the weights with the population therefore makes the data conform with the population more closely than it would in a complete dataset.

The subpopulation sizes are often available for the categories of several variables, but not for their combinations. It may be desirable to adjust the weights so that all sub-totals of the weights for the univariate margins agree with the corresponding subpopulation totals. This can be arranged by iterating the weight adjustments for one classification at a time, until the changes by an adjustment are small enough. This method is called *raking* [47].

A drawback of weight adjustment is that it is, effectively, a data reduction method, although the non-responding subjects are represented through the adjusted weights. The method relies on large subsample sizes within the groups, otherwise various anomalies may be encountered, such as very large weights. The subjects with such weights have an unduly large influence in most common estimators. Such estimators, although approximately unbiased, have inflated sampling variances. The problem can be resolved by trimming the weights, not allowing them to exceed a certain threshold. Although introducing some bias, the sampling variances of the estimators are usually reduced by trimming [172].

Weight adjustment is associated with a single (outcome) variable. For another variable, with nonresponse by different subjects, a different adjustment is appropriate. A compromise of the different adjustments is necessary in any multivariate analysis. This is difficult to arrange and, in the process, the rationale for the adjustment is difficult to sustain.

The original weights, set by design, are population quantities. After the adjustment, the weights are sample quantities because their calculation is based on the realised sample. In an estimator, such weights are random variables, and ignoring their sampling variation results in some distortion. The only protection at our disposal is to ensure that this variation is minute; in large-scale data, this can be achieved by defining adjustment categories with large subsample sizes. In other words, too detailed a poststratification may be counterproductive.

3.2.6 Regression imputation

Suppose variable Y is recorded with some values missing and variable Z is recorded completely. If Y and Z are associated, we may exploit their similarity by estimating (*predicting*) the missing values of Y. Suppose Y and Z are related by the model

$$Y = f(Z) + \varepsilon \, ,$$

Figure 3.1. Example of imputation using simple regression. Missing values of the outcome Y are marked by the symbol $\circ$, and the values imputed for them by $\times$.

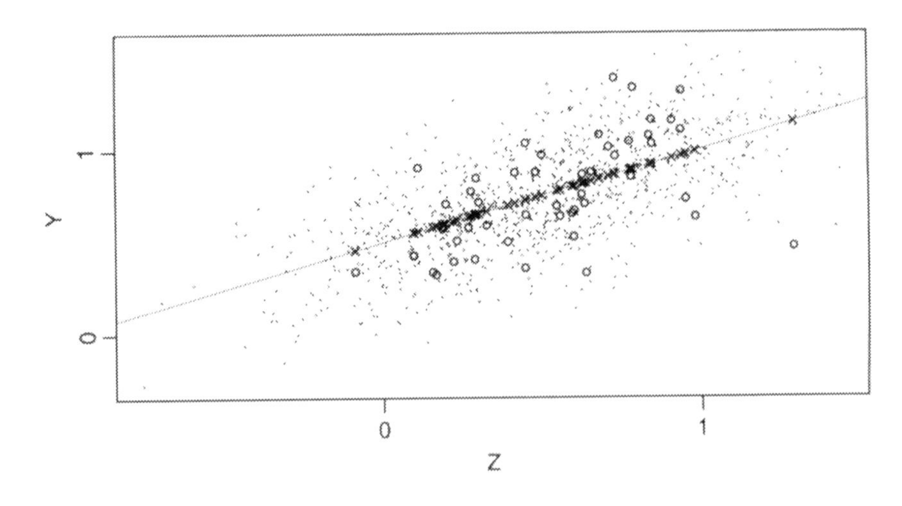

where f is a function, such as $f(z) = \beta_0 + \beta_1 z$, and ε a random variable with zero mean and a distribution known, except for some or all of its parameters, such as the centred normal, $\mathcal{N}(0, \sigma^2)$. If the function f were known

$$\hat{y}_j = f(z_j)$$

would be the obvious value to impute for the missing value y_j. By imputing $\hat{y}_j$, we reinforce the association of Y and Z because the pairs $(\hat{y}_j, z_j)$ satisfy the model more closely than (y_j, z_j) do. Also, the variation of y around z is distorted because the imputed deviation (residual) $\hat{\varepsilon}$ is equal to zero.

When f is not known, it (or its parameters) have to be estimated, and a further systematic 'error' is incurred as the estimated parameters ($\hat{\beta}_0$, $\hat{\beta}_1$ and $\hat{\sigma}^2$ for the simple regression) differ from their targets. The function f may involve several variables, it need not be linear, and the residual term need not be additive.

Regression imputation is illustrated in Figure 3.1. All the imputed values (marked by crosses $\times$) are on the regression line, here assumed to be known, whereas both the recorded values (dots $\cdot$) and missing values (circles $\circ$) are dispersed around the regression line. The sample residual variance is 0.0497, based on 1000 observations; its incomplete-data version, based on 950 observations is 0.0494, and its completed-data version is 0.470. The impact of the 50 (5%) imputed values with zero residuals is noticeable.

We could sacrifice the goal of fixing up the dataset by imputing $\tilde{y} = \beta_0 + \beta_1 z + \varepsilon$ instead of the prediction $\hat{y} = \beta_0 + \beta_1 z$. In this stochastic imputation we would need to know, in addition to β_0 and β_1, also the residual variance

σ^2, or use its estimate $\hat{\sigma}^2$. The values of y would not be 'estimated' optimally, but the dataset completed by $\tilde{y}$ would look more like what we might expect, as the values $\tilde{y}$ would be spread around the regression line as much as the recorded values y.

The model for y may involve several variables. If some of the regression variables themselves have missing values, the model may be fitted to the subsample of complete records. A compromise has to be sought between including more variables in the model, but basing the model fit on fewer observations, and including fewer variables but using more observations. With more variables, we improve our chances of an adequate model, but the model fit is associated with large sampling variation. With a less than adequate model, the model fit is associated with smaller sampling variation, but the model parameters are estimated with bias. Mean imputation can be regarded as a trivial case of regression imputation, with no regressors z.

For non-normally distributed variables y, we can formulate generalised linear models (GLM) [180]. Such models may yield predictions that are not admissible. For example, for binary data the prediction is converted to an estimated probability, $\hat{p}(z)$. In the spirit of estimating the outcome, we should round $\hat{p}(z)$, to zero or unity. By the stochastic version of this rule, a value is drawn from the fitted binary distribution $\mathcal{B}\{\hat{p}(z), 1\}$.

The problems with deterministic imputation schemes can be attributed to our failure to identify a model with negligible residual variation. The residual variation may be reduced by defining a model with many covariates. With the reduced estimated residual variance, the estimated sampling variance of the prediction $\hat{y}$ for an incomplete record would also be reduced. In most settings, this is not a realistic goal to aim for. The variation of the outcomes is inherent, and no attempt at its modelling is likely to account for its substantial part. When we do succeed, we should be wary of the increased sampling variation of $\hat{\sigma}^2$, especially when the number of degrees of freedom involved is greatly reduced.

3.2.7 Using experts' judgements

In surveys that collect a lot of information, in a variety of formats, formal rules for imputation are difficult to set. However, an expert knowledgeable about the population and the subject matter of the survey could propose a set of realistic values for the missing items after carefully studying the available part of the subject's record. Experts' guesses may be much more credible for imputation than using a simple or model-based imputation scheme. On the other hand, using experts is much more costly and time consuming, especially when only a few suitably trained and instructed experts are available.

Experts will impute typical values for the missing items, informed by the observed part of the record. Therefore, none of the imputed values will be unusual, even if idiosyncratic values can occasionally be found among the complete records. In brief, experts will make the database look more 'normal' than it should be. This deficiency is shared with regression imputation.

3.2.8 Data editing

The recorded data often contains obvious errors and conflicting values, such as employment status incompatible with age, unrealistic physical measurements, or a conflict of food consumed with declared dietary habit, such as being a vegetarian. In some cases, the data contains values, or sets of values, that are possible, but very unusual, so that it is reasonable to query them. The process of dealing with these certain or possible errors is referred to as *data editing.* It does not fall into the domain of missing data directly, but we can interpret a record with a likely error or a conflict as containing incomplete information. The value entered does not correspond to the information that we planned to collect. This idea is developed further in Section 4.6.

When there is an obvious way of correcting a value, the correction should be applied. A common example is the confusion of units, when sales, wages, or liabilities are given in units of currency (£) instead of multiples (£1000), as requested in the instructions. In some instances, incorrectness is identified straightaway, but the correct value is not. This should be regarded as a problem of imputation (with a positive probability of imputing the value entered originally. When numerous values of a variable are identified as incorrect (say, they are out of the realistic range of values), it is appropriate to regard as suspect even the values that do not appear erroneous. In the process of data recording, errors are committed that alter some of the appropriate values without making them unrealistic. For example, we may conclude that about 5% of the values of a variable are incorrect, but cannot identify any of them with certainty. No editing procedure can deal with this problem.

Editing shares with imputation the problem that the action taken may not restore the value or the record in the complete dataset. An item to be edited may be identified incorrectly and items that should be edited may not be flagged. And the change made (the *edition*) may be incorrect.

3.2.9 Single imputation. Summary

Completing the dataset is appealing to both the data constructor and the analyst because the result is an object in the same format as planned. If we do not distinguish between recorded and imputed data items the completed dataset pretends to contain more information than was collected by the survey. If we recovered all the missing values accurately the completed dataset would merely be a version of the observed data more convenient for the analysis.

With an inaccurate completion, we introduce errors in the data. Without distinguishing genuine and imputed values in the analysis, we end up under-estimating the sampling variation in our inferences. By how much? It depends on how much error has been introduced by the imputation, but also on the nature of the analysis. We show below that the extent of missing values is not always a good indicator of the extent of this underestimation, interpreted as an unjustified claim of precision. The inferences drawn may also be biased, especially when the imputation introduces a pattern in the survey data that is much stronger than among the recorded (genuine) observations.

If we draw a distinction between the recorded and imputed values we give up the original goal of relying on the complete-data tools and using them on a completed dataset as if it were the planned (complete) dataset. This suggests that the two goals — completing the dataset with efficiently estimated values of the missing items and promoting efficient analysis by complete-data tools — are in conflict. We cannot satisfy them simultaneously. What should be the data constructor's priority?

We regard as the principal purpose of the survey learning about the population (planned to have been) targeted by the survey. Therefore the data constructor's remit should be subordinated to the analysts' goals, and the former should aim to construct a database with which population inferences are relatively easy to make and are efficient and do not overestimate their precision (are 'honest'). A high-quality database, with imputation efficient for each value, is an intermediate product in the sequence connecting survey design and its analysis, and 'high-quality' should be interpreted as promoting efficient and 'honest' analysis, with the existing or reasonably expected resources and expertise. This confirms that the goals underlying single imputation, although well intended, aim to do the wrong thing.

3.3 Models for imputation

In the discussion of the single-imputation schemes, we have implied or stated directly that each of them is based on a model. In this section, we discuss such models in greater detail. By formulating the model explicitly, the case for more complex models and for reflecting the model's random variation becomes self-evident.

For LOCF with a categorical outcome variable, the model is

$$\mathrm{P}\left(X^{(k+1)} = X^{(k)} \,|\, X^{(k)} = x\right) = p\,, \tag{3.1}$$

where X denotes the outcome variable, the superscript k the time point, and the probability p is close to unity. In LOCF, we ignore the fact that $p < 1$ and act as if $X^{(k+1)} = X^{(k)}$ with certainty.

For a continuous variable, the model implied by LOCF is

$$X^{(k+1)} = X^{(k)} + \varepsilon^{(k)}\,, \tag{3.2}$$

with small residual variance $\sigma_k^2 = \mathrm{var}(\varepsilon^{(k)})$ for each k. In LOCF, we act as if $\sigma_k^2 \equiv 0$. The choices $p = 1$ and $\sigma_k^2 \equiv 0$ are convenient because they yield an obvious imputation. However, the observed data usually provide ample evidence that these extreme parameter values are inappropriate. Each imputed value is derived by a formula that is not satisfied by *all* the complete records.

This applies not only to (3.1) and (3.2), but to their various generalisations involving regression models. Regression imputation is appropriate only when the prediction is perfect and $\sigma^2 = 0$. When $\sigma^2 = 0$ and the regression function f contains a small number of parameters, f can be established without estimation error from a small number of complete records. When $\sigma^2 > 0$, not only f and σ^2 are estimated with sampling variation, but the deviation ε is not known either. Imputation would preserve *some* features of the incomplete dataset if f and σ^2 were known. By estimating them we do not preserve these features, merely attempt to do so.

3.3.1 Operating with uncertainty

Imputation schemes that aim to recover the value of a missing item by estimating it efficiently are suitable for recovering the values of any linear functions of the complete data. Let $f(\mathbf{x}) = b_1x_1 + \cdots + b_nx_n = \mathbf{b}^\top\mathbf{x}$ be a linear complete-data statistic with known coefficients $\mathbf{b} = (b_1, \ldots, b_n)^\top$. We can decompose it to its contributions from the recorded and missing values:

$$f(\mathbf{x}) = \sum_{i;R_i=1} b_ix_i + \sum_{i;R_i=0} b_ix_i \,.$$

As a complete-data statistic, $f(\mathbf{x})$ is associated with sampling variation — variation over the replications of the sampling design. With incomplete data, $f(\mathbf{x})$ is not a statistic because it involves values that are not available, namely, x_i for i such that $R_i = 0$. The value of $f(\mathbf{x})$ is *estimated*, even after the incomplete data is realised, by

$$\hat{f}(\mathbf{x}) = \sum_{i;R_i=1} b_ix_i + \sum_{i;R_i=0} b_i\hat{x}_i \,,$$

where $\hat{x}_i$ is the value imputed for x_i. Efficient estimation of each missing value x_i implies efficient estimation of $f(\mathbf{x})$. In particular, if each $\hat{x}_i$ is unbiased, then so is $f(\hat{\mathbf{x}})$. (For simplicity, we define $\hat{x}_i = x_i$ when x is recorded.) Here, efficient estimation of each missing value is in accord with efficient estimation of the statistic $f(\mathbf{x})$. This accord breaks down with any non-linear statistic.

Example 6

As a simple but instructive example, consider estimation of the quantity x^2 for a missing value x. Suppose the distribution of $\hat{x}$ is concentrated on -1, 0 and 1, with respective probabilities 0.1, 0.8 and 0.1, according to a suitable model, such as one implied by a hot-deck scheme. At first, it may be hard to find an argument against imputing zero; it is both the expected and modal value of the estimator $\hat{x}$. Zero is appropriate for imputing for x in any statistic that is linear in x, but imputing its square, also equal to zero, for x^2 does not seem to be rational. A small positive value is clearly better suited than zero, and imputing $\mathrm{E}(\hat{x}^2) = 0.2$ would eliminate the bias altogether. Similarly, for counting the number of positive values of x, 0.1 is the appropriate imputed value. □

This example shows that the substitution-estimator $f(\hat{\mathbf{x}})$ may not be suitable when f is not a linear function of $\mathbf{x}$. (Note that it is suitable for $f(x) = x^3$ in *this* example.) Estimating x^2 (with uncertainty) by $(\hat{x})^2$, or, more generally, $f(x)$ by $f(\hat{x})$ for any non-linear function f, may be inefficient, even when $\hat{x}$ is efficient for x. Without uncertainty, we can transpose the operations of substitution (for x) and evaluation (of a non-linear function). With uncertainty, we cannot transpose these operations. For an analyst not aware of this, or not aware of the uncertainty associated with the (imputed) values, this may appear as a contradiction: it is appropriate to use the value $x = 0$, but it is not appropriate to use $x^2 = 0$; $x^2 = 0.2$ is more appropriate, reflecting the uncertainty entailed.

This has several profound consequences. First, a dataset completed by (unbiased) efficient estimates of each missing value is a good basis for evaluating linear statistics but is not for non-linear statistics. For example, most estimators of sampling variances are quadratic functions of data. These require adjustments — an inflation to account for the uncertainty about the imputed values. Second, these adjustments depend on the actual uncertainty, which is not conveyed by the completed dataset. Third, each class of non-linear statistics requires a different adjustment. For example, $\mathrm{E}\{\exp(\hat{x})\} = (\mathrm{e}^{-1} + \mathrm{e} + 8)/10 = 1.109$ is greater than $\exp\{\mathrm{E}(\hat{x})\}$ by 0.109, whereas $\mathrm{E}\{(\hat{x})^2\}$ exceeds $\{\mathrm{E}(\hat{x})\}$ by 0.2.

In summary, we should estimate transformed quantities directly, and avoid transforming estimated quantities. It is impossible to adhere to this dictum all the time, but, whenever possible, we should. Estimating several population quantities and their sampling variances based on a single completed dataset is an example of ignoring this advice. Each non-linear transformation requires a different completion; if a single completed dataset is available each non-linear transformation requires a different adjustment to represent the uncertainty about the imputed values. The imputed values have to be flagged, and the information about the uncertainty implied by the imputation provided.

Multiple imputation, introduced in Chapter 4, addresses this problem by generating several completions, none of them aiming to recover the complete dataset, but representing the uncertainty about the missing values by the differences among the completions. By collating the results of the complete-data analyses, an estimator is defined that 'inherits' the good properties of the complete-data estimator and reflects the information lost due to missing values. To distinguish this approach, we refer to the methods discussed in this chapter as *single imputation*.

3.3.2 Models for the nonresponse process

The analyst's understanding of the studied processes in the population is but one contributor to the formulation of the models. The nonresponse process is another — it can inform the imputation process and the model it is based on. But it is difficult to learn about it from the observed data because, by definition, we fail to observe it. We may find out about it from sources external to the collected data; by contacting the respondents outside the remit of the survey, when this is possible, consulting the interviewers, from the survey and its predecessors, or from similar and related surveys. The best course of action is to organise the survey and set its details so that nonresponse would be reduced to minimum. The next best thing is to know about the reasons and motives for nonresponse, and how they are related to the data, missing or recorded, that we intended to collect. And further, what other information we could collect that would promote our understanding of the nonresponse process, and help us reduce its impact on the planned analyses.

The processes of sampling and nonresponse reduce the complete information about the population first to the complete (sample) dataset, and then to the incomplete (recorded) dataset. We assume that the two processes are independent (unconnected), as the subjects are either not informed about the sampling design or such information does not influence their willingness to cooperate. As nonresponse is a nuisance process, making inferences would become much simpler if we were able to deal with it separately from the sampling process. The key to such a separation is the assumption of MAR. MAR, or MCAR, is central to all common single-imputation schemes, although that is rarely stated explicitly. Without MAR, no claims can be made about good properties of the imputed values. The mechanism of MAR is qualified by the variables involved in conditioning. Inclusion of further variables in conditioning improves the chances that MAR is achieved, or reduces its deviation from MAR so much that the assumption of MAR is acceptable. NMAR contains all manner of idiosyncratic processes that are an obvious threat to inferences based on all data-reduction and completion schemes.

The models we have considered so far assume that certain features of the population appear also in the sample — an assumption supported by appropriate sampling design — and that they appear also among the incomplete records. The latter is not always a reasonable assumption. For example, subjects with a changed employment status in LFS, or those who have made a particular transition, such as from inactivity to employment, are more likely to be non-respondents. The observed data may not provide any clues about this, but that does not absolve us from disregarding such a possibility, especially if its consequence is a distortion of our inferences.

In practice, we have at most a limited insight into the nonresponse processes, and no simple model is likely to be adequate for their description. With a complex model, involving as many variables as is manageable, we improve our chances of including the appropriate model, or a model very close to it. (An appropriate model means that with it MAR applies; such a model need not be unique.)

We have highlighted the unsatisfactory nature of the model-based (single) imputation. The criticism is intended at single deterministic imputation, not at the use of the models. The use of the models is deficient because we pretend certainty where it is absent — for imputations we use the fitted values, even though they are less than perfect replacements. First, the collected data (observations) do not obey model formulas; second, the model parameters are not recovered from the available data accurately; and third, observations are oblivious to models, especially those constructed with convenience in mind, and to the conventions involved in the recorded versions of the variables that are aimed at simplifying the data-collection (interviewing or questionnaire completion) process and reducing the burden on the respondent.

3.4 EM algorithm

Many complete-data analyses use the individual data items only through a few data summaries. For example, the ordinary regression ($y = \mathbf{z}\boldsymbol{\beta} + \varepsilon$) requires only the totals of cross-products of all the variables involved, that is, y, $\mathbf{z}$ and the vector $\mathbf{1}$ (intercept). Let $\mathbf{X}^* = (\mathbf{1},\ \mathbf{Z},\ \mathbf{y})$ and $\boldsymbol{\theta} = (\hat{\boldsymbol{\beta}}^\top,\ \hat{\sigma}^2)$, the vector of all model parameters, and denote by $\hat{\boldsymbol{\theta}}$ its least squares estimator. Then

$$\hat{\boldsymbol{\theta}}(\mathbf{X}^*) = \hat{\boldsymbol{\theta}}\left\{\mathbf{t}(\mathbf{X}^*)\right\} ,$$

where $\mathbf{t}$ is the function that evaluates $\mathbf{X}^{*\top}\mathbf{X}^*$; the elements of $\mathbf{t}(\mathbf{X}^*)$ are called the *sufficient statistics* for $\boldsymbol{\theta} = (\boldsymbol{\beta}^\top, \sigma^2)$. They are all the sample quantities needed to evaluate $\hat{\boldsymbol{\theta}}$. The function $\mathbf{t}$ can be replaced by alternatives; $\mathbf{t}$ remains sufficient when we supplement it by some other statistics or when we apply a strictly monotone transformation to some of its components. By definition, even $\mathbf{X}^*$ is a sufficient statistic for $\boldsymbol{\theta}$. A set of sufficient statistics is called *minimal* if it can be recovered by transformations from any other set of sufficient statistics. For example, $\mathbf{X}^*$ is not minimal for ordinary least squares because it cannot be recovered from the matrix of totals of squares and cross-products $\mathbf{t}(\mathbf{X}^*)$. A set of (minimal) sufficient statistics is qualified by the estimators we wish to evaluate. A set of statistics may be sufficient for one set of estimators but not for another.

Why should we estimate each missing value when, for estimating a parameter vector $\boldsymbol{\theta}$, it suffices to estimate a set of minimal sufficient statistics for $\hat{\boldsymbol{\theta}}$? With complete data, $\mathbf{t}(\mathbf{X}^*)$ would be known; when it contains only a few items its estimation based on the incomplete dataset is a much simpler task than data completion. We have drawn a similar conclusion, motivated by the pursuit of efficiency, in Section 3.3.1.

The method of estimating the sufficient statistics is motivated by the EM (expectation–maximisation) algorithm. The EM algorithm is formulated for fitting models by maximum likelihood (ML). Likelihood is defined as the joint density of the observations, with the roles of the observed values $\mathbf{X}$ and (unknown) values of the model parameters $\boldsymbol{\theta}$ interchanged. Although many complete-data estimators for sample surveys are not ML, the principle of the EM algorithm carries over to our context.

Suppose the complete-data analysis maximises the log-likelihood function $l(\boldsymbol{\theta};\, \mathbf{X}^*) = \log\{L(\boldsymbol{\theta};\, \mathbf{X}^*)\}$. With incomplete data, ML amounts to maximising the log-likelihood function $l(\boldsymbol{\theta};\, \mathbf{X}) = \log\{L(\boldsymbol{\theta};\, \mathbf{X})\}$. This is related to the complete-data likelihood by the identity

$$L(\boldsymbol{\theta};\, \mathbf{X}) = \int L(\boldsymbol{\theta};\, \mathbf{X}^*)\, \mathrm{d}\mathbf{X}_{\mathrm{mis}}\,, \tag{3.3}$$

where $\mathbf{X}_{\mathrm{mis}}$ is the set of missing values of $\mathbf{X}^*$. The integral is with respect to the distribution of $\mathbf{X}_{\mathrm{mis}}$, that is, over the joint distribution of the missing data. Maximising (3.3) directly is often an intractable task, unless the integral can be expressed in a closed form. The second-order partial differentials of $l(\boldsymbol{\theta};\, \mathbf{X})$, required for the Newton-Raphson and Fisher scoring algorithms, are difficult to evaluate or even approximate, especially when missing values appear in a variety of patterns. The complete-data log-likelihood $l(\boldsymbol{\theta};\, \mathbf{X}^*)$ depends on the data only through a set of minimal sufficient statistics. It would be advantageous to relate the task of maximising $l(\boldsymbol{\theta}; \mathbf{X})$ to maximising $l(\boldsymbol{\theta}; \mathbf{X}^*)$, because the latter is the analysis planned at the outset.

The EM algorithm is an iterative procedure that combines the complete-data analysis with estimation of the sufficient statistics. Each iteration comprises two steps, E and M. In the E-step the sufficient statistics are estimated by their conditional expectations given the data and the current estimates of the parameters. A version of sufficient statistics is selected for which $l(\boldsymbol{\theta};\, \mathbf{X}^*)$ is their linear function. That is, the E-step estimates the complete-data log-likelihood. The sufficient statistics have to be estimated whenever they depend on missing values.

In the M-step, the complete-data analysis is applied, with the sufficient statistics replaced by their provisional estimates (conditional expectations) obtained in the preceding E-step. Iterations are necessary when the E-step depends on the parameter estimates because they have been updated in the preceding M-step.

An important practical advantage of the EM algorithm is that it makes use of the complete-data method, although the program implementing it has to be adapted. This requires some expertise in the complete-data method and programming skills to alter its implementation; the complete-data method cannot be applied as a black-box. Further, evaluation of the conditional expectations may be both tedious and difficult to program when many sufficient statistics have to be estimated and contributions evaluated from incomplete records with numerous response patterns. The EM algorithm requires iterations, and therefore much more computing time than the complete-data method. This is not a serious concern nowadays, even when the convergence is very slow.

In some situations, however, the changes by an iteration of the EM algorithm are very small, but getting smaller from one iteration to the next only fractionally. Then it may be difficult to judge when to stop the iterations, because substantial changes might accrue after a large number of subsequent iterations. The speed of convergence is related to the *fraction of the missing information*. .. Information about a quantity is defined as the reciprocal of the MSE of its efficient estimator. Of course, the dataset is an important factor in this definition. The missing information about a parameter is defined as the difference of the information contained in the complete and incomplete data sets, and the fraction of missing information is the ratio of this difference and the complete-data information.

Let $\mathcal{I}(\theta) = 1/\mathrm{var}(\hat{\theta}; \mathbf{X})$ and $\mathcal{I}^*(\theta) = 1/\mathrm{var}(\hat{\theta}^*; \mathbf{X}^*)$ be the reciprocal MSE's (precisions) of efficient estimators $\hat{\theta}$ and $\hat{\theta}^*$ of θ based on the respective incomplete and complete data. Then the fraction of missing information is

$$\frac{\mathcal{I}^*(\theta) - \mathcal{I}(\theta)}{\mathcal{I}^*(\theta)} .$$

Lower fraction of missing information is associated with faster convergence. The extent of missing data (the number of missing items) is not a reliable indicator of the fraction of missing information and the fraction is not the same for all the quantities estimated with the same dataset.

The EM algorithm can be applied without a reference to any likelihood. It suffices to define the sufficient statistics required for a particular complete-data estimator, and estimate these statistics, or the contributions to them made by the missing values. Without the reference to a likelihood, there is some ambiguity as to which version of a sufficient statistic should be estimated. Estimating $t(\mathbf{x})$ yields a result different from estimating $g^{-1}\{t^\dagger(\mathbf{x})\}$, where $t^\dagger(\mathbf{x}) = g\{t(\mathbf{x})\}$ and g is a non-linear strictly monotone function.

The term 'EM' was coined by [44] and they presented the algorithm as a general approach to dealing with missing values. The generality is further enhanced by defining certain problems in terms of incomplete (observed) data. These include measurement error and misclassification, rounding and censoring, using methods for balanced data when the observed data are not balanced, random-effect models and, more generally, complex models that would be much easier to handle if some of its terms were known. Although effective in many settings, the EM algorithm is a not well suited for a wide range of analyses because some of them require considerable development and programming effort in addition to implementing the complete-data analysis.

The methodological importance of the EM algorithm is that it exposes the weakness of the naive approach to data completion — single imputation breaks down when the imputed data are subjected to a non-linear transformation. The underlying problem is that the operations of a non-linear transformation and conditional expectation do not commute. (Estimation can be regarded as taking conditional expectation, as in the E-step.) In naive approaches, the estimates are transformed; in the EM algorithm, the transformations are estimated. In brief, it is preferable to estimate $g(\theta)$ by $\widehat{g(\theta)}$ than by $g(\hat{\theta})$, even when $\hat{\theta}$ is efficient for θ.

3.5 Suggested reading

The first part of [146] gives more background to incomplete data, with examples of small datasets from experiments and a more extensive discussion of single-imputation methods. Estimators derived by raking are studied by [21] and [18]. A generalisation of raking is developed by [46] and [47]. Reference [106] is a suitable entry point into literature on poststratification. An application of raking to dealing with nonresponse in a survey is presented in [17].

Variance estimators for statistics based on data completed by single imputation are developed in [221]. A similar goal is pursued by [142].

The subject of incomplete data was revolutionised by [44], who introduced the term 'EM algorithm'. Their general formulation draws on the solutions of specific problems in [97], [91], [92], [201] and [11]. Throughout the 1980's and 1990's, the EM algorithm has been developed in a multitude of directions, culminating in [188]. Two principal drawbacks of the EM algorithm are slow convergence and unavailability of an estimator of the sampling variance. The former is addressed, among others, by [186], [116], [127], [117] and [72]. Solutions to the latter include [169], [190] and [199]. A Bayesian version of the EM algorithm, known as data augmentation, is described in [269] and [284]. Reference [234] contains a summary of the developments and outlines several avenues for further research, some of them addressed by [188] and [117]. Reference [183] is a monograph on the EM algorithm and [184] deals with finite mixture models, a particular application of the EM algorithm. The setting of [147], with data comprising categorical and continuous (normally distributed) variables, covers a wide range of problems for which the implementation of the EM algorithm is feasible.

Probably the most prominent and high-profile problem in government statistics in the U.S.A. and the UK is the issue of the census undercount (referred to as underenumeration in the UK). This is a challenging missing-data problem, notwithstanding the small rate of nonresponse compared to most national surveys. See [15], [272] and [224].

3.6 Exercises

1. Generate a longitudinal dataset with at least 10 000 subjects, in which each subject starts, at time point 0, with the same value of the key variable, but at the next time point 1 the value increases by one with probability 0.1, decreases by one with probability 0.05 and remains unchanged with probability 0.85. At the following time points, the value increases by one with probability 0.25 and decreases by one with probability 0.30 if an increase or decrease, respectively, was registered also at the previous time point. Otherwise the probability of increase and decrease is 0.1 and 0.05, respectively. Suppose nonresponse occurs only at time points 4–7, with monotone patterns (by dropping out).

   Devise various nonresponse mechanisms that are MCAR, MAR or NMAR, at least one of each, and implement them. Aim to have at least 20% of the records incomplete. Apply LOCF to the incomplete data and compare the complete-data and completed-data distributions of the values at the time points 4–7 separately (by four univariate comparisons) and jointly (by a single multivariate comparison). For the multivariate comparison define suitable summaries of the quartets of values, so that the problem is manageable.
2. Repeat Exercise 1, using data reduction and a limited version of LOCF in which a value can be brought forward only one step (that is, only if it was recorded in the previous/donor time point).
3. Summarise the advantages of the hot deck as they relate to the setting of Exercise 1, and devise and implement a scheme to complete the data.

   Hints: Apply separate schemes for each response pattern (dropping out at points 4, ..., 7). Match on the entire available history for earlier drop outs, and on a latter part of it for later drop outs. Discuss the merits of imputing for the entire missing sub-vector (say, for time points 5–7) using a single donor, or using different donors for each time point.
4. Suppose the percentages of a population in sex-by-age groups are given by Table 3.1 for a country of 2.2 million inhabitants. Generate a small number of samples of size 2000 from this population (by SRS) and adjust the weights (originally constant) by raking. Compare the sets of weights across the samples. Assess the randomness associated with the adjusted weights.
5. Simulate a dataset by simple regression, $y = x + \varepsilon$, with the usual assumptions of normality and homoscedasticity, and the values of x drawn from a uniform distribution on $(0, 10)$. Use $\mathrm{var}(\varepsilon) = 1.0$. Delete about 25% of the outcomes y by MCAR and apply the regression imputation for them. Compare the model fit to the complete data, the completed data and the reduced data. Devise a sequence of NMAR mechanisms, by giving greater preference to deletion of outcomes y that exceed the predictor x, and compare the merits of the analyses based on the three datasets.

Table 3.1. Sex-by-age distribution of a population for Example 4.

	Age group (years)					
	0–15	16–24	25–39	40–64	65–	All
Men	10.4	5.2	10.8	18.2	4.5	49.1
Women	10.5	5.4	11.2	18.8	5.0	50.9

6. Apply a stochastic imputation scheme to the data generated in the previous example. Compare the analyses based on the complete and completed datasets and contrast them with the differences between the values of y that were deleted and the values imputed for them. Assess what is more important: to come close to the complete dataset or for the estimates to come close to the results of the complete-data analysis.
7. With a complete dataset generated in the previous exercise, add a 'measurement error' to each value of x, that is, generate $x^\dagger = x + \delta$, where δ is drawn at random from a centred distribution. Use $\delta \sim \mathcal{N}(0, 0.5)$ or δ uniformly distributed on $(-1.2, 1.2)$. Fit the simple regression model $y = a + bx + \varepsilon$ using the values of y and $x^\dagger$, and compare the results with the generating model ($a = 0$, $b = 1$, $\mathrm{var}(\varepsilon) = 1$) and the fit to the complete data. To compare the corresponding distributions, apply the data-generating and estimation processes in several replications.

4

Multiple imputation

The ideal solution of the problem of analysing incomplete data $\mathbf{X}$ would be its completion, to a dataset $\mathbf{X}_+$, for which the estimator $\hat{\theta}$ of the target θ is efficient and the estimator $\hat{s}^2$ of its sampling variance (approximately) unbiased, for a wide range of pairs of estimators $(\hat{\theta}, \hat{s}^2)$. As these estimators are considered for different datasets, it is essential to introduce a notation that indicates the dataset used. Thus, $\hat{\theta}(\mathbf{X}^*)$ and $\hat{s}^2(\mathbf{X}^*)$ are (complete-data) estimators of θ and $s^2 = \mathrm{var}\{\hat{\theta}(\mathbf{X}^*)\}$, respectively. We assume that $\hat{\theta}(\mathbf{X}^*)$ is efficient for θ and $\hat{s}^2(\mathbf{X}^*)$ (approximately) unbiased for $s^2 = \mathrm{var}\{\hat{\theta}(\mathbf{X}^*)\}$. In the ideal solution to the problem of data incompleteness, $\hat{\theta}(\mathbf{X}_+)$ would be efficient for θ and $\hat{s}^2(\mathbf{X}_+)$ (approximately) unbiased for $\mathrm{var}\{\hat{\theta}(\mathbf{X}_+)\}$. With the complete data $\mathbf{X}^*$, sampling (or data generation) is the only source of variation, whereas with the incomplete data both sampling and nonresponse contribute to the variation of any estimator. Therefore we are unlikely to find an estimator $\hat{s}^2$ that is unbiased both with $\mathbf{X}^*$ and with $\mathbf{X}_+$.

The standard error of an estimator or, more generally, any property of an estimator, depends on the replication scheme that would establish it. In particular, the distribution of an estimator with respect to the sampling process differs from the distribution with respect to the convolution of sampling and (nontrivial) nonresponse processes. A notation more complete than $\hat{\theta}(\mathbf{X})$ would include a reference to the replication scheme. We do not introduce such a notation, mainly for typographical reasons. The type of replication will either be obvious from the context or will be explicitly stated.

The EM algorithm and the arguments presented in Section 3.3.1 imply that the ideal of a single completion on which to base a multitude of inferences is unattainable. We can complete the dataset $\mathbf{X}$ so that $\hat{\theta}(\mathbf{X}_+)$ is efficient, but with the same completion $\mathbf{X}_+$, $\hat{s}^2(\mathbf{X}_+)$ is biased. Moreover, for an efficient estimator $\hat{\theta}'$ of a different quantity θ', $\hat{\theta}'(\mathbf{X}_+)$ may also be inefficient. If the completion $\mathbf{X}_+$ is such that a complete-data statistic $t(\mathbf{X}^*)$ is estimated by $t(\mathbf{X}_+)$ without bias, then a different complete-data statistic, $t'(\mathbf{X}^*)$, may be estimated by $t'(\mathbf{X}_+)$ with bias.

This chapter describes the method of multiple imputation as a resolution of the conflict between the desire for a single completion of the dataset and the use of complete-data estimators. Several completions are generated, but the complete-data estimators are applied without any alteration.

4.1 The consequences of imperfect imputation

Example 6 in Section 3.3.1 confirms the conclusion drawn from the EM algorithm. If we estimate each missing data item without bias and efficiently, we estimate a linear complete-data statistic $t(\mathbf{X}^*)$ without bias and efficiently, but not a quadratic (or some other non-linear) statistic $t'(\mathbf{X}^*)$. This has important repercussions on how a database constructor 'cleans' a survey dataset. The well-established practice is to complete the database as well as possible (imputation) and remove any unrealistic values or resolve any conflicts of the values (editing). The practice is appropriate so long as the uncertainty about each missing item is negligible. Otherwise, the cleaned-up data appears to contain more information than was collected. Analysts not acquainted with all the details of imputation and editing will analyse the dataset as if it were the observed data, not aware of the data clean-up or of its impact on the inferences. They are likely to draw inferences with greater estimated precision than is justified. But Example 6 implies that bias and loss of efficiency of the estimators used can also occur.

One solution to this problem is to inform the analysts about the importance of incompleteness (its impact on the inferences), and supply all the details relevant to it: how the missing data might be imputed; what is known or can reasonably be conjectured about the nonresponse process; and what other data sources might be useful in devising good imputation methods. In brief, to transfer all the know-how and information relevant to the analysis of incomplete data. The analysts would then deal with the incompleteness on their own. Providing information additional to the incomplete or completed dataset may involve references to other data sources. Logistic difficulties may arise when arranging access to them, or the access may be barred because of confidentiality concerns. As a result, the pursuit of good statistical practice is discouraged.

The problem is complex, its solutions are imperfect and highly contingent on available information and understanding of the underlying processes. A more effective way of dealing with the problem would be to stick to the current mode of operation and rely on the data constructors to address all problems that can be attributed to incompleteness. After all, they, or their organisations, conducted the survey and planned to collect a complete dataset. They have failed, not by their own fault, but a denial of the failure and of its consequences only compounds the problem. The constructors should not only complete the dataset, so that it would be amenable to any complete-data analysis, but enable their clients, (secondary) analysts, to draw inferences that are efficient, estimate the MSE of the estimators without bias, and yet require no specialised software or expertise beyond that for implementing the intended complete-data methods.

4.2 The method

The method of multiple imputation (MI) is motivated by the standard formulated in the previous section. It assumes that the database is to be analysed by several secondary analysts, with a wide range of inferential goals (population quantities as targets) and using a variety of statistical software tools and methods well suited only for complete data. In MI, a small number of alternative completions are generated, based on a model for nonresponse. The analyst applies the complete-data method to each completed dataset. The results are then averaged, with an appropriate inflation for the sampling variance that reflects the uncertainty about the missing values.

In the next four sections, we discuss each step in turn, starting with specifying and fitting models for missing values.

4.2.1 Fitting a model for missing values

This step entails specifying the joint distribution of the response indicator and the complete data, that is, $(\mathbf{R}, \mathbf{X}^*)$. Suppose $\mathbf{X}^*$ comprises a completely recorded vector $\mathbf{Z}$ and an incompletely recorded vector $\mathbf{Y}$; $\mathbf{X}^* = (\mathbf{Y}^*, \mathbf{Z})$ and $\mathbf{X} = (\mathbf{Y}, \mathbf{Z})$. The variables in $\mathbf{Y}$ and $\mathbf{Z}$ need not be the outcome variables and covariates, respectively, in any analysis. We can partition the joint distribution of the complete data $(\mathbf{R}, \mathbf{Y}^*, \mathbf{Z})$ as

$$(\mathbf{R}, \mathbf{Y}^*, \mathbf{Z}) \sim (\mathbf{R}, \mathbf{Y}^* \,|\, \mathbf{Z})\,(\mathbf{Z}) \,,$$

and then as either

$$(\mathbf{R}, \mathbf{Y}^* \,|\, \mathbf{Z}) \sim (\mathbf{R} \,|\, \mathbf{Y}^*, \mathbf{Z})\,(\mathbf{Y}^* \,|\, \mathbf{Z}) \tag{4.1}$$

or

$$(\mathbf{R}, \mathbf{Y}^* \,|\, \mathbf{Z}) \sim (\mathbf{Y}^* \,|\, \mathbf{R}, \mathbf{Z})\,(\mathbf{R} \,|\, \mathbf{Z})\,. \tag{4.2}$$

In (4.1), a complete-data model, $(\mathbf{Y}^* \,|\, \mathbf{Z})$, is specified together with a model for the response patterns, $(\mathbf{R} \,|\, \mathbf{Y}^*, \mathbf{Z})$. Models specified in this way are called *selection* models, because the conditional distribution of $\mathbf{R}$ given $\mathbf{X}^*$ describes a process that selects the items to be recorded (or missing). In (4.2), a different conditional distribution $(\mathbf{Y}^* \,|\, \mathbf{Z})$ is specified for each pattern $\mathbf{R}$; these models are called *pattern-mixture* models; they describe the joint distribution of the complete data as a mixture of distributions, one for each response pattern.

Each distribution in (4.1) and (4.2) is associated with a set of parameters. For instance, a more complete formulation of (4.1) is

$$(\mathbf{R}, \mathbf{Y}^* \,|\, \mathbf{Z};\, \boldsymbol{\zeta}, \boldsymbol{\psi}) \;\sim\; (\mathbf{R} \,|\, \mathbf{Y}^*, \mathbf{Z};\, \boldsymbol{\zeta})\, (\mathbf{Y}^* \,|\, \mathbf{Z};\, \boldsymbol{\psi})\,.$$

The parameter vectors $\boldsymbol{\zeta}$ and $\boldsymbol{\psi}$ are said to be *separated* when they are distinct and no constraints are imposed that involve some elements of both vectors. The nonresponse mechanism is called *ignorable* when it is MAR and $\boldsymbol{\zeta}$ and $\boldsymbol{\psi}$ are separated. The importance of ignorability is that the joint distributions in (4.1) and (4.2) do not depend on the missing values, $\mathbf{Y}_{\mathrm{mis}}$, and the log-likelihood has two unrelated summands, one depending on $\boldsymbol{\zeta}$ only and the other on $\boldsymbol{\psi}$ only. Then these parameter vectors can be estimated separately. In a selection model, $\boldsymbol{\zeta}$ can be estimated solely from $(\mathbf{Y} \,|\, \mathbf{Z}; \boldsymbol{\zeta})$, e.g., by maximum likelihood; it involves neither $\mathbf{R}$ nor $\boldsymbol{\psi}$.

When MAR applies, $\mathbf{Y}^*$ can be replaced by $\mathbf{Y}$ in both equations (4.1) and (4.2). For ignorable mechanisms, (4.1) and (4.2) coincide, but for non-ignorable models they differ substantially. The recorded data rarely provide any clues about the relative merits of the approaches based on selection and pattern-mixture models for NMAR mechanisms, and so an important criterion is how convenient it is to work with these models. That depends on the circumstances related to the data, but also on the analyst's preferences.

An advantage of the selection models is the connection to the complete data. Under MAR, the conditional distribution $(\mathbf{Y} \,|\, \mathbf{Z})$ does not depend on the pattern $\mathbf{R}$. So, the model fitted to the complete records applies also to each pattern $\mathbf{R}$. Without constraints on the parameters in $(\mathbf{Y} \,|\, \mathbf{R}, \mathbf{Z})$ and $(\mathbf{R} \,|\, \mathbf{Z})$, pattern-mixture models are not identified because, for incomplete patterns $\mathbf{R}$, they involve parameters that relate to values missing in $\mathbf{Y}$.

In practice, MAR is assumed and the parameters $\boldsymbol{\zeta}$ and $\boldsymbol{\psi}$ are separated. The model for nonresponse can then be fitted to the complete records; the same model applies to the records that are incomplete. The information about the nonresponse mechanism can be used more effectively by fitting the model using the EM algorithm. This is useful especially when there are many incomplete records, most of them with only one or a few items missing.

4.2.2 Generating plausible values

The fitted model can be regarded as an instrument for generating replacements for the missing values. As an example, suppose univariate Y and Z are related by simple regression,

$$Y \;=\; \beta_0 + \beta_1 Z + \varepsilon\,, \tag{4.3}$$

with the usual assumptions of normality, independence and homoscedasticity. The regression parameters $\boldsymbol{\beta} = (\beta_0\,, \beta_1)^\top$ are estimated by least squares applied to the complete records $(Y,\, Z)$. The estimator $\hat{\boldsymbol{\beta}} = (\hat{\beta}_0\,, \hat{\beta}_1)^\top$ has sampling variance $\sigma^2 \left(\mathbf{Z}^\top \mathbf{Z}\right)^{-1}$, where $\sigma^2 = \mathrm{var}(\varepsilon)$ and $\mathbf{Z} = (\mathbf{1}, \mathbf{z})$ is formed by attaching the intercept column of ones to the vector of the values of Z.

In MI, the replacements for the missing values are generated not from the fitted model, but from a *plausible* model. A plausible model is based on a plausible set of parameters $\tilde{\sigma}^2$ and $\tilde{\boldsymbol{\beta}}$ drawn from the (approximate and/or estimated) sampling distribution of the parameter estimates. Thus, for the simple regression example in (4.3), we draw first $\tilde{\sigma}^2$ by the following scheme:

1. draw u from χ^2_{n-2};
2. set $\tilde{\sigma}^2 = (n-2)\hat{\sigma}^2/u$.

(n is the sample size.) This is derived by inverting the distributional identity

$$(n-2)\frac{\hat{\sigma}^2}{\sigma^2} \sim \chi^2_{n-2} \,.$$

As an alternative, $\tilde{\sigma}^2$ can be generated as the $(n-2)/\hat{\sigma}^2$-multiple of u.

With a generated value of $\tilde{\sigma}^2$, a plausible vector of regression parameters $\tilde{\boldsymbol{\beta}}$ is obtained by a draw from

$$\mathcal{N}\left\{\hat{\boldsymbol{\beta}},\, \tilde{\sigma}^2 \left(\mathbf{Z}^\top\mathbf{Z}\right)^{-1}\right\} \,.$$

The key feature of the plausible parameters is that they reflect the uncertainty involved in their estimation. The *plausible values*, used for imputation of the missing values, are generated from the plausible model. For (4.3) with $\tilde{\boldsymbol{\beta}}$ and $\tilde{\sigma}^2$, a set of plausible values for $\mathbf{Y}_{\mathrm{mis}}$ is generated as

$$\mathbf{Y}_{\mathrm{mis}} \sim \tilde{\beta}_0 + \tilde{\beta}_1 \mathbf{Z}_{(\mathrm{Y;mis})} + \boldsymbol{\varepsilon} \,,$$

where $\mathbf{Z}_{(\mathrm{Y;mis})}$ is the vector of values of Z associated with the observations that have missing values of Y and $\boldsymbol{\varepsilon}$ is a random sample from $\mathcal{N}(0, \tilde{\sigma}^2)$, with an element for each missing value of Y.

The plausible values are generated with randomness that reflects the uncertainty about the missing values, given a plausible model. In most settings, this involves drawing a set of plausible parameters in the model for nonresponse. They are drawn from the estimated distribution of the corresponding estimators. Plausible values are then drawn from the plausible model, given by the plausible parameters. By conditioning on a plausible model, we would pretend that we know the model parameters. Without such conditioning, the variation of the plausible values reflects the uncertainty about the missing values, given the (general) model in (4.3).

MI requires several sets of plausible values. To obtain another set, the processes of generating a plausible model and plausible values based on it are replicated. Setting the number of sets of plausible values, denoted by M, is discussed later; five sets are sufficient in most settings. The sets of plausible values entail two sources of variation: within a set, the consequence of uncertainty resulting from the stochastic nature of the plausible model, and among sets, the consequence of uncertainty about the model parameters.

4.2.3 Analysis of each completed dataset

In the next step, the complete-data analysis is applied to each dataset constructed by completing the observed dataset $\mathbf{X}$ with a set of plausible values. The resulting datasets are called *completed*. The completion is illustrated in Figure 4.1. There are three missing items in the example, all for variable D, and the $M = 5$ sets of plausible values are given in the columns M1, ..., M5. The completed datasets are denoted by $\mathbf{X}_1, \mathbf{X}_2, \ldots, \mathbf{X}_M$. Suppose $\hat{\theta}^* = \hat{\theta}(\mathbf{X}^*)$ is an efficient complete-data estimator of θ and $\hat{s}^2(\mathbf{X}^*)$ an unbiased estimator of $\mathrm{var}(\hat{\theta}^*)$. The mth completion of $\mathbf{X}$ yields the completed-data estimate $\hat{\theta}_m = \hat{\theta}(\mathbf{X}_m)$ and the estimate of the associated sampling variance $\hat{s}^2_m = \hat{s}^2(\mathbf{X}_m)$. Each estimator $\hat{\theta}_m$ is unbiased for θ, and each $\hat{s}^2_m$ is unbiased for the complete-data estimator of the sampling variance $s^2\{\hat{\theta}(\mathbf{X}^*)\}$. However, $\hat{s}^2_m$ underestimates the sampling variance of $\hat{\theta}_m$ when the variance is evaluated over both sampling and imputation (completion).

4.2.4 The MI estimator

The MI estimator of θ is defined as the average of the completed-data estimators,

$$\hat{\theta}_{\mathrm{MI}} = \frac{1}{M} \sum_{m=1}^{M} \hat{\theta}_m ;$$

it is unbiased for θ. Its sampling variance is estimated, with small or no bias, by

$$\hat{s}^2_{\mathrm{MI}} = \overline{\hat{s}^2} + \frac{M+1}{M} \hat{B} ,$$

where

$$\overline{\hat{s}^2} = \frac{1}{M} \sum_{m=1}^{M} \hat{s}^2_m$$

$$\hat{B} = \frac{1}{M-1} \sum_{m=1}^{M} \left(\hat{\theta}_m - \hat{\theta}_{\mathrm{MI}} \right)^2 .$$

The MI estimator of the sampling variance, $\hat{s}^2_{\mathrm{MI}}$, is aimed at the variance of $\hat{\theta}_{\mathrm{MI}}$ in replications of the sampling *and* nonresponse mechanisms.

4.2.5 The lost information

The average completed-data sampling variance estimator $\overline{\hat{s}^2}$ is an unbiased estimator of the complete-data sampling variance $s^2(\mathbf{X}^*)$. The between-imputation sample variance $\hat{B}$ is an unbiased estimator of the between-imputation variance B, the variance attributable to the missing data. If an

Figure 4.1. Multiple imputation. An illustration.

Observed data

Id.	A	B	C	D
1	•	•	•	?
2	•	•	•	•
3	•	•	•	•
4	•	•	•	?
5	•	•	•	•
6	•	•	•	•
7	•	•	•	?

Plausible values

Id.	Var.	M1	M2	M3	M4	M5
1	D	$i11$	$i12$	$i13$	$i14$	$i15$
4	D	$i21$	$i22$	$i23$	$i24$	$i25$
7	D	$i31$	$i32$	$i33$	$i34$	$i35$

Datasets completed by imputations

	Completed dataset 1				Completed dataset 2				Completed dataset 3				Completed dataset 4				Completed dataset 5			
Id.	A	B	C	D	A	B	C	D	A	B	C	D	A	B	C	D	A	B	C	D
1	•	•	•	$i11$	•	•	•	$i12$	•	•	•	$i13$	•	•	•	$i14$	•	•	•	$i15$
2	•	•	•	•	•	•	•	•	•	•	•	•	•	•	•	•	•	•	•	•
3	•	•	•	•	•	•	•	•	•	•	•	•	•	•	•	•	•	•	•	•
4	•	•	•	$i21$	•	•	•	$i22$	•	•	•	$i23$	•	•	•	$i24$	•	•	•	$i25$
5	•	•	•	•	•	•	•	•	•	•	•	•	•	•	•	•	•	•	•	•
6	•	•	•	•	•	•	•	•	•	•	•	•	•	•	•	•	•	•	•	•
7	•	•	•	$i31$	•	•	•	$i32$	•	•	•	$i33$	•	•	•	$i34$	•	•	•	$i35$

infinite number of imputations were applied (that is, as $M \to \infty$), the MI estimator $\hat{\theta}_{\text{MI}}$ would have the sampling variance $s^2 + B$. So, B/M represents the loss of efficiency brought on by using only M imputations.

As $1/M$ converges to zero rather slowly, the first few imputations reduce the sampling variance of $\hat{\theta}_{\text{MI}}$ substantially and later imputations make only small contributions to the precision of $\hat{\theta}_{\text{MI}}$. The difference of the sampling variances of $\hat{\theta}_{\text{MI}}$ based on M and $M+1$ imputations is $B/\{M(M+1)\}$, a decreasing function of M. Suppose $B = s^2/5$; then $M = 2, \ldots, 5$ are associated with respective sampling-and-nonresponse variances $1.3s^2$, $1.27s^2$, $1.25s^2$ and $1.24s^2$, and with $M = \infty$, the variance would be $1.2s^2$. So, the inflation of the sampling variance caused by using only $M = 5$ imputations, as compared to infinitely many, is about 3.3%. This would be halved if we used $M = 10$ imputations.

The missing data brings about the inflation of the sampling variance of $\hat{\theta}_{\mathrm{MI}}$ over $\hat{\theta}$ from s^2 to at least $s^2 + B$. It is natural to define $B/(s^2 + B)$ as the fraction of the information lost (due to missing data). Note that, for a fixed dataset, this fraction depends on the target.

4.2.6 Assumptions and properties

The key assumptions of MI are that the complete-data estimator $\hat{\theta}$ is unbiased and efficient, its sampling variance is estimated by $\hat{s}^2$ without bias, the complete dataset is large, and the model for missing data is correct. All but the last assumption are natural, and usually raise no difficulties. The large sample size is a technical assumption; the proofs require that the sampling variance of $\hat{s}^2$ be of lower order of magnitude than s^4. Further, the modelling and simulation steps have to be *proper*. The qualifier 'proper' (proper imputation) means that the within- and between-imputation variances of the completed datasets accurately reflect the uncertainty about the missing values ([233], Section 4.2).

With these assumptions, the MI estimator $\hat{\theta}_{\mathrm{MI}}$ is unbiased and its variance, with respect to sampling and nonresponse, is estimated by $\hat{s}^2_{\mathrm{MI}}$ with at most a small bias.

4.3 Conditional distributions

Regression models are the obvious candidates for the first step of MI, especially for (incompletely) recorded continuous variables. When several variables are recorded incompletely, multivariate models have to be applied. Linear regression models for normally distributed data are related to models that describe the joint distribution of all the variables involved. In such a setting, plausible values are generated from a plausible conditional distribution of the missing sub-record given the observed part of the record. In this section, we give formulae for the conditional distribution for normally distributed and categorical variables. The applicability of the models for normally distributed data is widened by transformations and extensions to generalised linear models.

4.3.1 Normally distributed data

For normally distributed variables $\mathbf{x} = \left(\mathbf{x}_1^\top, \mathbf{x}_2^\top\right)^\top$, partitioned to their recorded a missing sub-vectors, let $\boldsymbol{\mu} = \left(\boldsymbol{\mu}_1^\top, \boldsymbol{\mu}_2^\top\right)^\top$ be the conforming partitioning of the vector of expectations, and

$$\boldsymbol{\Sigma} = \begin{pmatrix} \boldsymbol{\Sigma}_1 & \boldsymbol{\Sigma}_{12} \\ \boldsymbol{\Sigma}_{21} & \boldsymbol{\Sigma}_2 \end{pmatrix}$$

the variance matrix, also partitioned conformably. The conditional distribution of $\mathbf{x}_2$ given $\mathbf{x}_1$ is normal,

$$(\mathbf{x}_2 \,|\, \mathbf{x}_1) \sim \mathcal{N}\left(\boldsymbol{\mu}_2 + \boldsymbol{\Sigma}_{21}\boldsymbol{\Sigma}_1^{-1}(\mathbf{x}_1 - \boldsymbol{\mu}_1),\, \boldsymbol{\Sigma}_2 - \boldsymbol{\Sigma}_{21}\boldsymbol{\Sigma}_1^{-1}\boldsymbol{\Sigma}_{12}\right) . \qquad (4.4)$$

The least squares estimator can be derived from these equations by replacing each (co-)variance with its sample estimator, and each expectation with the corresponding sample mean. An outstanding property of the conditional distribution in (4.4) is its constant variance; the variance reduction, by the non-negative definite matrix $\boldsymbol{\Sigma}_{21}\boldsymbol{\Sigma}_1^{-1}\boldsymbol{\Sigma}_{12}$, can be attributed to the information about $\mathbf{x}_2$ contained in $\mathbf{x}_1$. The connection of (4.4) with linear regression suggests that the assumption of normality can be relaxed to (component-wise) variance homogeneity.

Having estimated $\boldsymbol{\mu}$ and $\boldsymbol{\Sigma}$, a plausible value of $\mathbf{x}_2$ is generated by the following steps. First, a plausible variance matrix $\tilde{\boldsymbol{\Sigma}}$ is drawn, by the multivariate version of the procedure described in Section 4.2.2. That is, $\tilde{\boldsymbol{\Sigma}}$ is drawn from the Wishart (matrix-χ^2) distribution and scaled appropriately. The plausible parameter vector $\tilde{\boldsymbol{\mu}}$ is then drawn from the estimated multivariate normal distribution of $\hat{\boldsymbol{\mu}}$, with $\tilde{\boldsymbol{\Sigma}}$ substituted for $\boldsymbol{\Sigma}$. And finally, a plausible value of $\mathbf{x}_2$ is drawn from (4.4) assuming that $\mathbf{x} \sim \mathcal{N}(\tilde{\boldsymbol{\mu}}, \tilde{\boldsymbol{\Sigma}})$. A set of plausible values is based on the same plausible distribution $\mathcal{N}(\tilde{\boldsymbol{\mu}}, \tilde{\boldsymbol{\Sigma}})$, and different sets on independent plausible distributions, with independently drawn replicates of $\tilde{\boldsymbol{\mu}}$ and $\tilde{\boldsymbol{\Sigma}}$.

4.3.2 Categorical variables

The joint distribution of two categorical variables, A and B, with h_{A} and h_{B} categories, respectively, is given by an $h_{\mathrm{A}} \times h_{\mathrm{B}}$ matrix $\mathbf{P}$ of probabilities, with non-negative entries such that $\mathbf{1}^\top\mathbf{P}\mathbf{1} = 1$. The marginal distributions of A and B are given by the respective vectors $\mathbf{P}\mathbf{1}$ (column) and $\mathbf{1}^\top\mathbf{P}$ (row). The conditional distribution of B given $A = a$ is obtained by standardising the row $\mathbf{p}_{a\cdot}$ corresponding to $A = a$:

$$(B \,|\, A = a) \sim \frac{1}{\mathbf{p}_{a\cdot}\mathbf{1}}\mathbf{p}_{a\cdot} \,, \qquad (4.5)$$

assuming that the marginal probability $\mathbf{p}_{a\cdot}\mathbf{1}$ is positive.

When A is recorded and B is missing a plausible category of B is drawn from the plausible conditional distribution of B given A. This plausible distribution is derived by the following steps. Suppose the joint distribution of $\mathbf{P}$ is estimated, by $\hat{\mathbf{P}}$, from a random sample of subjects with complete data on A and B. Then $\hat{\mathbf{P}}$ is unbiased for $\mathbf{P}$ and its sampling variance matrix is proportional to $\mathrm{diag}(\mathbf{p}) - \mathbf{p}\mathbf{p}^\top$, where $\mathbf{p}$ is the vector of the elements of $\mathbf{P}$. When each combination of the categories of A and B occurs several times (say, more than ten times), the normal approximation to the multinomial sampling distribution is adequate and a plausible distribution $\tilde{\mathbf{P}}$ can be drawn from the naive approximation to this distribution;

$$\tilde{\mathbf{P}} \sim \mathcal{N}\left[\hat{\mathbf{p}}, \frac{1}{n^{\dagger}}\left\{\mathrm{diag}(\hat{\mathbf{p}}) - \hat{\mathbf{p}}\hat{\mathbf{p}}^{\top}\right\}\right], \tag{4.6}$$

where $n^{\dagger}$ is the sample size, appropriately adjusted. The plausible conditional distribution $(B \mid A = a)$ is defined by substituting $\tilde{\mathbf{P}}$ in (4.5) and a plausible category of B is drawn from this multinomial distribution.

Plausible values may be required for A, B or both categorical variables. In the procedure for generating a plausible category of A, with the category of B known, the roles of A and B are interchanged. When neither A nor B are recorded, plausible categories of A and B are drawn from the plausible distribution $\tilde{\mathbf{P}}$ directly. A set of plausible values has to be based on the same plausible distribution $\tilde{\mathbf{P}}$ and different sets of plausible values on mutually independent draws of $\tilde{\mathbf{P}}$.

Of course, missing values may occur for several categorical variables. Any set of p categorical variables, with h_1, h_2, ..., h_p categories each, can be represented as a single categorical variable with $h_1 \times h_2 \times \cdots \times h_p$ categories. Therefore, the categorical variables with recorded values can be identified with A and the complement with B, and the problem of imputation for B treated as if there were two categorical variables. This approach is suitable only when the cross-tabulation of the categorical variables comprises a small or moderate number of categories. Otherwise many cells in the cross-tabulation contain very few (or no) subjects. Then not only the normal approximation in (4.6) is inadequate, but the draws of many plausible values are made from very dispersed and poorly estimated distributions.

4.3.3 Categorical and continuous variables

The joint distribution of a vector of continuous variables $\mathbf{X}$ and a categorical variable A is defined by the set of conditional distributions $(\mathbf{X} \mid A = a)$, one for each category a, and the (marginal) distribution of A, given by the probabilities of each category. Denote the densities of these category-specific distributions by $f_a(\mathbf{x})$ and the marginal probabilities by p_a.

When each component of $\mathbf{X}$ is recorded, but the category of A is not, a plausible category is drawn from the plausible conditional distribution of A. The distribution is given by the probabilities

$$\mathrm{P}(A = a \mid \mathbf{X} = \mathbf{x}) = \frac{p_a f_a(\mathbf{x})}{\sum_{a'} p_{a'} f_{a'}(\mathbf{x})}, \tag{4.7}$$

where the summation in the denominator is over all the categories of A. Each plausible distribution $\tilde{f}_{a'}$ is drawn from the distribution obtained by substituting plausible values of the parameters in $f_{a'}$. When these parameters are separated (do not involve any constraints that span the category-specific distributions f_a), the estimators are mutually independent across the categories of A, so plausible parameter values can be drawn separately for each a.

When the entire vector $\mathbf{X}$ is missing and A is recorded, $A = a$, $\mathbf{x}$ is drawn from the distribution with a plausible density $\tilde{f}_a$. When neither $\mathbf{X}$ nor A is recorded, a category of A is drawn first from a plausible marginal distribution of A, followed by a draw from the conditional distribution given by density $\tilde{f}_a$.

When only some of the continuous variables are recorded plausible values for the missing items are generated from the plausible conditional distribution given the recorded continuous values, and the category of A if it is also recorded. If the continuous variables are normally distributed, (4.4) is applicable, conditionally on A; if A is not recorded its application has to be combined with (4.7). In brief, a draw from a conditional distribution can be made in stages, according to the distributional identity

$$g(\mathbf{X}_1 \,|\, \mathbf{X}_2 = \mathbf{x}_2) \sim \sum_a g\left(\mathbf{X}_1 \,|\, \mathbf{X}_2 = \mathbf{x}_2, A = a\right) \, g\left(\mathbf{X}_2 \,|\, A = a\right) ,$$

where g stands for a (generic) density implied by its arguments.

4.3.4 Multivariate and multi-stage imputation

A comprehensive model formulation for nonresponse posits a particular joint distribution for a record $\mathbf{x}$. A deterministic imputation scheme would use the conditional expectation (median or mode) of the missing sub-record $\mathbf{x}_{\mathrm{mis}}$ of this distribution given the observed sub-record $\mathbf{x}_{\mathrm{rec}}$. A stochastic scheme uses a random draw from this distribution and MI draws at random from a plausible distribution.

Two profound difficulties are encountered in any direct implementation of MI. First, the joint distribution has to be estimated. The second, model specification, is much more complex in practice because, with few exceptions, multivariate distributions with a wide range of dependence structures are difficult to specify. The multivariate normal and categorical distributions are notable exceptions. Their conditional distributions remain within the class of distributions (normal and categorical, respectively), and the classes contain distributions with very general dependence structures. The advantages of the normal distribution extend to distributions that are component-wise transformations of the normal, such as the multivariate log-normal distribution. They can be defined conveniently by the underlying normal distribution and the transformations applied.

Other multivariate distributions are much more difficult to handle. A general strategy is to specify the joint distribution in terms of some lower-dimensional (conditional) distributions. In this way, an unmanageable task is replaced by a number of tasks that are manageable. This may come at the cost of reduced flexibility and realism, as the range of the feasible dependence structures is reduced. In MI, this strategy is implemented by generating plausible values for missing items within sub-records. Having generated a completion for one sub-vector, we proceed to complete the next, and so on. This way of generating plausible values (specifying models, imputing, and the like) is called *multi-stage*. In general, multi-stage imputation is not proper because some auxiliary information is ignored in the process of generating plausible values, and the uncertainty in one stage is not reflected fully (or at all) in the subsequent stages.

4.3.5 Imputation with monotone response patterns

Proper multi-stage imputation procedures can be devised when the response patterns are monotone. Suppose X_0, X_1, ..., X_K are the variables in the non-increasing order of response. The joint distribution of a complete-data record, expressed as

$$(X_0)\,(X_1 \,|\, X_0)\,(X_2 \,|\, X_1\,, X_0)\;\ldots\;(X_K \,|\, X_{K-1}, \ldots, X_0)\,, \tag{4.8}$$

suggests a procedure starting with a completion of X_0, followed by generating plausible values of X_1 when it is missing, using recorded or imputed values of X_0, then plausible values of X_2, using recorded or imputed values of X_0 and X_1, and so on, concluding with generating plausible values of X_K by conditioning on the (recorded or imputed) values of all the variables $X_0, X_1, \ldots, X_{K-1}$. If the plausible values are properly generated at each stage, then the set of all plausible values is also properly generated. Without monotone response patterns, and the appropriate order of the variables, such a procedure would not be proper because, for instance, imputation for X_k would fail to draw on information in X_h for some $k < h$. With monotone patterns, there is no such information.

The advantage of imputation for data with monotone response patterns is that plausible values are generated by univariate models. When these patterns are monotone for most of the subjects, and would become monotone if a few additional items were deleted, the sequence of univariate imputations can be applied after such deletions, and the temporarily deleted values either restored or combined with their plausible counterparts. With the restoration, the correlation structure of the variables is affected, and in some extreme cases, combinations of values may occur that are not feasible.

When the number of variables is very large it may be advantageous to reduce the number of stages, or to organise the imputations in stages at two or more levels. Thus, each stage at one level may itself comprise a multi-stage procedure. For example, at stage 1, plausible values are generated for a vector of variables $\mathbf{X}_0$, using only information contained in these variables; at stage 2, they are generated for $\mathbf{X}_1$, using information from $\mathbf{X}_0$ and $\mathbf{X}_1$, and so on, in analogy with the imputation implied by (4.8). The sets of variables $\mathbf{X}_0$,

$\mathbf{X}_1, \ldots, \mathbf{X}_K$ are said to have group-monotone response patterns if any set of variables $X_0, X_1, \ldots, X_K$ from them (X_k from $\mathbf{X}_k$, $k = 1, \ldots, K$) has monotone patterns with the same ordering of the variables, from most-observed X_0 to least-observed X_K. The variables in either set $\mathbf{X}_k$ need not have monotone patterns themselves. With the vector version of the partitioning in (4.8), each stage involves a multivariate imputation problem, but its dimensionality is much lower than for the entire list of variables. If the imputation at each stage is proper, then so is the multi-stage imputation procedure. At each stage k, the procedure may itself be multi-stage.

4.3.6 The method of chained equations

The Gibbs sampler ([75] and [76]) is a general method for drawing samples from a multivariate distribution when draws cannot be generated from the distribution directly. For a K-variate distribution, the method uses the K conditional univariate distributions $(X_k \,|\, \mathbf{X}_{-k})$, where $\mathbf{X}_{-k}$ denotes the vector $\mathbf{X}$ with its kth component removed. From an initial solution $\mathbf{x}^{(0)}$, its first component is updated by a draw from the conditional distribution $\left(X_1 \,|\, \mathbf{X}_{-1} = \mathbf{x}_{-1}^{(0)}\right)$. In the kth updating step, kth component of $\mathbf{x}$ is updated by drawing from the distribution $\left(X_k \,|\, \mathbf{X}_{-k} = \mathbf{x}_{-k}^{(k-1)}\right)$. The draws from the conditional distributions are mutually independent. The set of K updating steps is repeated. The main theoretical result about this procedure is that as the number of repeats (iterations) of the sets of K updatings increases, the distribution of $\mathbf{x}$ approaches the joint distribution of $\mathbf{X}$, irrespective of the initial vector $\mathbf{x}^{(0)}$, so long as $\mathbf{x}^{(0)}$ is in the interior of the support of the distribution of $\mathbf{X}$. Also, $\mathbf{x}^{(0)}$ has to be connected to the support, that is, any possible realisation of $\mathbf{X}$ has to be accessible by the updating steps.

The Gibbs sampler motivates the following method of generating plausible values, due to [23]. First, a 'default' completion $\mathbf{X}^{(0)}$ is defined for $\mathbf{X}$. Then the missing values of the first variable in $\mathbf{X}^{(0)}$ are replaced by random draws from a plausible conditional distribution of the first variable given the remaining variables. The conditioning is on the recorded or imputed values of the variables 2, ..., K, so that it is a univariate imputation task. Next, the missing values of the second variable are imputed by random draws from a plausible conditional distribution of the second variable given the remaining variables 1, 3, 4, ... K, followed by the similarly defined imputation steps for the third and consecutive variables. The set of K imputation steps is replicated several times, and the concluding completion $\mathbf{X}_+$ is adopted as a single draw from the conditional distribution of $\mathbf{X}^*$ given $\mathbf{X}$.

The method can be applied to incomplete data with any response pattern, so long as sufficiently many replications are used for generating every set of plausible values. For data with monotone response patterns, one replication is sufficient, and therefore the convergence in distribution is likely to be fast when the patterns are monotone but for a few exceptions. The method is particularly appealing when there is a natural default value for the initial imputation, such as zero, or there is another obvious deterministic single imputation.

4.3.7 From MAR to NMAR models

NMAR comprises a much greater variety of response mechanisms, and so both their specification and identification are much more complex. A NMAR mechanism can be specified by the departures of the pattern-specific distributions $(\mathbf{X} \,|\, \mathbf{R} = \mathbf{r})$ of the records from the distribution of completely observed records $(\mathbf{X} \,|\, \mathbf{R} = \mathbf{1})$. The variety of possible combinations of departures is extremely wide, and identifying any particular combination, or narrowing down their range is usually not possible.

This may appear to be a strong argument against applying MI; however, the threat of NMAR is present in simple single-imputation schemes, although there it is compounded with the patently improper nature of the imputation, and by the simplicity of the underlying models. With more extensive conditioning, we improve the chances that MAR is applicable, or that the departure from it is insubstantial.

4.4 From theory to practice

This section addresses some issues that commonly arise in the application of MI and when deciding whether to apply MI or a single-imputation approach.

4.4.1 Organising MI

The first step of MI, specifying and fitting a model for missing values, is by far the most difficult. Although it can be carried out at a range of levels of complexity, from a straightforward adaptation of a common single-imputation procedure to employing multivariate or generalised linear models with many covariates, complexity is in general rewarded by greater protection from the excesses of NMAR. Of course, complexity brings about increased uncertainty about the model parameters, and that imposes a limit on our ability to combat NMAR. The second step, generating plausible values, is much simpler, but is best executed in connection with the first step. The third and fourth steps, completed-data analysis and averaging, rely on complete-data tools, and their execution requires only minimal computational expertise (dealing with the plausible values) and simple instructions, in addition to what is required for the complete-data analysis.

It is therefore natural to assign the tasks to the parties that are appropriately equipped for them. The data constructor, such as a national statistical agency, where computational expertise and software are available, is better suited for the complex tasks. The quality of the modelling can be greatly enhanced by the information about the nonresponse processes, both from the analysed survey and from other surveys of similar populations, using similar instruments and similar methods of data collection. Here, complexity may be rewarded by more appropriate imputations.

The modelling and simulation steps have to be conducted only once; the sets of plausible values carry all the information about the nonresponse process, in the sense that any MI-version of an efficient complete-data estimator used by a secondary analyst will be efficient, so long as the plausible values have been generated properly. Thus, the analyst can focus on the research problem at hand, without any distraction caused by the imperfect conduct of the survey. The cost incurred is, in effect, M-fold increase in computing, but the programming effort additional to the complete-data analysis is minimal. The underlying rationale is that computer equipment and computer time are much less costly than personnel with the relevant analytical and programming skills.

With appropriate flagging, missing values can be indicated in the database supplied to the secondary analysts, so they can apply other methods for dealing with missing values or, indeed, apply their own MI procedures, or other methods for dealing with incompleteness.

In a typical database, the incomplete data form a rectangular array (matrix), with appropriate codes for the missing values. The sets of plausible values can be formatted as another rectangular array, with $M + 1$ columns; the first column locates the missing value and the following M columns contain the corresponding plausible values. If an ordering of the locations is defined without any ambiguity, the first column can be dispensed with. In this setting, the database comprises two arrays, the incomplete data and the plausible values, one set in each column.

In many databases, most of the variables are recorded completely and imputations are required only for a few variables. Then each completion can be represented as another variable in the database. This arrangement is not very economic for storage because the recorded values are repeated $M+1$ times (once in the original version of the variable). However, the cost of storage and the added complexity in handling a bigger database may be offset by the convenience of the completed-data analysis.

In some environments, it may be more practical to supply the computer program for generating sets of plausible values, or even the program that combines the modelling and simulation steps of MI. Of course, the details of the model to be fitted in the first step could be fixed and hard-coded, avoiding a duplication of the analytical effort.

4.4.2 Validity of the assumptions

The theoretical properties of MI are contingent on correctly specifying the model for missing data. In most settings, the options are restricted to a class of MAR mechanisms, even though their validity cannot be tested formally. The problematic nature of the assumption of MAR is often quoted as the reason for not applying MI. Here we argue that this is an unintended consequence of the clear statement of the assumptions associated with MI and the properties of the MI estimator. In contrast, single-imputation methods appeal for validity either to the optimal way of reconstructing the complete dataset (not a relevant goal), or to enabling the use of complete-data methods with *approximate* validity of the inferential statements. The approximation breaks down under NMAR *and* estimators that are distinctly non-linear functions of the data. Single-imputation methods are simpler to apply, but that is hardly a point of any substance, given that, for a secondary analyst, MI requires in essence the same software equipment. The cost and effort of generating sets of plausible values is substantial, but it should be pro-rated over the numerous analyses to which the database is subjected.

A model for nonresponse is easily identified with most single-imputation methods, and upon a critical evaluation each would be found wanting. That has been the substance of our assessment of the schemes discussed in Chapter 3. It is essential to judge the alternative approaches by the same yardstick. MAR is equally essential for both single- and multiple-imputation procedures. MAR-based procedures can be adjusted for known or estimated departures from MAR by adaptations that are identical for both types of imputation procedures. We argue below for MI indirectly, by pointing out how commonly applied single-imputation schemes can be improved, by making the (implied) model for missing values more realistic, by incorporating the uncertainty about the missing values (at least approximately), and by an integrated way of exploring the impact of certain departures from the assumed model for the missing values.

4.4.3 MI adaptation of LOCF

LOCF implements the imputation of missing values for X_2 based on the (recorded) values of X_1 according to the usually inappropriate model which states that $X_2 = X_1$ when X_2 is not recorded. A more realistic model is that the two variables coincide with a large probability. For variables X_1 and X_2 with support on consecutive integers, such as $1, 2, \ldots, H$, this can be formulated as

$$\begin{aligned} \mathrm{P}(X_2 = X_1 \,|\, X_1 = x) &= p \\ \mathrm{P}(X_2 = X_1 + 1 \,|\, X_1 = x) = \mathrm{P}(X_2 = X_1 - 1 \,|\, X_1 = x) &= \frac{1-p}{2}\,, \end{aligned}$$

with suitable provisions for $x = 1$ and $x = H$. More complex models allow for differences $X_2 - X_1$ by two or more points (with decreasing probabilities), and for probabilities that depend on x.

When the values of X_1 and X_2 are categories without any ordering the probabilities may depend on the values of X_1 and X_2, although some constraints on these probabilities can be imposed. For example, the probabilities may be symmetric:

$$\mathrm{P}(X_2 = x_1 \,|\, X_1 = x_2) \;=\; \mathrm{P}(X_2 = x_2 \,|\, X_1 = x_1)$$

for any pair of values x_1 and x_2. Further, the probabilities may depend on the distance defined as a positive function of x_1 and x_2. The distance can be defined for each point x as its neighbourhood with layers. The kth layer contains points x' that are in distance k from x.

For continuous variables X_1 and X_2, a model more realistic than $X_1 = X_2$ that underlies LOCF is that $(X_1 - X_2 \,|\, X_2)$, or the difference after a suitable transformation, has a distribution centred around zero. The distribution may be symmetric, $(X_1 - X_2 \,|\, X_1 = x_1) \sim (X_2 - X_1 \,|\, X_1 = x_1)$, and may depend on the value of x_1. The probability that LOCF is appropriate may be positive; this can be represented as $(X_1 - X_2 \,|\, X_1 = x_1)$ being a mixture of a continuous distribution and the degenerate distribution with all its mass at zero.

Except for anomalous settings, LOCF is not valid because the variation from one time point to the next (or, more generally, the variation of $X_2 - X_1$) is ignored, and because it is assumed that there is no trend; $\mathrm{E}(X_2 - X_1) = 0$. Both problems can be resolved for specific complete-data estimators by defining more general models for the missing values (such as regression) and by estimating the contributions to the sufficient statistics. This can be accomplished by various adjustments, such as estimating x_2^2 by $\hat{x}_2^2 + \hat{\sigma}^2$, where $\hat{x}_2$ is the (efficiently) imputed value for x_2 and $\hat{\sigma}^2$ the estimate of the residual variance $\sigma^2 = \mathrm{var}\{X_2 - \mathrm{E}(X_2 \,|\, X_1)\}^2$. However, each class of non-linear transformations requires a different adjustment.

4.4.4 MI-proper hot deck

Hot deck is a general imputation method in which missing sub-records are completed by sub-records of (more) completely recorded subjects. We describe hot deck first for the setting with one incompletely and one completely recorded variable. Let these variables be X_1 and X_2. A special case of hot deck is the nearest-neighbour imputation. For an incomplete record $(?,\, x_2)$, a complete record $(x_1',\, x_2')$ is found, such that the distance $|\, x_2 - x_2' \,|$ is as small as possible. The distance need not be based on the absolute value. The value x_1' of the selected record is substituted for the missing value in $(?,\, x_2)$. The record $(?,\, x_2)$ is called the *recipient* and $(x_1',\, x_2')$ the *donor*. In case of a tie, either a random draw is made from the candidate donors or further criteria are introduced, such as small distance on other (completely recorded) variables. Ties are likely to occur for categorical variables in particular.

In hot deck, a pool of donors is identified for each recipient, and the missing sub-record for the recipient is completed by the corresponding sub-vector of a randomly selected donor. For example, the pool of donors for an incomplete record $(?,\, x_2)$ may be defined by a match on x_2; that is, the pool comprises all the complete records that share the value of x_2 with $(?,\, x_2)$. For a continuous variable X_2, the pool may be defined by an interval $(x_{2,\mathrm{L}},\, x_{2,\mathrm{U}})$ that contains x_2. The interval may be defined for each x_2 separately, or the range of values of x_2 may be partitioned by points $x_2^{(1)} < \ldots < x_2^{(H-1)}$ to intervals that define H pools of donors. The apparent disadvantage of such a set of donor pools is that a recipient $(?,\, x_2)$ with x_2 in the left-hand neighbourhood of $x_2^{(h)}$ will be donated a value x_1' that is very likely paired with $x_2' < x_2$.

For a categorical variable X_1, the imputed value x_1' is a random draw from the multinomial distribution defined by the values of X_1 in the donor pool. A replication of the sampling and nonresponse mechanisms would yield a different donor pool, both comprising different subjects and leading to different multinomial probabilities. The replicate donor pools have a common underlying multinomial distribution, the conditional distribution of X_1 given X_2. This distribution can be estimated from a single realisation. When the sampling design is simple random the multinomial probabilities $\mathbf{p}$ are estimated by the sample probabilities $\hat{\mathbf{p}}$, with the sampling variance matrix

$$\mathrm{var}(\hat{\mathbf{p}}) = \frac{1}{n}\left\{\mathrm{diag}(\mathbf{p}) - \mathbf{p}\mathbf{p}^\top\right\}, \tag{4.9}$$

where n is the size of the pool. For large pools of donors, the sampling distribution of $\hat{\mathbf{p}}$ is approximately normal with the variance matrix given by (4.9).

For datasets with several categorical variables and many response patterns, it is practical to define donor pools separately for each combination of response pattern and pattern of scores on the observed sub-records. Variables that are not involved in the definition of the donor pool need not be recorded completely for the donor pool. A missing value on a variable not in this subset may be part of the criterion for inclusion in the donor pool. Thus, some incompletely observed records may also appear in the donor pool. Also, imputations may be necessary only for a subset of the incompletely recorded variables.

Hot deck is not a proper imputation method because it pretends that the probability of a particular completion of a recipient's record is fixed in replications. This deficiency can be resolved by drawing the distinct values of x_1' not by the estimated probabilities $\hat{\mathbf{p}}$ but by their plausible counterparts, drawn from the estimated distribution of $\hat{\mathbf{p}}$. In most settings, the normal approximation is applicable, so the plausible probabilities are drawn from $\mathcal{N}\left[\hat{\mathbf{p}}, n^{-1}\{\mathrm{diag}(\hat{\mathbf{p}}) - \hat{\mathbf{p}}\hat{\mathbf{p}}^\top\}\right]$, obtained by naive estimation of the distribution in (4.9).

Multivariate hot deck

In hot deck, recipients are usually matched with donors according to the values of several variables. This cannot be regarded as a genuinely multivariate feature because in most applications a single variable can be constructed from the original variables, and the matching would yield the same result.

Donors may provide values of several variables. It is essential that a single (randomly drawn) donor provides values for all the variables that are missing in the recipient's record. If a different donor is used for each variable, or for sub-vectors of the missing part of the record, the donated values are independent and the correlation structure of the variables is not maintained.

Pools of donors may be defined based on the response patterns (in addition to other criteria). If the pools are disjoint (have no overlap), some efficiency is lost because some records suitable for several pools can be included in only one of them. On the other hand, the multinomial distributions associated with overlapping pools are not independent, and so the uncertainty about them is more difficult to reflect accurately. While this problem does not have a practical solution, assuming independence is far superior to ignoring the uncertainty altogether. Of course, when the pools are large, even the uncertainty about the multinomial probabilities can be ignored. However, the hot deck should still be applied M times, to reflect the uncertainty associated with the underlying (*fixed*) multinomial distribution.

4.4.5 Propensity scoring

Propensity score methods can be motivated as hot deck with donor pools defined by a regression model. Suppose dataset $(\mathbf{Z}, \mathbf{X})$ has only two response patterns; $\mathbf{Z}$ is observed completely and $\mathbf{X}$ is recorded completely for a subset of the sample and not recorded at all for the complement. Let R be the binary variable that indicates whether $\mathbf{X}$ is recorded. A model is formulated for R in terms of $\mathbf{Z}$ and the plausible values of the probability that $R = 1$ are classified into a number of categories. Within each category, hot deck is applied to impute for missing values of $\mathbf{X}$. Propensity scoring is particularly attractive when, possibly with a few exceptions, only two response patterns occur. In some applications, long sub-records are imputed, such as responses to whole pages or sections of a questionnaire.

A practical choice for the model for $(R \,|\, \mathbf{Z})$ is logistic regression, although alternative link functions can also be applied. The model fit is described by the vector of estimates $\hat{\boldsymbol{\beta}}$ of the regression coefficients in

$$\mathrm{P}(R = 1 \,|\, \mathbf{z}) = \mathrm{logit}^{-1}(\mathbf{z}\boldsymbol{\beta}) \,,$$

where $\mathrm{logit}(p) = \log(p) - \log(1-p)$ is the logit function; its inverse is $\mathrm{logit}^{-1}(u) = 1/\{1 + \exp(-u)\}$. The sampling variance matrix of $\hat{\boldsymbol{\beta}}$ is estimated by the matrix of the weighted totals and cross-products of the variables in $\mathbf{Z}$, with weights $\hat{p}(1-\hat{p})$, where $\hat{p} = \hat{\mathrm{P}}(R = 1 \,|\, \mathbf{z})$ is the fitted probability of response. A plausible vector $\tilde{\boldsymbol{\beta}}$ is drawn from the estimated (asymptotic) distribution of $\hat{\boldsymbol{\beta}}$, that is, $\mathcal{N}\left\{\hat{\boldsymbol{\beta}}, \widehat{\mathrm{var}}(\hat{\boldsymbol{\beta}})\right\}$, and it defines the plausible probabilities $\mathrm{logit}^{-1}(\mathbf{z}\tilde{\boldsymbol{\beta}})$. These probabilities are grouped into (propensity) intervals

$[0, p^{(1)})$, $[p^{(1)}, p^{(2)})$, ... , $(p^{(H)}, 1]$, and they define the groups of recipients and pools of donors. Donors are *similar* to a recipient if their values of $\tilde{p}$ fall into the same propensity interval, and the recipient is donated a completion from a randomly selected similar donor. Note that a replication yields a different plausible vector $\tilde{\boldsymbol{\beta}}$, and so the composition of the propensity intervals differs across the replications. This is an important source of between-replication variance that reflects the uncertainty about the model for R.

Propensity scoring cannot deal with a wide variety of response patterns, but is well suited for settings in which entire blocks of variables have missing values. When such a pattern is spoilt by relatively few subjects, the values of some of the variables may be overwritten, kept unchanged, or a random decision may be made. In general, overwriting introduces inefficiency by discarding recorded values, but the replacement by a proper imputation introduces no bias. In contrast, keeping the values unchanged introduces bias without inflating the sampling variance. Overwriting will help to maintain the associations among the variables, whereas by retaining a recorded value we maintain data item correctness but fail to maintain the associations. A mix of the two strategies may be a good compromise, although in some settings overwriting has to be restricted, so that some incompatibilities in the completed data are avoided.

4.5 NMAR and sensitivity analysis

So far, we have considered only models for ignorable nonresponse, that is, MAR with its model parameters separated from the parameters in the complete-data model. Specification of an appropriate NMAR model is much more difficult. MAR is characterised by identical associations in the complete and incomplete records. Any way of departing from this identity corresponds to a NMAR mechanism. The wide range of such departures illustrates the wealth of NMAR mechanisms. It is instructive to think of the departures as classified by their *direction* and *extent*, so that they are partially ordered by the extent within a direction. A practical method of generating plausible values according to a NMAR mechanism is by adjusting the sets of MAR-generated plausible values for the departure from MAR. For example, each plausible value of a variable may be increased (additively or multiplicatively) by a constant. This constant (and the way it is applied), together with the (original) MAR mechanism, describes the NMAR mechanism.

In most settings, there is no one or a narrow range of NMAR mechanisms that are applicable. A more practical proposition is to find out how far could the nonresponse mechanism depart from MAR, in one or a few directions, without altering the conclusions substantially. *Sensitivity analysis* is a general term for exploring the impact of an assumption, input, or setting, on the outcome of the analysis. The desirable outcome of a sensitivity analysis is that the result of the analysis is changed appreciably only when the input is altered from the original setting to an extent generally regarded as not feasible. In such a case, we would declare that the estimator (analysis) is not sensitive to (the details of the setting of) the input. Sensitivity analysis is qualified by the assumption that is being subjected to scrutiny. As the assumption of MAR cannot be tested, it is a prime candidate for sensitivity analysis.

The variety of ways (directions) in which a mechanism can depart from MAR is usually so vast that sensitivity with respect to each of these ways cannot be established. A practical implementation of sensitivity analysis specifies one or a few directions that are explored. For each direction, sets of plausible values are generated for models that assume a specific extent of the deviation from MAR.

For illustration, suppose the model for missing values of a variable y is based on ordinary regression, $y = \beta_0 + \beta_1 x + \varepsilon$, and a set of plausible values $\tilde{\mathbf{y}}_{\text{mis}}$ has been generated. A simple NMAR mechanism can be introduced by assuming that, for each missing value, $y = \beta_0 + \Delta + \beta_1 x + \varepsilon$, where $\Delta \neq 0$. For a given Δ, the corresponding plausible values $\tilde{\mathbf{y}}'_{\text{mis}}$ can be generated by the same adjustment $\tilde{\mathbf{y}}_{\text{mis}} + \Delta$ of the MAR-based plausible values. The complete-data analysis is then applied to the datasets completed by the sets of plausible values with this adjustment, and the association of Δ with the MI estimate $\hat{\theta}_{\text{MI}}$ explored. Instead of an additive deviation, the plausible slope $\tilde{\beta}_1$ can be adjusted, or the plausible value of the residual variance $\text{var}(\varepsilon)$ increased, or these alterations combined.

Sensitivity is likely to depend on the target θ. In general, it is difficult to gain an understanding for which estimators, and which targets, are resistant (insensitive) to deviations from MAR, and in which directions.

An effective way of conducting sensitivity analysis is to define the deviation from NMAR with the intention to undermine the conclusion of a specific analysis. Suppose the target is the difference of the means for two groups, A and B, and the estimate is positive. This result is undermined most effectively by reducing the plausible values for A and increasing them for B. The simplest way of implementing this is to change each plausible value by $\pm\Delta$, with the sign dependent on the group. Other schemes are not much more complex (e.g., multiplicative adjustment), and may be more natural in the specific context.

Sensitivity analysis is not specific to dealing with incompleteness, to MI or to the concern about NMAR. For the latter, it can, in principle, be applied with single-imputation schemes, using the same adjustments of the MAR-based imputed values as in MI. A common application of sensitivity analysis is in model-based estimation, when the impact of some elements of the model specification has to be explored.

4.6 Other applications of MI

Although MI was originally designed to deal with missing values, it is applicable to all problems that can be formulated as incomplete-data analysis. It is up to the analyst's ingenuity to relate a particular complex estimation task to an artificial complete-data problem that is relatively easy to solve by an available method. For example, the complete-data method may be non-iterative, whereas the direct implementation of the incomplete-data method would be either iterative or would require an extensive analytical or programming effort. For the data that represent the missing information, the difference between the complete and incomplete data, sets of plausible values are generated in such a way that the uncertainty about the missing values is appropriately reflected. After generating sets of plausible values, no programming effort other than to implement the complete-data method is required.

In this section, we discuss three generic applications, connected with measurement error, misclassification and coarse data, and outline some others, involving random-effect models, changed classification and observational studies.

4.6.1 Measurement error

Measurement, assessment and other kinds of error are common in data collection processes. An ideal version X^* of a variable is defined, but it is recorded, as X, subject to error. The measurement-error (ME) process is defined as a class of conditional distributions $(X \mid X^*)$. Usually the class is defined by one or a few parameters and their ranges. A common example of a ME process is

$$X = X^* + \varepsilon \,, \tag{4.10}$$

where ε is distributed according to $\mathcal{N}(0, \sigma_e^2)$, with unknown variance σ_e^2, and is independent of X^*. The realisations of ε are usually mutually independent, although they may be correlated, for instance, when measurements take place within sets or clusters of units, or the order in time induces some dependence. Normality of the deviations $X - X^*$, although analytically convenient, need not be an appropriate assumption. Its scope is extended somewhat by transformations; that is, the normal measurement-error model may be appropriate for $f(X)$ and $f(X^*)$.

The variance of ε may be a function of some variables. In the simplest version of such a model, ε has variance $\sigma_{e,k}^2$, depending on the value k of a categorical variable Z. Care should be exercised in specifying parametric forms for $\mathrm{var}(\varepsilon)$; in particular the variance should be positive for all feasible values of the parameters. In the multivariate version of the model in (4.10), the components of the error $\boldsymbol{\varepsilon} = \mathbf{X} - \mathbf{X}^*$ may be correlated, although in many settings they are independent. The variances in $\boldsymbol{\Sigma} = \mathrm{var}(\boldsymbol{\varepsilon})$ need not be constant. When the components of $\boldsymbol{\varepsilon}$ are independent and have unrelated variances, separate univariate models can be specified for each component.

As with a nonresponse mechanism, we can define the complete data and their complete-data analysis, the analysis that would have been applied had there been no measurement error. The applications of MI to nonresponse and measurement error share the difficulty that the nuisance process involved (nonresponse or measurement) cannot be stripped away, so that the sampling would be left as the sole source of the inferential problem.

Unlike the nonresponse mechanism, the measurement error is usually 'planned' — it is anticipated, as a result of the human or technological imperfections of the measurement and other instruments used to obtain the values of X. The measurement process can be studied in advance, by applying the instruments (repeatedly) in a setting as close to the survey as possible. The obvious difficulty is that the subject of the measurement may be conditioned by the process, and so the second and subsequent applications cannot be regarded as replicates. If this problem does not arise, or is overcome, inferences about the measurement process can be made, with accuracy limited only by the available resources.

Suppose $\mathbf{Z}$ comprises the variables that involve no measurement error and, for simplicity, suppose they are recorded completely. Formally, we may regard $(\mathbf{Z}, \mathbf{X}^*, \mathbf{X})$ as the complete data and $(\mathbf{Z}, \mathbf{X})$ as the incomplete data. The fact that $\mathbf{X}$ is not used in any complete-data analyses is incidental. A model for the 'missing' data $\mathbf{X}^*$ is a class of conditional distributions $(\mathbf{X}^* \,|\, \mathbf{X})$. These are obtained from $(\mathbf{X} \,|\, \mathbf{X}^*)$ by the Bayes theorem:

$$g(\mathbf{x}^* \,|\, \mathbf{x}, \mathbf{z}) = \frac{g(\mathbf{x} \,|\, \mathbf{x}^*, \mathbf{z})\, g(\mathbf{x}^* \,|\, \mathbf{z})}{g(\mathbf{x} \,|\, \mathbf{z})}, \tag{4.11}$$

where g denotes a generic density function. This provides a prescription for generating plausible values of $\mathbf{X}^*$, as draws from $g(\mathbf{x}^* \,|\, \mathbf{x}, \mathbf{z})$. Uncertainty about this density is addressed by using a plausible density $\tilde{g}$. To obtain it, a parametric form of g is posited, its parameters estimated and a vector of parameters is drawn from their estimated sampling distribution.

The identity in (4.11) requires the marginal distributions of $\mathbf{X}$ and $\mathbf{X}^*$ conditional on the covariates $\mathbf{Z}$ and the conditional distribution of $\mathbf{X}$ given $\mathbf{X}^*$. The latter distribution can be estimated directly in an experiment in which the value of $\mathbf{X}^*$ is under our control. When such control cannot be exercised, information about the measurement process can be collected by observing a non-informatively selected sub-sample of subjects twice or several times, with independent realisations of the measurement error.

For example, with the model in (4.10), the difference of a pair of replicate measurements of X^*, $X_1 - X_2$, has centred normal distribution with variance $2\sigma_e^2$. The measurement-error variance can therefore be estimated from a sample of such differences for J subjects,

$$\hat{\sigma}_e^2 = \frac{1}{2J} \sum_{j=1}^{J} (x_{j,1} - x_{j,2})^2 ,$$

and $J\hat{\sigma}_e^2/\sigma_e^2$ has χ^2 distribution with J degrees of freedom. The distribution of X can be estimated from the sample. The values of X^* are not observed, so their distribution has to be estimated indirectly. Suppose X is distributed according to $\mathcal{N}(\mu, \sigma_x^2)$. Then X^* is distributed according to $\mathcal{N}(\mu, \sigma_x^2 - \sigma_e^2)$, derived by assuming that X^* and ε in (4.10) are independent.

Any population considered is finite, so the values of any variable in it could not have any continuous distribution, such as the normal. Although the assumption of normality is not valid, it is constructive when it provides a good approximation. Without normality, the mean and variance of X^* remain μ and $\sigma_x^2 - \sigma_e^2$, respectively, but there is no simple way of drawing samples from its distribution, or distributions derived from it. A particular advantage of the normal distribution is that it is closed with respect to 'reversing' the conditioning by (4.11).

$$(X^* \,|\, X) \sim \mathcal{N}\left(\mu \frac{\sigma_e^2}{\sigma_e^2 + \sigma_x^2} + X \frac{\sigma_x^2}{\sigma_e^2 + \sigma_x^2}, \frac{\sigma_e^2 \sigma_x^2}{\sigma_e^2 + \sigma_x^2}\right) . \tag{4.12}$$

The conditional expectation, or its naive estimator, can be interpreted as a shrinkage estimator of the realisation of X^*; the observation X is pulled toward the mean μ, with the extent of shrinkage dependent on the relative sizes of the variances σ_e^2 and σ_x^2.

The distribution in (4.12) applies when X^* is observed by X only once. When H (replicate) observations, $X^{(1)}, \ldots, X^{(H)}$, are made, (4.12) applies with X replaced by the sample mean $\overline{X} = (X^{(1)} + \cdots + X^{(H)})/H$, and the variance σ_e^2 by σ_e^2/H, that is, as if the mean $\overline{X}$ was the sole observation made, but with greater precision.

Single imputation schemes may estimate X^* by the corresponding observation X. The analyses based on this imputation scheme are deficient because $\mathrm{var}(X) > \mathrm{var}(X^*)$. For example, the simple regression of an outcome Y, applied to X as a covariate, is biased for $(Y \,|\, X^*)$. Using the conditional expectation $\mathrm{E}(X^* \,|\, X)$ introduces a different bias, as its variance, $\mathrm{var}\,\{\mathrm{E}(X^* \,|\, X)\} = \sigma_x^4/(\sigma_x^2 + \sigma_e^2)$, is smaller than σ_x^2. The shrinkage in (4.12) could be reduced so that the sample variance of the estimates matches σ_x^2, but then other summaries would be estimated with bias.

MI generates replicates of the sets of estimated conditional distributions of $(X^* \,|\, X)$ for each observation X and draws the plausible values at random from each distribution. Estimation of the measurement-error distribution(s) is possible only when replicate measurements are made. An important design issue is how many replicate measurements to make. More replicates lead to a more precise estimation of the measurement-error distribution but, with limited resources, fewer observations of $(X, \mathbf{Z})$ are then made. The analytical solution of this optimisation problem depends on the variances σ_x^2 and σ_e^2. When these are not known the problem is best resolved by considering a range of plausible scenarios.

For some simple analyses, the EM algorithm can be applied. For example, the ordinary regression fit

$$\hat{\boldsymbol{\beta}} = \{\widehat{\mathrm{var}}(\mathbf{X}^*)\}^{-1}\, \widehat{\mathrm{cov}}(Y, \mathbf{X}^*)$$

can be evaluated by estimating the complete-data (co-)variance matrices $\widehat{\text{var}}(\mathbf{X}^*)$ and $\widehat{\text{cov}}(Y, \mathbf{X}^*)$. With the standard normality assumptions, the E-step estimates $\widehat{\text{cov}}(Y, \mathbf{X}^*)$ by $\widehat{\text{cov}}(Y, \mathbf{X})$ and $\widehat{\text{var}}(\mathbf{X}^*)$ by $\widehat{\text{var}}(\mathbf{X}) - \widehat{\text{var}}(\mathbf{X} - \mathbf{X}^*)$. In this case, the EM algorithm requires only one iteration.

In principle, any distributions can be specified for $(X \mid X^*)$ and X (or X^*), although distinct computational advantage is attained with normal distributions for both. Specification by mixtures of normal distributions may be necessary when the exact value of X^* is recovered with positive probability. Mixtures of two normal distributions are useful when substantial errors occur with a small probability or when the error distribution is asymmetric.

4.6.2 Misclassification

Misclassification can be motivated as the discrete version of the measurement error. Instead of a categorical variable X^*, its error-prone version X is recorded. Usually X^* and X have the same range of values. The misclassification process is described by the square matrix $\mathbf{T}$ of probabilities of 'transition' from X^* (rows) to X (columns). The rows of this matrix comprise the conditional distributions of X given values of X^*. The Bayes theorem (4.11) is applicable, with discrete density functions g (that is, vectors of probabilities that add up to unity).

There are advantages to characterising misclassification processes with parsimony, by fewer model parameters. This can be achieved by imposing a structure on the matrix $\mathbf{T}$. For example, the probability of correct classification, $\text{P}(X = X^* \mid X^* = x)$ may be constant and the probabilities of transitions between categories symmetric: $\text{P}(X = x \mid X^* = x^*) = \text{P}(X = x^* \mid X^* = x)$. Further, a structure can be imposed on the categories. For ordered categories, the natural structure is defined by the distance (absolute difference) and a model for $\mathbf{T}$ in which the transition probabilities are a function of the distance. More generally, layers of neighbourhoods can be defined around each category, and the transition probabilities set constant in each layer. The transition to the same state is associated with the highest probability, followed by the top layer (close neighbourhood), and the bottom layer (the most distant categories) is associated with the lowest probability of transition. Separate matrices $\mathbf{T}$ may be defined for strata of subjects, or the transition probabilities may be functions of one or several (continuous) variables. Of course, the dependence on these variables $\mathbf{Z}$ has to be such that the transition probabilities are positive for any combination of $\mathbf{Z}$.

As in Section 4.6.1, repeated classifications are essential for estimating $\mathbf{T}$, although the ideal way of collecting information about $\mathbf{T}$ is by classifying subjects with known values of X^*. The marginal distribution of X is estimated from the observations directly, and the distribution of X^* is estimated using an estimate of $\mathbf{T}$.

Measurement error and misclassification are two examples in which elementwise estimation of the 'missing' items X^* would lead to inefficient estimators of most targets. In most settings, the singly recorded value X is the obvious estimator of X^*. Therefore, any analysis with this single imputation would disregard the difference between X^* and X. Linear regression on X would not correct for attenuation, and estimators in other complex models would also be biased. The sampling variation would be underestimated because a replacement of X^* by X is bound to result in a loss of information that is not acknowledged by the single-imputation approach.

4.6.3 Coarse data and rounding

Exact values of the variables are desirable in any analysis, but attempts to obtain them may be counterproductive. Subjects may refuse to respond because the recovery of the value may require recall of many mundane details, consultation of personal records, calculations, or an effort of some other kind that they may deem as not worth the cause. Also, the definition of the (ideal) variable may be ambiguous or difficult to convey, and so its value could not be elicited easily in an interview, especially when subjects are not highly motivated to respond and better cooperation can be promoted by keeping the interview short and uncomplicated. In brief, an effort to obtain the precise values of variables may result in collecting less information overall.

Coarsening is a term used for any known transformation of a variable, $c(X^*) = X$, that is not one-to-one. The function c may be subject-specific, but is known for every subject. Common examples of coarsening are rounding or, more generally, classifying the values of X^* to intervals delimited by points $u_1 < u_2 < \ldots < u_H$. The location and number of these cut-points, and intervals, may differ from subject to subject, may be infinite, but their values are known.

Common examples of coarsening are sets of income-bands presented as response options, such as less than £5000, £5000–10 000, £10 000–20 000, and so on. The cut-points may provide an important cue for the respondent who may readily identify the relevant category. Average time spent watching television, commuting to work, and on other everyday activities are conventionally recorded in hours or its fractions (quarters), and the number of miles travelled by a car in a year in thousands of miles or kilometres. Rounding to a uniform precision need not be the most convenient way of coarsening. For example, age of children may be rounded to years if they are over three years of age or so, but for younger children the respondent (mother or carer) may give the age in fractions of a year (halves or quarters), and for children younger than one year, the number of months or even weeks might be given.

The obvious single imputation scheme estimates each value of X^* by the centre of the interval in which X is found. The centre may be calculated after some transformation. When X^* has a continuous distribution the coarsened values X do not reproduce it well, and it is easy to find non-linear summaries of them that differ substantially from the corresponding summaries of X^*.

In MI, sets of plausible values of X^* are generated as random draws from the plausible conditional distributions of X^* given X. The main difficulty is in defining a suitable (marginal) distribution of X^*. In some cases, uniform distribution is appropriate, but often no reasonable hypothesis can be formulated, other than, perhaps, unimodality. Sensitivity analysis provides a solution in principle, by exploring a range of candidate distributions of X^*. The selected distribution of X^* has to be compatible with the distribution of X, that is, its coarsened version should have probabilities similar to the empirical distribution of X.

The conditional distribution $(X^* \mid X)$ is derived by normalising the restriction of the density to the appropriate X-interval. Plausible values are drawn from a plausible version of this distribution.

Example 7

We generated a random sample of size 800 from the bivariate normal distribution with mean $(0,0)^\top$ and variance matrix $\begin{pmatrix} 2 & 4 \\ 4 & 10 \end{pmatrix}$. The first component is coarsened using the cut-points $-2, -1, 0.5, -0.25, 0, 0.25, 0.5, 1, 2$. The values smaller than -2 are coded as -2.5, those greater than 2 as 2.5, and the remaining values are assigned the centre of the interval into which they fall. As an alternative, a less detailed coarsening is considered, based on the cut-points $-1, -0.5, 0, 0.5, 1$, with ± 1.75 used for the original values outside the range $(-1, 1)$, and the centers of the intervals otherwise.

The sample variance matrix of the original values is $\begin{pmatrix} 2.05 & 4.05 \\ 4.05 & 9.94 \end{pmatrix}$, so that the sample correlation of the two variables is 0.897. The variances of the less and more coarsened variables are 1.86 and 1.58, respectively, and their correlations with the second original variable are 0.873 and 0.834, smaller than the correlation of the original variables ($4/\sqrt{20} = 0.894$). Thus, any estimator for which the variances or covariances (sums of squares or cross-products) involving the coarsened variable are sufficient statistics is likely to be biased.

Censoring is an example of coarsening relevant to survival analysis in particular. Uncensored observations are recorded exactly, and for censored observations only an interval, such as $(t, +\infty)$, is recorded. Direct maximum likelihood methods are available only for a restricted range of models such as the Cox proportional hazards regression, [36] and [38].

Checklists

A checklist is a long sequence of questions with the same lead-in passage (preamble) and the same list of response options. A common example of a checklist is a frequency questionnaire, in which the subject is asked to respond to each item by a frequency selected from the options, such as 'Never', 'Once a year', ..., 'Every day'. A likely problem is that the negative response option ('Never') is sometimes overlooked and no response is given. This may be caused by a momentary lapse or a misunderstanding of the instructions. Often a typical subject responds positively to only a few items. Imputing the negative option for each nonresponse is an attractive proposition in such a case, supported by the conjecture that many instances of nonresponse were meant for a negative answer.

With MI, a posited MAR mechanism assumes that there is no excess of negative responses among the missing items. This can be adjusted by overwriting the MAR-generated values by zeros with a certain probability, or a probability drawn from a distribution that reflects our hypothesis about it, akin to a Bayes prior.

It can reasonably be assumed that subjects misjudge the frequency. For example, a non-trivial proportion of the positive responses may be borderline cases, some of which are bound to be misclassified, if the 'ideal' frequency were well defined. Such misjudgement can be represented by a misclassification process. This process can accommodate bias in the judgement due to social (un-)desirability.

The frequencies are not well suited for many analyses. Their lower-dimensional summaries would be much more convenient. To obtain such summaries, each frequency for an item is associated with a value (score or quantity), and these values are added up. For example, in food frequency questionnaires, each frequency is 'converted' to quantities of nutrients, such as protein, carbohydrates, and the like. Such a deterministic conversion does not allow for any variation in the consumption among the subjects who declared a particular category. Its application fails the criteria of efficiency and unbiased assessment of the precision, even when the analysis planned for the exact quantities of nutrients satisfies them.

If the complete-data analysis involves the quantities underlying the frequencies declared by the subjects, plausible quantities have to be generated for each questionnaire item. This is a complex task that involves the intermediate step of generating plausible (ideal) frequencies. The declared frequencies can be regarded as the ideal frequencies affected by misclassification. In the absence of any replication, no inference can be drawn about the misclassification process. Replication may be useful, although its timing has to be chosen carefully. If the time between the two administrations of the questionnaire is too short some subjects may lose motivation and others may remember some of their responses from the earlier administration. If the time elapsed is too long, the inconsistency of subjects' judgements (misclassification) is compounded with the non-trivial changes in the frequencies (diet).

Thus, we may have to resort to an educated guess about the misclassification process. By ignoring the issue of subjects' inconsistency we assume that their responses are consistent (equal to the ideal frequencies), so a guess may still be preferable because consistency represents the extreme choice. Each questionnaire item is associated with an unknown distribution of the underlying quantities. The uncertainty about this distribution can, in principle, be represented by plausible distributions. For a given plausible frequency, the plausible quantity is drawn from the conditional distribution given that the quantity is in the interval that delineates the declared frequency. Thus, the sets of plausible values differ in the plausible frequencies, in the conditional distributions given a frequency, and in the draws from this distribution. An analyst may be concerned that too much variation is introduced in this way, for instance, because it is not introduced in similar analyses. However, without an appropriate representation of the imperfections in the data, we are deceiving ourselves by gross inferential dishonesty, and the key estimators are biased and do not refer to suitable (ideal) variables.

An advantage of MI is that the two (or several) sources of incompleteness can be dealt with one at a time. A weakness of the approach is that each questionnaire item is dealt with separately (independently). However, defining a multivariate distribution for the quantities underlying all the items, or for suitably defined blocks, is too complex a task.

Altered classification

Definitions of categorical variables such as administrative regions, occupational codes and income bands, are frequently altered. After the change they may be more appropriate, but a link with the old classification is difficult to maintain — comparisons over a time span that includes the change is possible only for the categories that have not been altered. Suppose an outcome variable Y is recorded, on independent samples, at time points t_1 and t_2. A classification X^* is recorded at time t_1 and an altered classification X at time point t_2. The target of inference is the difference of the population means of Y, or of another pair of summaries, for each category x^* between t_2 and t_1. This problem would be easy to solve if the classification X^* were available for the sample at time t_2. Establishing it for every subject in the sample at t_2 may be too great a burden on the survey operation. Instead, it is established only for a random (or non-informative) sub-sample. The design of such a sub-survey may be stratified, omitting categories that have not been altered and sub-sampling more densely in categories that have been defined by more substantial or intricate changes. An example of such a change is when a 'new' category is composed of subsets of several 'old' categories.

We consider (Y, X, X^*) as the complete information, and completely recorded (Y, X) together with partially recorded X^* as the incomplete information. Information about the values of X^*, when missing, is available from the cross-tabulation of X and X^* on the sub-sample of subjects at t_2. Alternatively, such a cross-tabulation can be obtained from a separate survey, on subjects selected independently of those at time points t_1 and t_2. The cross-tabulation estimates the joint distribution of (X^*, X). Single imputation might choose the value of X^* with the highest (estimated) probability, but then rare combinations of X and X^* would be under-represented. In MI, a plausible category of X^* is drawn from a plausible conditional distribution of X^* given X.

How many subjects should be classified by both X and X^*? There is no single solution to this design problem. When the categories are completely redefined, so that many categories of X involve several categories of X^* each, information is required about each cell in the cross-tabulation of X^* and X. When the sub-survey can be focussed on a relatively few cells in the table $X \times X^*$ that are sparse but not empty, the sub-survey is more effective.

Budget surveys and imputation by experts

A budget survey inquires about the subject's distribution of a particular resource, such as income or time. Income is declared by the subject, so it may be subject to an error, but everybody has available 24 hours a day. Diet diaries can be regarded similarly, as the energy intake should roughly match the energy expenditure, and that can be estimated from the information about the subject's lifestyle and basic physiological measurements. Any resource can be regarded as the basis, 100%, and responses then may be given in percentages. This is not a practical format for subjects not comfortable with the calculations involved.

Budget surveys usually have extensive questionnaires, similar to checklists, that inquire about a wide range of activities or items. For any one subject, many of the questions are not relevant, and the appropriate answer to them is 'Never' or 'None'. Such a response is easily confused with nonresponse (choosing no option), especially in self-administered questionnaires. If many such questions are presented in a sequence, one for which a positive answer should be given is easily missed. Also, subjects' perceptions of social desirability and other momentary impressions, not necessarily generated by the questionnaire, may influence the responses.

When processing records from such surveys electronically it is easy to identify records in which the responses to the options do not add up to the declared, estimated or universal total (income, nutritional requirement or time, respectively). The discrepancies arise because of subject's misjudgement or selective recall, some activities or items not listed among the options (and not recalled by the subject), or because of rounding or incorrect (declared or estimated) total. Survey organisations use experts or computer software to edit the records that contain discrepancies and to impute for missing values. The experts' remit is to fix up the records as best as they can, given their judgement, possibly informed by the records that are complete and consistent.

The quality of the expert's work can be judged by asking them to edit records that were deliberately altered by a third party, without leaving any trace, or in which some items were deleted. Closer match of the experts' guesses to the original records would be judged as higher quality. Such an assessment is concerned with recovery of the complete (consistent) dataset, and is not in concert with the standard of efficient inferences and unbiased assessment of their precision. The experts probably fix up the database better than anybody else could, given the information at their disposal. However, they are unlikely to 'venture' and impute some unusual quantities even though such quantities (or their combinations) do occur among the consistent records. As a consequence, the database is made more homogeneous by editing, and has fewer idiosyncratic combinations of values than would be appropriate.

The expert judgements could be made more useful if the uncertainty about them were incorporated in the database and in the subsequent analyses. Without recognising the imperfection of their judgements, we pretend to have more information than was collected, and the complete-data analyses are not honest. If the imputations are without bias (that is, are correct on average), estimators that are non-linear statistics are biased.

The quality-control process of the experts' judgements provides an opportunity to learn about the quality and consistency of the expert judgements. This can be represented by the distribution of the differences between the judgement and the underlying value. These have to be considered jointly for all the items, because their entries and judgements about them are correlated.

The MI solution considers the conditional distribution of the vector of queried values (that are subject to an expert's review) given the values regarded as correct and the expert's judgement, and it draws (plausible) values from a plausible version of this distribution. The contribution of the experts can be assessed by discarding their judgements in this conditioning. If the judgements contribute little to the precision of the MI estimators, the experts can be replaced by an MI scheme, although they still have to be retained for quality control.

Observational studies

In many settings, it is not feasible to implement a probability sampling design because no sampling frame is available, the members of the population have, and exercise, the right to decline any cooperation, and identifying and recruiting subjects relies on agents who do not necessarily get in touch with a good representation of the studied population. Sampling is particularly difficult from populations of sufferers from medical conditions, those with particular consumer habits, experiences, or preferences. Similar difficulties are encountered when studying populations of events, such as electronic or business transactions.

Any sample $\mathcal{S}$ obtained without a sampling design (that is, with an unknown sampling design) can be conceived as a simple random sample $\mathcal{S}^*$ affected by (informative) unit nonresponse. Sample $\mathcal{S}^*$ can be regarded as the complete information and $\mathcal{S}$ as incomplete. In this formulation, plausible records (subjects) have to be generated for the complement of $\mathcal{S}$ in $\mathcal{S}^*$. Without any information about the nature of informativeness of $\mathcal{S}$, this cannot be accomplished. However, regarding the sample obtained as simple random, or applying estimators and quoting their (estimated) properties that are based on simple random sampling, is not appropriate either. Bias may be a substantial component of uncertainty and, unlike sampling variance, it is not reduced with increasing sample size, unless the sample is a large fraction of the population. The deviation of the sample from good representation is referred to as *selection bias*.

MI offers a solution in principle, but this can be implemented effectively only with a suitable method for generating plausible records. In most settings, there is no cast-iron background information that would enable this, although experts may have some realistic conjectures about the selection bias in $\mathcal{S}$. Sensitivity analysis can be applied to explore the range of feasible selection biases. A selection bias can be represented using a stratification of $\mathcal{S}$. Each stratum $\mathcal{Q}$ is supplemented, from $\mathcal{S} \bigcap \mathcal{Q}$ to $\mathcal{S}^* \bigcap \mathcal{Q}$, by drawing a random sample from $\mathcal{S} \bigcap \mathcal{Q}$, with replacement. The stratification and the within-stratum probabilities (or, more generally, sampling designs) are the factors that specify such a *sample-completion design*. The outcome of a sensitivity analysis is not a statement in the conventional format of an estimate and the associated estimated standard error, but a collection of such statements, one for each completion design, of which the extreme ones should be highlighted to indicate the uncertainty due to convenience (unknown) sampling design.

Data editing

Data editing refers to procedures for reconciling implausible values and conflicting combinations of values. Most univariate procedures check that the values of each variable are in a specified range, and multivariate procedures deal with records that have inconsistencies involving several variables, such as unemployed and age below 16 years or vegetarian diet and consumption of meat. Typical procedures overwrite the values of one or several variables, so that they no longer involve any conflicts, while making as few and as small changes as possible. The rules applied may be informed by the process that might have caused the conflict, such as misprints, misplacing decimal points, using units different from the instruction, entering responses in wrong columns, and the like.

Such procedures pursue the standard of efficient estimation of each data item. Even when this goal is accomplished for the flagged items, the standard is not adhered to with any rigour because some errors in the data may not result in detectable conflicts. If a variable is involved in many conflicts and its values are correctly identified as having to be altered by editing (the new value need not be correct in all cases), some other values of the variable are bound to be incorrect without causing any conflicts. Inferences with data subjected to editing lack honesty if they are regarded as the complete dataset. Editing does not always recover the correct values and it does not identify all the incorrect values.

MI addresses this problem by assuming that a (small) proportion of the 'consistent' (non-conflict) records are incorrect, and specifying a process that generates the errors in them. This may combine elements of measurement error and misclassification, with processes that capture the conjectured ways of how the errors arise. Univariate and multivariate outliers can be treated similarly. MI allows us to incorporate the uncertainty about the outlier status of an item or a record; it is overwritten with a certain (estimated) probability by a plausible value, and left intact otherwise.

Random-effect models

Missing information can take on the form of model parameters or other model-related quantities. Models that are easy to fit may be found wanting because they do not accommodate a particular feature of the data or of the modelled processes. The extended model, possibly more appropriate, may be difficult to fit, requiring some analytical development and complex programming.

With the EM algorithm and MI, we can take advantage of the methods (estimators) for the simpler model by adopting them for the complete-data analysis. The E-step in the EM algorithm is concerned with estimating the complete-data sufficient statistics, or the contributions made to them by the missing quantities. The data constructor's tasks in MI are to generate sets of plausible values of these quantities, or of the parameters that constitute the missing data, drawn from their estimated distributions.

We illustrate the general idea on a class of simple random-effect models. They are defined as

$$y_{ij} = \mathbf{x}_{ij}\boldsymbol{\beta} + \delta_j + \varepsilon_{ij} \tag{4.13}$$

for elements (individuals or subjects) i in groups (clusters) j; $j = 1, \ldots, n^{(2)}$ and $i = 1, \ldots, n_j$. The elementary-level sample size is $n = n_1 + \cdots + n_{n^{(2)}}$. The respective elementary- and group-level deviations, ε_{ij} and δ_j, are mutually independent and normally distributed with variances σ_1^2 and σ_2^2.

If the deviations δ_j were known the model in (4.13) could be fitted by ordinary least squares applied to the model

$$y'_{ij} = \mathbf{x}_{ij}\boldsymbol{\beta} + \varepsilon_{ij}\,, \tag{4.14}$$

where $y'_{ij} = y_{ij} - \delta_j$. Given the data $\mathbf{U}_j = (\mathbf{y}'_j, \mathbf{X}_j)$ for group j and the parameters $(\boldsymbol{\beta}, \sigma_1^2, \sigma_2^2)$, δ_j has the conditional distribution

$$\delta_j \sim \mathcal{N}\left(\frac{\omega}{1+n_j\omega}\mathbf{1}_{n_j}^{\top}\mathbf{e}_j\,,\ \frac{\sigma_2^2}{1+n_j\omega}\right), \tag{4.15}$$

where $\omega = \sigma_2^2/\sigma_1^2$ is the variance ratio and $\mathbf{e}_j = \mathbf{y}_j - \mathbf{X}_j\boldsymbol{\beta}$ is the vector of model deviations for group j, comprising elements $e_{ij} = y_{ij} - \mathbf{x}_{ij}\boldsymbol{\beta}$, so that $\bar{e}_j = n_j^{-1}\mathbf{1}_{n_j}^{\top}\mathbf{e}_j$ is the average of the deviations e_{ij}.

The sufficient statistics for the complete-data analysis, fitting (4.14), are the totals of cross-products $\mathbf{U}^{\top}\mathbf{U}$, where $\mathbf{U} = (\mathbf{y}', \mathbf{X})$ is formed by vertical stacking of $\mathbf{U}_j$, $j = 1, \ldots, n^{(2)}$. The E-step of the EM algorithm estimates the contributions to these cross-products made by the deviations δ_j. They are linear and quadratic functions of δ_j, and their estimates can be derived from the conditional mean and variance of δ_j given by (4.15).

Single imputation would rely on the estimate of the conditional mean in (4.15), $\hat{\bar{e}}_j n_j \hat{\omega}/(1 + n_j \hat{\omega})$, with an estimate substituted for ω and the average within-group residual $\hat{\bar{e}}_j = n_j^{-1}(\mathbf{y}_j - \mathbf{X}_j \hat{\boldsymbol{\beta}})^\top \mathbf{1}_{n_j}$ based on an estimate of $\boldsymbol{\beta}$.

MI is based on the plausible values of δ_j, drawn from their plausible conditional distributions. A difficulty in implementing MI is that the distributions of $\hat{\boldsymbol{\beta}}$ and $\hat{\omega}$ depend on ω, which is often not estimated with high precision. If $\mathrm{var}(\hat{\omega})$ is estimated naively, the error in estimating ω is committed again when estimating $\mathrm{var}(\hat{\omega})$.

In fact, the model in (4.13) and some of its generalisations can be fitted directly by maximum likelihood; see Section 7.2 and 7.3. But EM algorithm and MI can be applied to models that are extensions of these. They may contain non-linearities, several random effects, or random effects with distributions different from normal.

For example, the algorithm for direct maximisation of the likelihood for the model with crossed random effects,

$$y_{ijk} = \mathbf{x}_{ijh}\boldsymbol{\beta} + \delta_{ih} + \gamma_{jh} + \varepsilon_{ijh},$$

with mutually independent random samples δ_{ih}, γ_{jh} and ε_{ijh}, presents considerable difficulties when numerous groups i overlap with several groups j. Further, some of the variables in $\mathbf{x}$ may be recorded subject to a measurement error.

4.6.4 Summary

MI, and the missing-information principle underlying it, is a general approach to dealing with nuisance features of the data. Missing values are but one example of such nuisance; measurement error and other forms of contamination, erosion of detail (by coarsening or rounding) are others that are frequently encountered in practice. The impact of ignoring them can be established by simulations, but simple theoretical arguments may be just as convincing: methods, models and analyses intended for the ideal data are bound to be optimistic (dishonest) because they do not recognise that the data submitted to the analysis is of lower quality than assumed.

Taken literally, this proposal may lead us down the path of unending simulations, taking care of each source of imperfection in the data, and each analytical difficulty in model fitting. A sound and constructive approach identifies and attends only to the principal sources of the contamination of the data, so that the analytical operation is of manageable complexity and the biases incurred are only slight.

4.7 Suggested reading

The theoretical background to MI is laid out in [233]. It is formulated from a Bayesian perspective, but it readily translates to the frequentist paradigm, as the quality of the estimators is assessed by a reference to replications. A wealth of practical experience with modelling and computing is conveyed in [243]. Alternatives to MI that do not compromise on the quality of the estimators, but are less universal than MI, are discussed in [146]. These include direct maximisation of the likelihood and EM algorithm. Models for nonresponse and their impact on the incomplete-data analysis are studied in [143], [144], [145] and [148]. A slightly different terminology for incomplete data and nonresponse mechanisms is used by [48]. Reference [171] is an extensive collection of contributions on all aspects of incomplete data in large-scale surveys.

The rationale for MI and its advantages are presented in [237]. References [66] and [221] discuss methods for variance estimation based on single imputation. The properties of MI when its assumptions are not satisfied are explored by [187]. References [135], [136] and [191] present algorithms for combining the completed-data test statistics, or nominal p values, for significance testing. Reference [99] presents an application of MI based on the hot deck.

An application of MI to coarse data is presented in [100]. Altered classifications are handled by MI in [247] and [29]. Several applications of MI in U.S. health-care surveys are discussed in [238] and [8]. Propensity score methods are discussed in [240] and a case study is described in [39]. MI is applied to incomplete data in opinion polling and election data in [239] and [78]. Reference [28] describes a numerical study of the data augmentation method for complex random-effect models, in which a set of random effects is regarded as missing information. Two important monographs on models for data subject to measurement error are [73] and [25]; see also [32]. They make no mention of MI.

Methods for direct maximum likelihood estimation with incomplete binary data are developed by [70] and [71]; [111] and [112] extend these models to nonignorable mechanisms; see also [193]. Censored data are handled by MI in [202], [108] and [64]. Sensitivity analysis is applied by [34] to explore the departures from good representation in observational studies.

4.8 Exercises

1. Prove the identity in (4.4).
   Hint: Use the identities for the inverse and determinant of a partitioned matrix:

$$\det \begin{pmatrix} \mathbf{\Sigma}_1 & \mathbf{\Sigma}_{12} \\ \mathbf{\Sigma}_{21} & \mathbf{\Sigma}_2 \end{pmatrix} = \det(\mathbf{\Sigma}_1)\det(\mathbf{G})$$

$$\begin{pmatrix} \mathbf{\Sigma}_1 & \mathbf{\Sigma}_{12} \\ \mathbf{\Sigma}_{21} & \mathbf{\Sigma}_2 \end{pmatrix}^{-1} = \begin{pmatrix} \mathbf{\Sigma}_1^{-1} + \mathbf{\Sigma}_1^{-1}\mathbf{\Sigma}_{12}\mathbf{G}^{-1}\mathbf{\Sigma}_{21}\mathbf{\Sigma}_1^{-1} & -\mathbf{\Sigma}_1^{-1}\mathbf{\Sigma}_{12}\mathbf{G}^{-1} \\ -\mathbf{G}^{-1}\mathbf{\Sigma}_{21}\mathbf{\Sigma}_1^{-1} & \mathbf{G}^{-1} \end{pmatrix},$$

where $\mathbf{G} = \mathbf{\Sigma}_2 - \mathbf{\Sigma}_{21}\mathbf{\Sigma}_1^{-1}\mathbf{\Sigma}_{12}$, assuming that $\mathbf{G}$ is non-singular.

2. Describe the MI versions of the imputation schemes used in Examples in Chapter 3. Implement the MI versions for some of the examples by adapting the code for the single imputation. Compare the additional amount of work (programming) needed to do this.
3. Alter the MI algorithms constructed in the previous example by omitting the step that generates plausible values of the parameters of the model for nonresponse. What impact does this change have on the results?
4. Repeat the application of the nonresponse mechanism in one of these examples, but make it NMAR by deliberately altering the probabilities of deletion according to the value in the complete dataset. Compare the performances of the single- and multiple-imputation schemes. Conduct a sensitivity analysis specific to the complete-data analysis. In doing this, make sure that the alterations made at the data deletion stage and in the sensitivity analysis do not cancel out.
5. Suppose (household) ownership y of a computer is related to the annual household income x (in thousands of UK£), in a given year and a specified population, by the logistic regression

$$\operatorname{logit}\{\mathrm{P}(y=1)\} = \operatorname{logit}(-5.0 + 0.25x).$$

Suppose the log-incomes have the normal distribution with mean 2.98 and standard deviation 0.15. Generate a dataset (income x and ownership y) with sample size of at least 10 000 according to this model. Classify the income into suitably selected bands so that each of them contains 5–15% of the sample, and choose a 'representative' income $x^\dagger$ for each band. Apply the logistic regression with the representative incomes, and compare the results with the regression on the exact incomes. Try to alter the representative incomes so that the results would agree more closely.
6. For the dataset generated in the previous example, apply MI to the representative incomes first assuming the distribution $\mathcal{N}(2.98, 0.15)$, and then trying to guess it by trial and error or by estimating it. Apply the MI logistic-regression estimator. How much information is lost by coarsening the income?
7. Inspect a survey questionnaire (e.g., obtained from an organisation that conducts population surveys), and discuss:
   a) what provisions are made in the questionnaire to reduce nonresponse;
   b) which variables are collected principally as auxiliary variables;
   c) what (additional) provisions you would introduce to address nonresponse either directly (to reduce it) or indirectly (to make imputation more efficient).

8. Write a computer code, in the environment of your choice, for the secondary analyst's tasks in MI (imputation and averaging). Do it for various arrangements of the plausible values: as columns in the original dataset, as a separate dataset, or as a programme that generates them.

5

Case studies

This chapter describes four case studies in which MI is applied. The first three address the issue of missing data in large-scale national population surveys and the fourth uses MI to deal with inconsistency in the data comprising assessments by expert surveyors.

5.1 The UK Labour Force Survey

The UK Labour Force Survey (LFS) is an important source of information about the labour market in the UK. The key targets in the analysis of LFS data are the rates of unemployment in the whole country and its regions, cross-classified by gender and age groups. The sampling frame used is the Small-User Postal Address File compiled by the UK Post Office. It contains all the addresses in the UK where mail is delivered. Businesses and institutions, identified as addresses that receive on average more than 25 items of mail per day, are excluded from the list. The list is supplemented by the accommodation provided by the National Health Service. A different sampling design and interview arrangements apply in the north of Scotland; the population of this area is less than 0.1% of the population of the UK.

LFS is conducted continually, although the data collected in a quarter (a period of 13 weeks) is regarded as survey on its own. The survey has a rotating panel design. An address included in the sample at a particular time point, say, in spring (March–May) 2002, is kept in the sample for one year, till spring 2003, so that its adult occupants are (planned to be) subjected to the initial interview in spring 2002, and then to shorter interviews three, six, nine and twelve months later. The first interview is conducted face-to-face; the other four interviews are conducted by phone whenever possible. The five occasions are referred to as *waves* I–V; the addresses (or their occupants) selected at a time point are referred to as a *cohort* identified by the date (e.g., spring 2002). The addresses (or subjects) contacted in a given survey are called the survey subjects (e.g., in spring 2003). The sample size at any time point is about 140 000, comprising about 20% of subjects from each wave I–V.

A two-stage clustered sampling design for the first inclusions (wave I) is used. In the first stage, a random sample of postal sectors (typically a street) is selected, and in the second a systematic sample (with a random start) of addresses within each selected postal sector is contacted. For all purposes, the systematic sample is regarded as being simple random. At a contacted address, an interview is planned with every adult occupant, although responses by proxy, of one adult for another, are permitted. Adults respond on behalf of the children (aged 15 or younger) in the same household. Note that some addresses comprise several households.

Intended interviews may not take place for a variety of reasons. First, a representative of the household may respond by an *active refusal* to the first contact by a letter informing about the intention to interview the occupants of the household. Such a household is not contacted any more. One or several occupants at an address may refuse to cooperate with the survey, in a particular wave or in all consecutive waves, in variance with the remaining occupants. Further, the interviewer may fail to contact an address. At that time, it may not be known whether anybody resides at the address. Contact may be made, but one, several or all residents may refuse to respond to some or to all the questions. One or several subjects may be absent, with no-one willing to act as a proxy respondent for them. Each interview has to take place in a relatively narrow time interval. One week is designated for each address and the next week is kept in reserve.

A residential address may be unoccupied at the time of the planned interview, its occupants may move out and others move in. Also, the household(s) at the address may be altered by one member moving in or one moving out. Conceivably, several such moves may take place, although that is less likely. An address may change its residential status and some dwellings are demolished and others are newly built. Care has to be taken in distinguishing between nonresponse and change in the population, due to migration, births and deaths, formation of new households and alteration and dissolution of existing ones.

The public release database distributed to the clients comprises files that contain the records of subjects in one survey (e.g., in spring 2003). One completely recorded variable identifies the wave for the subject (wave I for a subject at an address included for the first time and wave V for a subject at an address that was included a year ago).

We discuss details of the database for spring 2001, but the features explored are likely to be present in each survey. The database for spring 2001 contains values of about 700 variables for 138 796 subjects. These subjects are residents at the addresses on the panel at the time with whom an interview was conducted, either directly or through a proxy. The database comprises 29 845 subjects in wave I in spring 2001, 28 568 subjects in wave II, 27 319 subjects in wave III, 26 695 subjects in wave IV and 26 369 subjects in wave

V. These numbers decrease not as a consequence of the planned sampling design (the numbers of addresses added in each survey were approximately constant), but because of attrition. Addresses in the sample that wish no longer to participate, or end up not participating in the survey for some other reason, are omitted from the database. We refer to this type of (unit) nonresponse as *absence* from the database. Some subjects in the sample have incomplete records. Their presence at the address has been established, but the values of some of the variables, and the employment status in particular, have not been. We refer to this type of (item) nonresponse as *incompleteness* (of the record).

Absence from the database can be explored by extracting the datasets for a given cohort. We discuss the cohort of spring 2000; its subjects are in wave I in the database for spring 2000, in wave II in the database for summer 2000, and so on, in wave V in spring 2001. These five datasets contain 35 656 unique subjects, but only 21 341 (60%) of them are present in every wave. The remaining 40% can hardly be accounted for by migration, births and deaths. Failure to contact the address and unavailability are likely to be the causes in a majority of the cases.

For each subject in the cohort, we define the pattern of presence by a quintet of digits 0/1, indicating the absence or presence in the corresponding database. Thus, pattern 01100 stands for presence in waves II and III and absence in waves I, IV and V. The complete pattern 11111 does not indicate perfect cooperation with the survey because it does not exclude incompleteness of the record. Conversely, an incomplete pattern, such as 00111, does not indicate imperfect cooperation because the subject may have moved to the address between waves II and III.

There are $2^5 - 1 = 31$ possible patterns of presence. (The pattern 00000 is not possible.) They can be classified as perfect (11111), drop-out (10000, 11000, 11100, 11110), drop-in (00001, 00011, 00111, 01111), almost perfect (10111, 11011, 11101), imperfect drop-out (01000, 01100, 10100, 10110, 11010), imperfect drop-in (00010, 00101, 00110, 01011, 01101), and other (e.g., 00100). The drop-out and drop-in patterns are by far the most frequent, accounting for 834–3709 subjects each and 12 768 subjects in total (89% of those with incomplete patterns of presence). Drop-outs account for 7927 and drop-ins for 4841 subjects. The next most frequent patterns are 01000, occuring for 372 subjects, and 00100, for 210 subjects. For sixteen patterns, the number of subjects is smaller than 100 each (191 subjects in total). Nonresponse is bound to be the reason for most of the absence in the records with these patterns.

We discuss imputation for employment status of the subjects present in the database and imputation of records for absent subjects separately, and focus on the former. The latter requires a much greater analytical and information gathering effort. The definition of the employment status by the International Labour Organisation (the ILO status) is used in the survey. A person is unemployed if he or she is without employment (on the day of the

Figure 5.1. Percentages of records with missing and imputed values, as functions of age; waves of the cohort spring 2000.

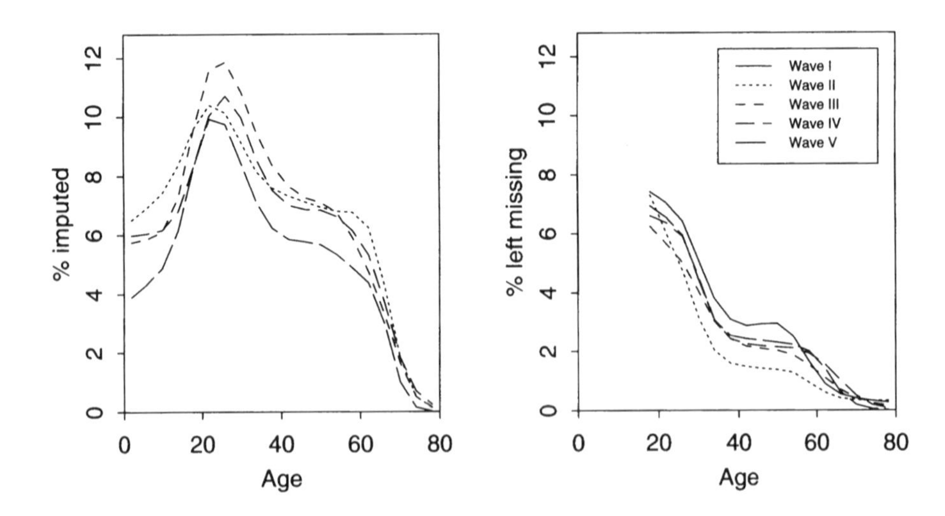

interview), and is both available for and actively seeks work. A person who is not employed and does not seek work is said to be economically inactive. The classification is applied only to adults (aged 16 or over).

For subjects present in a database, ILO status is missing when the subject, known to reside at the address, was not available for the interview or failed to answer the relevant question and no other occupant was willing to act as a proxy and disclose the status of the subject. In the operation, a limited form of LOCF is applied. For the missing ILO status in a wave II–V, the status of the same subject from the previous wave is imputed, unless the subject is absent from the wave, that status is also missing or has itself been imputed. For example, in wave V of the spring 2000 cohort, ILO status was imputed for 1418 subjects (5.4% of the sample), and was left missing for 562 subjects.

The frequency of missing values is strongly associated with age. Figure 5.1 shows that missing data occur and imputations are used most frequently for subjects in their twenties, and least frequently for the elderly. The percentages are plotted for four-year age groups (0–3, ..., 76–79), separately for each wave. The left-hand panel summarises the imputed values and the right-hand panel the values that are left missing (all missing values in wave I and missing values in cases when the value was not recorded in the previous wave either). Smoothing is applied in both graphs. The curves in the right-hand panel start with the age-group 16–19; the ILO status for children is always imputed when their age (date of birth) is known.

On the one hand, the imputations, when applied, inject unjustified optimism because they are not correct with certainty, yet are meant to be used

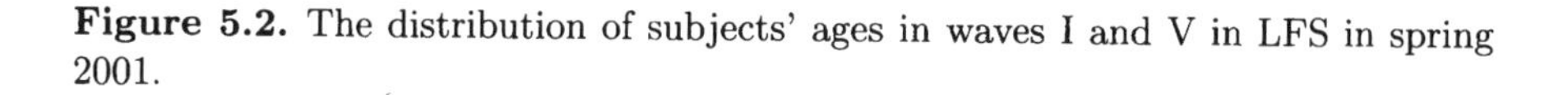

Figure 5.2. The distribution of subjects' ages in waves I and V in LFS in spring 2001.

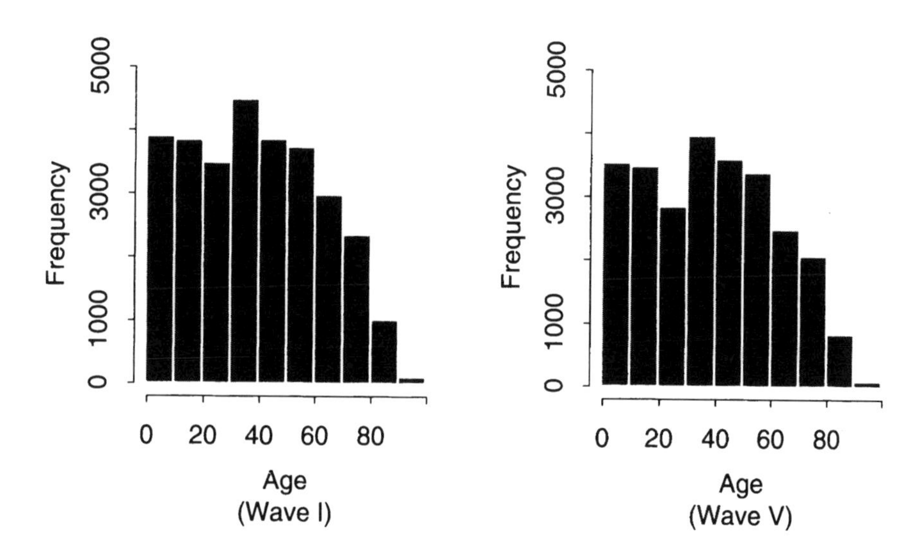

as if they were. On the other hand, the imputations do not deal with a large fraction of the missing values. Admittedly, there is more uncertainty about these values because we have less recent, or no, information (history of ILO status in particular) about the subjects concerned.

Young adults have disproportionately many incomplete records. They are also frequent absentees. The database for spring 2001 contains fewer subjects in the age group 20–29 than the population at large. This is shown in the histograms for waves I and V in Figure 5.2. The age group 20–29 has a much smaller realised sample size than its neighbours. This age group contains a greater proportion of unsettled members of the labour force than any other. Many young adults explore the available career options by changing jobs, having spells of unemployment and economic inactivity, for instance, as students. On the one hand, LOCF is used for them much more than for any other age group; on the other hand, it is least appropriate for them because they tend to change their ILO status more often than others.

5.1.1 From LOCF to hot deck

In LFS, LOCF aims to recover the complete dataset, although completeness is interpreted in a limited way: ignoring the absentees and imputing only when the perceived level of uncertainty about the missing value is low. We seek improvements on LOCF in three directions: imputing for all missing values of ILO status of subjects present in the database, applying more realistic models and representing the uncertainty about the imputed values, without introducing any complex schemes that may be optimal in some circumstances, but are associated with some assumptions that are difficult to verify.

Greater realism

The employment status of a typical subject does change on occasions, and so a more appropriate complete-data model is that transitions from each status to the other states take place with small probabilities. These probabilities vary with age, marital status and other socio-demographic variables, but depend also on the employment history, as captured by the recorded employment status in the previous waves.

Representing the uncertainty

As the transition probabilities differ from zero and unity, their uncertainty would be described by a multinomial distribution, if the distribution were known. Not knowing this distribution is another component of the uncertainty. By applying a more detailed conditioning, the former component is reduced but the latter is inflated because some multinomial probabilities are then estimated from small subsamples. Therefore, too zealous a pursuit of the 'correct' model is not necessarily rewarded by better imputation. If model selection is applied a useful reality check is to apply it also in other surveys and their waves, to realise that the model selection itself is subject to uncertainty and each dataset yields a different selected model. Continuity suggests that similar (or identical) models should apply to each of these datasets, especially when they are separated by not more than a year or two.

Operational robustness

Smaller but certain improvement should be given preference to the potential for optimality because, after implementing the imputation process operationally, the expertise may not be readily available to deal with minor problems that would hold up the delivery of the survey products to the clients. Also, the general ideas of MI may be easier to understand with a simpler model. When the staff who construct the database and the sets of plausible values are comfortable with the implemented model they will recognise the potential of more complex models and will weigh it against the difficulties that may arise. Jumping from the trivial to the possibly optimal is neither good science nor good practice of statistics, because the implementation is bound to be treated like a black-box and the theoretical advantages of MI will not be fully exploited.

Hot deck

Hot deck is a flexible method of imputation for one or a set of variables. Its simplest version defines a single pool of donors, the subjects with complete sub-records on the incompletely recorded variables. When several pools of donors are defined, each recipient is associated with a pool, for instance, by the values of one or several matching variables. The hot-deck adaptation of LOCF for LFS defines donor pools using the employment status in the previous wave as the sole matching variable. For example, the donor pool for a recipient whose previous employment status is 'employed' (EM) comprises all the subjects whose previous employment status is also EM, and their current status is recorded. LOCF corresponds to the trivial donor pool in which the current status of every subject is EM. Hot deck is more realistic and flexible because the imputed status for the recipient is drawn from a multinomial distribution given by the probabilities of transition from EM to the other two states, UN (unemployed) and IA (economically inactive). Let these probabilities be $\hat{\mathbf{p}}^{(\mathrm{EM})} = \left(\hat{p}_{\mathrm{EM}}^{(\mathrm{EM})}, \hat{p}_{\mathrm{UN}}^{(\mathrm{EM})}, \hat{p}_{\mathrm{IA}}^{(\mathrm{EM})}\right)^{\top}$. They are estimates of the population probabilities of the same transitions. The superscript of $\hat{\mathbf{p}}$ indicates the value of the matching variable, the status three months ago. Hot deck is a stochastic imputation scheme; if replicated with the same donor pool the donated value (as well as the donor) for the recipient may be different. Further, in a replication of the survey and hot-deck imputation, a different donor pool is formed and the probabilities $\hat{\mathbf{p}}^{(\mathrm{EM})}$ are different.

Thus, hot deck represents the uncertainty due to the probabilities $\hat{\mathbf{p}}^{(\mathrm{EM})}$, but fails to represent the uncertainty about the underlying $\mathbf{p}^{(\mathrm{EM})}$. This representation is necessary to make the imputation method proper. A remedy for this is quite straightforward. We draw a random sample from the fitted distribution of $\hat{\mathbf{p}}^{(\mathrm{EM})}$. Unless the pool is very small, the normal approximation

$$\tilde{\mathbf{p}}^{(\mathrm{EM})} \sim \mathcal{N}\left[\hat{\mathbf{p}}^{(\mathrm{EM})}, \frac{1}{n^{(\mathrm{EM})}-1}\left\{\mathrm{diag}(\hat{\mathbf{p}}) - \hat{\mathbf{p}}\hat{\mathbf{p}}^{\top}\right\}\right]$$

is adequate. ($n^{(\mathrm{EM})}$ is the size of the pool.) Thus, a plausible value for the recipient is generated in two steps. A plausible multinomial distribution $\tilde{\mathbf{p}}^{(\mathrm{EM})}$ is drawn first, followed by a draw from this distribution. Several recipients may share the same donor pool. A set of plausible values for these recipients is drawn from the same plausible distribution $\tilde{\mathbf{p}}^{(\mathrm{EM})}$, and different sets of plausible values are based on replicate draws of $\tilde{\mathbf{p}}^{(\mathrm{EM})}$.

Many donor pools

LFS has a large sample size, so a more detailed matching is warranted in hot deck. Earlier discussion in this section suggests that matching on age groups may be useful, as may be on the employment status from waves earlier than quarter a year ago, when available. For example, subjects who have not changed their employment status over several waves are perhaps less likely to have changed their status between the previous and the current wave. Each donor pool is associated with an (estimated) trinomial distribution. For a set of plausible values for the entire dataset, the probabilities in these trinomial distributions are meant to be drawn from their joint distributions. The draws can be made separately for each distribution when the pools of donors do not overlap. Having disjoint pools of donors conveys therefore a considerable advantage. In samples drawn by a complex design, including clustering, there is some (weak) dependence among the subjects, and therefore some weak dependence among non-overlapping pools of donors. In practice, this can be ignored, and the pools regarded as independent.

The details of a hot-deck scheme for LFS are given in [164]. It comprises separate schemes for each wave and pattern of presence in the database. A hierarchy of the matching variables is defined, and matching criteria specified according to the wave and pattern of presence. In the hierarchy, the previous employment status is at the top, followed by the earlier states, age groups, sex and marital status. Variables for matching are selected with a view to have donor pools that are not too small, preferring variables from the top of the hierarchy. Instead of matching on the status at each previous wave, subjects are classified according to the number of changes in status (most of them have none), although the immediately previous status is matched throughout.

For subjects in wave V, there are many patterns of presence, and so less detailed conditioning is applied. Subjects in wave I have no recorded employment history, so the imputations for them can be based on very detailed matching of subjects' attributes (all the matching variables, with several age groups). No claims can be made that a particular scheme is optimal. Some cosmetic improvement can be achieved by defining the matching that yields donor pools with sizes almost exactly as desired. Other variables, such as income, education and housing and household circumstances may be included in the scheme.

However, the complexity is not warranted if it delays the replacement of LOCF because of various technical difficulties, uncertainties about defining the donor pools, and a need for occasional improvisation. For example, LOCF was applied for a few subjects in the hot-deck scheme because no suitable donors were found for them. Although statistical theory is preoccupied with optimality, the best (solution) may in practice be a potent enemy of good. Poor statistical practice may linger on because none of the several obvious ways of improving it can be identified as superior.

5.1.2 Results and discussion

This section discusses the results of applying the MI scheme and compares the LOCF, hot-deck and MI estimates.

Five sets of plausible values were generated for LFS in spring 2001. The uncertainty about missing values can be summarised by the proportions of subjects who have quintets of plausible values that are not constant. Extreme uncertainty is indicated by the proportion of quintets that contain all three employment codes. Since the plausible values are generated by a random mechanism, it is not meaningful to interpret them for any particular subject, or a small group of subjects, as an indicator of any feature associated with them. However, the exploration need not be confined to the entire set of incomplete records. In particular, it is instructive to explore the plausible values for young people and subjects for whom LOCF was applied or not. In a particular realisation for the 5537 incomplete records, 4236 (76.5%) of quintets have the same code, 1098 involve two codes and 203 involve all three codes. A disproportionate contribution to the non-constant quintets is from the 1165 young adults (16–24 years of age). Only 638 (55%) have constant quintets, 418 quintets involve two different codes, and 109 involve all three codes. For the 2780 subjects with ILO status not imputed by LOCF, only 828 (30%) have constant quintets. Among the 892 young adults in this group, the uncertainty is much greater; only 14% of them have constant quintets of plausible values.

The impact of MI

From a purely empirical perspective, if MI estimates differ little from the corresponding LOCF-based estimates, MI is redundant. On the other hand, having implemented MI, we need not sit on the edge every time a secondary analyst evaluates another estimator using the dataset completed by LOCF, hoping that it is not deficient and its precision not overstated.

The estimates of the respective rates of UN and IA in spring 2001 are 3.62% and 21.30% based on LOCF and 3.62% and 21.47% based on MI. The estimated standard errors are also very similar: 0.066% (LOCF) and 0.067% (MI) for UN and 0.146% for IA with both methods. Based on this comparison, the effort to implement MI is difficult to justify. The argument that LOCF underestimates the standard error and MI estimates *its* standard error without bias is moot.

Our motivation of MI suggests that a stronger case for it may be presented by comparing the estimators of the UN and IA rates for young adults. Table 5.1 lists the estimates and estimated standard errors for them, classified by age and sex. To conserve space, results are given only for even years of age. Three estimators are compared: LOCF, a single application of the hot deck and MI based on the same hot-deck procedure. The estimates for the hot deck vary more than what is indicated by their standard errors, because a replication of the hot deck would yield a different completed dataset; this source of variation is ignored. In contrast, the MI estimator is 'honest'; it includes the between-imputation variance, both in terms of different imputed values and different multinomial probabilities. The latter source is negligible, though. The largest differences between LOCF and MI estimates are for UN rates of the 16-year-olds and IA rates of the 24-year-olds. Of course, doubts

Table 5.1. Estimates of the sex-by-age rates of unemployment and economic inactivity in the LFS in spring 2001.

	LOCF		Hot deck		MI		
Age	Estimate	Stand. error	Estimate	Stand. error	Estimate	Stand. error	% Missing information
Unemployment – Men							
16	7.55	0.89	7.33	0.88	7.57	0.99	17.9
18	9.90	1.08	10.21	1.05	9.99	1.09	6.0
20	8.92	1.06	9.36	1.02	9.11	1.18	21.3
22	7.95	1.04	7.85	0.99	7.95	1.21	27.8
24	6.16	0.96	7.05	0.94	6.56	1.01	11.7
Unemployment – Women							
16	6.83	0.86	6.92	0.85	6.94	0.94	13.5
18	6.37	0.91	6.41	0.88	6.25	0.95	11.2
20	6.30	0.89	6.11	0.85	6.11	0.87	5.1
22	3.86	0.72	3.99	0.69	3.89	0.72	5.5
24	5.41	0.88	5.73	0.85	5.47	0.87	3.1
Economic inactivity – Men							
16	59.12	1.65	59.43	1.62	59.87	1.69	6.7
18	27.08	1.60	26.57	1.56	27.16	1.63	7.2
20	27.16	1.65	27.04	1.58	27.30	1.67	8.5
22	22.83	1.61	22.62	1.54	23.08	1.61	6.8
24	10.90	1.24	11.51	1.25	12.43	1.39	15.4
Economic inactivity – Women							
16	56.83	1.69	57.60	1.66	57.41	1.85	15.9
18	31.72	1.73	31.64	1.70	31.88	1.78	6.9
20	34.32	1.74	34.66	1.68	34.76	1.82	12.5
22	32.88	1.74	34.15	1.70	34.02	1.75	4.6
24	23.91	1.65	26.12	1.63	25.64	1.68	5.0

about the quality of the model implied by the hot deck may be appropriate, but these are substantially magnified when the model implied by LOCF is held up to a similar examination.

How many imputations?

The right-hand column of Table 5.1 gives the estimated percentage of missing information defined as $\hat{B}/\left(\bar{\hat{s}}^2 + \hat{B}\right)$; see Section 4.2.5. It is highest for the UN rate of 22-year-old men, nearly 30%. The information lost because we use only $M = 5$ imputations is approximately 6% and it would be reduced to about 5% by another set of plausible values. When 10% of the information is missing, only 2% is lost with $M = 5$ imputations. Thus, little additional precision would be achieved by using more than five imputations, and the choice of their number is not crucial.

High percentage of missing information is not associated with large differences between LOCF and MI. Simply, the contribution from the incomplete records does not alter the estimate. Conversely, small proportion of missing values does not preclude a large difference. A case in point are the estimates of the rates of economic inactivity for the 24-year-old women. Discussion of the results has to be qualified by the uncertainty due to estimation of the standard errors. For example, the hot-deck estimated standard error for 24-year-old women exceeds its LOCF counterpart, by 0.01%. However, the hot deck is based on more observations, so its standard error is smaller. The seeming contradiction arises because the estimates of the two standard errors, functions of $p(1-p)$, are based on different (their own) estimates of the probability p.

Concerns about NMAR

On the one hand, more extensive conditioning improves the chances that MAR applies; on the other, the extent of conditioning is limited by insisting on sufficiently large pools of donors. Inasmuch as hot-deck imputation is a generalisation of LOCF, the concern about NMAR is much more acute with LOCF. Scenarios can be devised in which LOCF is poorly suited. For example, more of the non-responders may be unemployed than would be expected according to MAR. More detailed conditioning is likely to reduce its impact although it does not necessarily account for it completely.

The quality of the hot-deck scheme can be assessed informally by exploring the distributions of employment status within the pools. Variation in these distributions is a sign of having selected suitable matching variables. For example, using age groups is supported by observing that there are many transitions among the young, that most elderly women are economically inactive, and that the middle-aged tend to change their status much less frequently than others. Transitions between states are more frequent among the single, and, for the young, among men. A better choice of the matching variables, their categorisation, hierarchy, and other details may improve the scheme, but most of the gains are realised by using the obvious matching variables.

Inconsistencies in the estimates

For a frozen population, a population quantity is absolute and incorruptible. Although not known, it could be established, in principle, if sufficient resources were available. On the other hand, the efficiency of an estimator is relative. To maintain our professional edifice, we have strong incentives to claim that our estimators cannot be improved. An appropriate way of qualifying this is by a reference to the sources that were available to us at the time of the analysis.

Identifying suitable data sources and collecting intelligence and information is unambiguously assigned as the analyst's responsibility. Three months later, after the next wave, we have a new data source, and possibly better understanding of the processes associated with the housing and labour markets, interviewing processes, and the like. For example, an address not contacted in wave I has now been contacted, and it has been established that the household has not been altered in the last three months. A quick check may establish that 'incorrect' information was imputed, say, in four of the five sets of plausible values of the ILO status. (For example, in one imputation, the address is not occupied.) What to do now? Should we prefer the consistency and insist that the report from three months ago is 'correct'? Or humbly admit the need for an 'adjustment' (the official's euphemism for an error). Neither is an appropriate reaction. With more information we are 'wiser' and no humility is needed to justify the adjustment. The commitment to exploit all the available information should take precedence over cosmetic considerations and the appearance of the estimates as if they were population quantities.

For comparison across time, such an adjustment is useful, but generating plausible values for several past surveys is too great a burden on the database constructor, so some compromise has to be found. But consistency in the sense described is neither a scientifically well-founded goal, nor a sign of quality of the database.

5.1.3 Imputation for absentees

The survey intended to collect the relevant information from all subjects residing at the selected addresses. Addresses at which no contact was made are not represented in the database because at the time of the database construction it is not known whether the address is occupied or not and, if known to be occupied, whether its composition has remained unchanged, was altered by a member leaving or joining (or by several such changes) in the last three months, or is occupied by a different household. For multi-household addresses, the range of possibilities is even wider.

A comprehensive application of MI would deal also with the absence from the database. This task is much more complex than imputation for missing ILO status of subjects in the database. It is best organised in stages. First the address status (occupied or empty) is imputed. Next, for occupied addresses, their occupants are imputed. In wave I, there is little information to go on, other than characteristics of the area or neighbourhood. In waves II–V, a list of occupants in the previous wave may be available. In waves III–V, we have some information about the extent of changes in the composition of the household(s) at the address. And finally, we impute an employment status for each occupant.

Each stage requires a model, and the first step in constructing it is to identify the relevant characteristics that inform about the values of the missing items. We consider first addresses that have not been contacted before. The interviewers are not meant to gather any intelligence about an address, other than, perhaps, whether the address is residential. A sign that the property is for sale or to be let may suggest that the address is not occupied. Observing that the mail and other items delivered to the address have not been collected, inquiries with the neighbours, and the like, are regarded as invasion of privacy and the recording and use of such information is not appropriate. However, publicly available information about the area or the neighbourhood, about the housing market in particular, may be very useful. Where a lot of properties are for sale or for rent and many residents are highly mobile (single young professionals in particular), it is more likely that a non-contact is due to a move. Larger single-household properties tend to change occupants much less frequently than smaller properties. There is probably more migration in the cities than in rural areas. The time of the year may also be a factor. For addresses that are occupied, the number and composition of their occupants may be inferred from the information about the neighbourhood.

For imputing the values of the variables for a set of plausible occupants, multivariate hot deck is well suited, using a donor from the same neighbourhood or from a neighbourhood of the same type. For addresses that have been contacted in the past, it is very likely that no change among the occupants has occured. The probabilities of the changes of various types, and of a wholesale move, are small, possibly varying with the household size and composition. This suggests an extensive programme of information gathering about all the neighbourhoods in the country. Conducting it thoroughly is not a realistic goal, neither logistically not economically. A more constructive strategy is to pick-and-choose sources that are available, easy to use, and have a potential to inform about the occupancy of the addresses.

Identifying the relevant sources of such information, extracting the relevant data, and formulating models for each stage is a non-trivial task. The pursuit of a comprehensive model should be discouraged because it is an open-ended and never-ending task. Consistency, in the form of using the same model over a long period of time, is not an indication of good choice, because changes are warranted as sources become (more) accessible and our expertise in them is enhanced. Appreciation of the imperfection and the temporary nature of such models goes hand-in-hand with the understanding of the substantial uncertainty about the predicted values.

In generating one set of plausible values, a given address may be marked as (plausibly) unoccupied, in which case, it is not represented in the database. In another set, it may be marked as occupied; then the next stage generates its plausible composition (ages, incomes, and the like). As a consequence, the sets of plausible values have unequal dimensions, as do the completed datasets.

In LFS, about 30% of the selected addresses are not contacted. Imputation for them is a substantial task rewarded by greater integrity of the database — reflection of the uncertainty about the missing values for individual items, whole records and sets of records that correspond to households. With such a large-scale imputation, the threats of NMAR have to treated more seriously, and so sensitivity analysis has an important role. Complex multi-stage imputation implies a wide variety of departures from MAR that should be explored. In practice, their exploration has to be rationed by the available resources and focussed on the most relevant concerns. Of course, such concerns may develop and drift over time. As sensitivity analysis is specific to the complete-data analysis, it has to be carried out by the secondary analysts, although the data constructor can apply it to a strategically selected set of analyses. The importance of sensitivity analysis should be disseminated to the secondary analysts. However, it should not be presented to them as a burden specific to MI; it is equally applicable to single-imputation schemes for which NMAR schemes can also be defined and implemented.

5.2 The National Survey of Health and Development

The Medical Research Council National Survey of Health and Development (NSHD) commenced in 1946 and includes subjects born in the week of March 3rd–9th, 1946. All single legitimate births to wives of non-manual or agricultural workers and a 25% simple random sample of the single legitimate births to wives of manual workers were included in the study. The subjects were followed up regularly through their childhood, adolescence, and in less frequent intervals in their adulthood. Information was collected about their physical and cognitive development, health, education, professional careers, and the like.

The original sample comprised 5362 subjects, but by the 19th follow-up in 1989, it has been reduced to 3262 (61%). The causes of the losses were refusals (12%), emigration from Great Britain (11.5%), loss of contact (9%), and death (7%). The analyses are commonly reduced to the cooperating subjects (3262 in 1989), or even further by discarding incomplete records. A cooperating subject may refuse to respond to some isolated questions, blocks of questions, or terminate the interview prematurely. Following the interview, the subjects may be left to complete and return a questionnaire — there is scope for further incompleteness.

We assume that the original sample was a good representation of the population of interest. Over time, this population may have shifted slightly. For instance, the population is reduced by death and emigration but, depending on its definition, it may be boosted by immigration. Thus, only losses of the sample by failure to trace affect representation. Deaths do not, and emigrants from Great Britain become members of the population of interest only when they return. Of course, there may be deaths among those with whom no contact is maintained.

The dominant response pattern is that of dropping out at a follow-up, although there are subjects who skipped one or several follow-ups. Within a follow-up, drop-out from the interview is also possible, as well as isolated missing items or their contiguous segments. Further, dropping out occurs within a block of questions, when the subject is no longer willing to answer any questions on the theme of a particular block, but would be happy to respond to questions in the next block.

Imputation in this setting is not a realistic proposition for all the waves of the survey. Given this state of affairs, it is important to appreciate that all analyses share a source of uncertainty, both in terms of bias and variation in excess of what is estimated, due to the loss of representativeness. Further losses are incurred if we reduce an analysis to the complete records. In this section, we discuss a MI scheme for a self-completion questionnaire in 19th follow-up conducted in 1989 when the subjects were 43 years old.

The subjects were requested to record in a diary all the food and drinks they consumed during a designated week. The week started the day before the interview and each contacted subject was requested to recall all the food and drinks they consumed on that day and on the day of the interview, including their quantities or volumes. In this way, each subject would have no problem following the instructions during the remaining five days. The interviewer took a copy of the diary for the first two days for the record and left a self-addressed envelope for the subject to mail the completed diary at the end of the week. Completing a diary for a week (or five days) requires a substantial commitment on the part of the subject. To some extent, this is strengthened by maintaining a contact between the Survey management and the subjects over many years. Nevertheless, only 2002 subjects (61%) returned completed diaries for all seven days. Most of the remaining subjects (970, that is, 30%) completed only the two days with the visiting interviewer. No diary records were obtained from 97 subjects; in most of these cases, the interview was terminated before reaching the point when the diary would be introduced. In total, of the $3262 \times 7 = 22\,834$ diary-days only 18 290 were recorded.

The percentage of missing diary days, about 20%, is not a good reflection of the information lost. We can illustrate this on two extreme examples. If each subject completed only 80% of the diary, little information would be lost because most middle-aged people have a set diet with relatively little variation, much of it due to a different pattern of activities on weekdays and weekends. Thus, imputation for the day or two, when the diary was not completed, would entail relatively little uncertainty. In contrast, if 20% of the subjects contributed with no diary data, and 80% with complete diary records, imputation would entail much more uncertainty because of the substantial variation in the diet among the subjects. Our setting is halfway between these two examples. Most incomplete diaries have records for two days. Assuming a MAR mechanism, we can learn from the 'diligent' subjects how consistent each subject's diet is. Little information would be lost if each subject had a regular daily diet.

Interruptions of keeping the diary influenced by the diet itself are an example of NMAR. Consumption of alcohol is a case in point. For instance, excessive consumption may bring about incapacity, illness, distraction from the everyday routine, and the like, and with it a failure to complete the diary.

Completing the diaries by imputation for the subjects who failed to follow the instructions is essential because the recorded items and their quantities are converted to nutrients and other components of food. Zero quantity, even for a day, is not a realistic value, and data reduction methods lead to a substantial loss of information. We discuss imputation for the quantities of alcohol consumed by the subjects in the survey. This is of interest for epidemiology — alcohol is a cause and a contributor, confirmed or suspected, to several diseases, and for family studies and related areas — alcohol is frequently quoted as a cause of marital problems, social dysfunction, domestic violence, low productivity and poor management of personal and family's financial affairs. For statistical methodology, the example is instructive because it exploits information in related variables.

5.2.1 Eliciting information about alcohol consumption

Diary is regarded as the gold standard for collecting information about the consumption of food and drink. If diligently completed, the diary is reckoned to be much more precise than any form of recall. However, of interest is consumption not in a particular week or a similar period of time, but over several years or even decades, for example, when studying the association of diet and diseases, such as cancer and heart disease. Only diaries completed on several occasions can inform about this, because a consistency of dietary habits over a long period of time cannot be assumed. We analyse the diary records only from one follow-up, so we cannot address this problem.

The subjects were also requested to recall their consumption of alcohol in the immediately preceding week. This was done by a set of three questions with a common lead-in passage

> 'In the last seven days, how many of the following drinks have you had? (*Do not count non-alcoholic drinks.*)'

relating to three types of alcoholic beverages:

> A. Spirits or liqueurs (e.g., whisky, gin, brandy, vodka) — measures;
> B. Wine, sherry, martini or port — glasses;
> C. Beer, lager, cider or stout — half pints.

For brevity, we refer to these categories as spirits, wine and beer. Further, subjects were asked the following four questions, called CAGE, following [61]:

> C. Have you ever felt you ought to <u>c</u>ut down on your drinking? (*Do not include dieting.*)
> A. Have people ever <u>a</u>nnoyed you by criticising your drinking?
> G. Have you ever felt bad or <u>g</u>uilty about your drinking?
> E. Have you ever had a drink first thing in the morning to steady your nerves or to get rid of a hangover (<u>e</u>ye opener)?

These questions refer to any time in the past. Any positive response was followed up by the question whether it happened last year. A measure of spirits, a glass of wine and half a pint of beer contain approximately 7900 mg of net alcohol each. In the diaries, details of the beverage consumed are often given, and the conversion to the quantity of alcohol consumed is more precise.

The diary and recall have complementing strengths as questionnaire instruments. The diary is more detailed but is bound to contain more missing values because the recall questions can be responded in a matter of a minute or two, after a brief reflection. But some subjects may not recall each instance of alcohol consumption, and their totals are then understated. This is easy to confirm with the NSHD data. Only 1532 subjects have complete records for both diary and recall; 877 of them (57%) declared greater consumption in the diaries than in the response to the recall questions. Of course, some differences are expected because the diary and recall refer to different weeks, although approximately the same number of them should be positive and negative. Only eight subjects declared consumption greater by at least 150 g (about $9\frac{1}{2}$ pints of beer or equivalent) by recall than in the diary. In contrast, 93 subjects declared consumption greater by at least 150 g in the diary than by recall.

The recall questions contain many missing values, many more than might be expected for a relatively simple task. Only 2456 subjects (75%) have complete records, but only 87 subjects (3%) have empty records on all three questions. The 806 subjects with incomplete records share 1436 missing values. A plausible explanation for this pattern is that zeros and leaving a blank response have been confused when completing the questionnaire. On the one hand, combinations of zeros and blanks are very rare; there are only 14 such cases among the 719 partial records. On the other hand, zeros are quite frequent responses. There are 4407 zeros and 3943 positive values among the $3 \times 3262 = 9786$ items. In summary, missing values in the recall questions are mainly due to imperfect conduct of the interview, whereas in the diaries they are due to subjects' imperfect cooperation.

The responses to the CAGE questionnaire are conventionally dichotomised. No or a single positive response are classified as 'no problem' and two or more positive responses as 'a problem'. There are missing responses even to CAGE questions; here we regard them as negative responses, although one could explore the sensitivity of this assumption. Only 265 subjects (8%) have scores 2–4.

We address incompleteness of the diaries by using the recall data as conditioning variables that both promote MAR and yield better prediction. As the recall is not recorded completely, we have to impute for its missing values. For this purpose, we formulate a model that draws on some of the obvious correlates of alcohol consumption: sex, smoking habit (a dichotomous variable), the logarithm of body mass, and recent history of problems with alcohol (CAGE). Even the body mass is missing for some subjects, so it is multiply imputed using a linear regression of the logarithm of height.

We organise the imputations in stages, starting with the body mass, followed by the recall and the diary data. The model for body mass and height assumes that they have a joint log-normal distribution. The distribution is fitted by the EM algorithm, in which the nonresponse mechanism is assumed to be MAR. The two variables are highly correlated, so it is essential to model them jointly.

The values of the recall variables and daily diary quantities have distributions that can be described as mixtures of zeros and log-normal distributions. That is, the positive values of each variable have a log-normal distribution. Imputations for each of these variables comprise two steps; imputing the sign (zero or positive) and imputing the quantity when the sign is positive.

The model for the sign of the recall conditions on the CAGE score, sex and smoking habit. Whenever missing, smoking habit is imputed singly as 'non-smoker'. The impact of this departure from MI is diluted in the stages of imputation that follow. The model, a two-way table with the (eight) combinations of signs for the three recall questions and the combinations of all the values of the conditioning variables, is fitted by the EM algorithm described in Section 3.4. The outcome of the analysis is a two-way table of (fitted) probabilities and an estimate of their sampling variance matrix. From this, a plausible set of probabilities is drawn, followed by draws from the appropriate plausible marginal probabilities.

The sets of imputations of the signs are not constant for all subjects. This complicates the imputations for the quantities because the response pattern has to be combined with the pattern of the signs, the latter changing from one imputation to the next. To avoid this problem, we define the *hypothetical* quantity; it is equal to the complete-data quantity when positive (irrespective of whether is it recorded or not) and otherwise to a positive value that will turn out to be irrelevant. Positive quantities are imputed first for all values that are either missing or equal to zero. Then each of them is overwritten with zero if the corresponding imputed or realised sign is zero. In this way, we operate with trivariate outcomes throughout, the assumption of multivariate log-normality for them is appropriate, and a trivariate regression model can be specified for the 'missing' values. In this setting, 'missing' combines nonresponse and no consumption. The regression model conditions on sex, smoking habit and log-body mass. Plausible values of the hypothetical quantities are drawn from the estimated sampling distribution of the matrix of regression coefficients and the 3×3 residual variance matrix. The high correlations in this matrix (0.65–0.85) support the rationale for the joint modelling of the three recall variables.

The imputation of signs for the daily diary quantities proceeds in the time order, starting with the signs for the first diary day of the 97 subjects with empty diaries, followed by the signs for the second day for these and additional 14 subjects who completed the diary for the first day only, and so on. A few diary days of data are discarded, so that the response patterns are monotone, and the procedure is proper if the posited model is appropriate.

For the first day, the model for missing signs conditions on sex, smoking habit, CAGE score, sign of the recall total and the day of the week (weekday, Monday–Thursday, or weekend, Friday–Sunday). To avoid any iterative procedures, the conditioning is on the entire cross-classification of these variables. This is equivalent to including all the interactions in the model. (More parsimonious models can be fitted with logistic regression.) In a few instances, categories that are similar have to be aggregated to avoid cells containing very few subjects. For the second day, the model conditions on the same variables as for the first day, but the sign of the first day is added to them. For the third and subsequent days, it is not practical to condition on all the previous days, so only the two immediately preceding days are included in the model.

A seven-variate model is defined for the hypothetical daily diary quantities. The dimensionality of the problem is reduced by totting up the quantities consumed over the four types of beverages. (Unlike by recall, the quantities of beer and cider are derived from the diaries separately.) The regression model conditions on sex, smoking habit, CAGE score, the day of the week (seven categories) and the log-body mass. In the EM algorithm used for fitting this model, both zero and missing quantities are regarded as 'missing' information. The algorithm starts by fitting the model for the 194 subjects who declared positive quantities on every one of the seven days. The conditional distributions of the missing sections of the records are evaluated and the M-step executes the complete-data analysis with the sufficient statistics replaced by their conditional expectations. Fast convergence, after 25 iterations, indicates that the amount of information missing due to nonresponse and zero quantities is not overwhelming.

The described procedure is rather complex, although each of its elements is easy to program, involving standard statistical algorithms, implemented as complete-data methods in an EM algorithm. Some short-cuts are unavoidable in this procedure. For example, the sampling variation of each EM estimator is difficult to derive, so a compromise between the complete-data and the reduced-data sampling variance matrices is used. The outcome of the procedure is a set of plausible values for the amount of (net) alcohol consumed on each diary day.

5.2.2 Excessive alcohol consumption

Consumption of alcohol in small or moderate quantities is assumed to have no long-term effects on the health or mental capacity. In contrast, excessive consumption is generally regarded as harmful and undesirable. Standard approaches to assessing alcohol consumption are based on estimating the population mean consumption, from which the extent of excessive consumption is inferred indirectly. This is problematic because the inference is predicated on a fixed distribution of the quantities consumed in moderation, including the proportion of abstaining members of the population.

We prefer to estimate the proportion of excessive consumers directly, by specifying a threshold for excessive consumption and estimating the proportion of the population who exceed it. It is impossible to define a universally acceptable threshold quantity, so we estimate the proportions for a range of realistic values of the threshold. Variations on this theme include defining thresholds that depend on the body mass and estimating the proportions as functions of the body mass. In these cases, the complete-data analysis is elementary, so conducting it several times creates no difficulties. Although plausible values are generated for many items, the amount of missing information in these analyses is quite modest. To see this, consider an incomplete record that indicates excessive consumption on the first two days and has missing values for the next five days. If the consumption over the first two days exceeds the threshold, then so does the consumption over the week. If the recorded consumption is close to the threshold, then the consumption over the whole week is very likely to exceed it, especially when the recorded part is from weekdays. However, two recorded days of no consumption provide only weak evidence of moderate (or no) consumption over the whole week. All discussion of examples below refers to $M = 7$ sets of plausible values.

For example, subject 1 completed the diary only for the first two days, declaring no consumption on day 1 and consumption of 107 g on day 2. The septet of imputed totals ranges from 156 g (little consumption on the five days with missing diary data) to 475 g, with substantial consumption on most of the five days. Subject 3 also completed the diary only for the first two days, declaring no consumption on either day. With one exception, 139 g, the plausible totals of net alcohol consumed during the week are very small; two plausible values are equal to zero, and the remaining four values are between 3 g (less than quarter a pint of beer) and 29 g (about two pints). The plausible values indicate that this subject very likely drinks in moderation, or not at all, but a higher consumption is not ruled out altogether. Subject 7 declared identical amounts of alcohol consumed on the first two days, 55.1 g, and failed to continue the diary for the next five days. The lowest of the seven plausible values for the total consumed is 235 g, indicating that the subject consumed a lot of alcohol also on the diary days 3–7. The highest of the plausible totals is 576 g, an excessive amount by any standards.

In the analysis, reported in greater detail in [166], seven sets of plausible values were generated. This turned out to be somewhat of an overkill because the fraction of the missing information is much smaller than the fraction of the missing items. It is a consequence of a lot of regular (habitual) alcohol consumption and extensive modelling of missing data, exploiting the high correlation of the daily quantities consumed. However, the amount of computing additional to the setting of $M = 5$ plausible values is insubstantial and requires no intervention by the analyst.

The estimate of the population percentage of those who consumed more than 400 g of alcohol in the reference week is 4.22%, with estimated standard error 0.37%. The contributions to the estimated sampling variance are $\bar{s}^2 = 0.124$ and $\hat{B} + \hat{B}/M = 0.014$; see Section 4.2.5. The estimated fraction of the missing information in this analysis is 10.1% and only about 1.5% is a result of using only finite number ($M = 7$) of sets of plausible values.

The uncertainty about the missing values can be exposed by the counts of subjects with excessive (plausible) consumption in each completed-data analysis. Among the complete records there are 82 positive and 1920 negative cases. Among the 1260 incomplete records, all seven plausible values are smaller than 400 g for 1099 subjects and greater than 400 g for 16 subjects. Further eight subjects have consumption in excess of 400 g in six of the seven sets of plausible values, six subjects in five sets each, seven is four sets, 17 in three sets, 24 in two sets and 73 in one set each, so that 233 subjects are in the pool of plausibly excessive consumers. Yet, in the seven completed-data analyses, the numbers of excessive consumers are in the range 132–144. No single-imputation method could represent this uncertainty.

The estimated threshold-specific proportions of excessive consumers are summarised by Figure 5.3, together with the estimated proportions for men and women. The thick lines of the three types indicated in the legend are for the estimates and the thin lines for the upper and lower 95% symmetric confidence intervals. The diagram confirms that excessive consumption is much more common among men than among women, not a surprising finding, although it conveys much more detail about the extent of excessive consumption.

In research on abuse of alcohol, it is recognised that men tend to consume more alcohol, and so, as a rule of thumb, a threshold lower by 25% is defined for women than for men, such as 300 g for women and 400 g for men. This rule makes little difference to the disparity in the rates of excessive consumption among men and women.

5.2.3 Sensitivity analysis

The models for missing values contain many opportunistic features — they are not based on any theory, merely attempt to make use of the available information, in a form that is amenable to analysis. At the same time, intuition suggests that some of the model assumptions, especially in the earlier stages of imputation, are less important. A comprehensive review of these assumptions is beyond what any analyst can be reasonably expected to accomplish. However, an indication of their importance can be gauged by altering one of them, replacing it with an assumption that is clearly more restrictive or less realistic. If this leads to no appreciable differences in the results of the conducted analyses, we can 'down-grade' the caveat associated with the non-response model. (Recall that in a single imputation, the caveat refers to the imputed values themselves.)

One assumption that can rightly be questioned is that the recall values are missing at random. A credible alternative is that most of the missing

Figure 5.3. The estimates of the percentages of excessive consumers of alcohol for thresholds in the range 250–500 g per week.

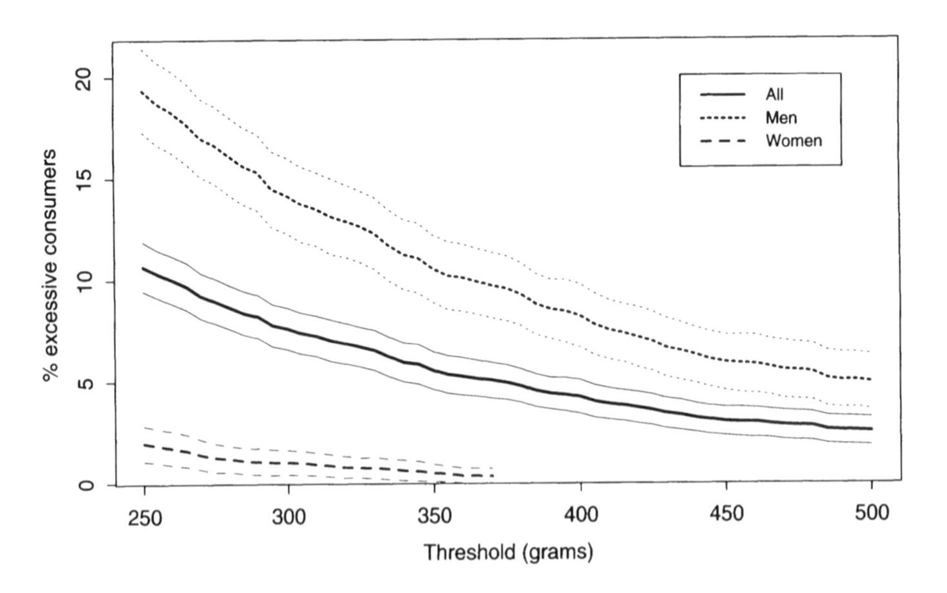

quantities are equal to zero, reflecting subjects' expectations that the absence of a response would be interpreted as no consumption. The sensitivity of the results with respect to this assumption is assessed by defining alternative plausible values for missing recall. Simply, each missing value for recall is replaced by zero, and the imputations for daily diary consumption are based on the same model as in the last stage of the original imputation procedure.

This change has only a slight impact on the results. The estimated percentages of the excessive consumers are altered by 0.10% for the threshold of 300 g (from 7.61% to 7.71%) and by 0.01% each for 400 g and 500 g. The estimated standard errors are also altered only slightly, e.g., from 0.32 to 0.30 for the threshold of 500 g. The problem with such an assessment is that the multitude of analyses planned, intended or improvised, can at best be represented only by a selection.

A sensitivity analysis can be targeted for a specific estimator, such as the difference in the percentage of excessive consumers between men and women. For such an analysis, the plausible values generated with the MAR assumption are reduced for men and increased for women. Additive change is not realistic because zero quantities would never be imputed for women and a substantial change represents different quantities for an abstainer and an excessive consumer. Multiplicative change is not suitable either because it does not alter zero plausible values. A realistic scheme combines either additive or multiplicative change, or both, with overwriting by zero.

5.3 The International Social Survey Programme

The International Social Survey Programme (ISSP) began in 1985, and in 1999 it had more than thirty member countries in which social science surveys with similar designs, protocols and questionnaire instruments were conducted. This section describes an implementation of MI for the surveys conducted in 1995 in 23 countries. The national surveys used similar sampling designs, adapted for the circumstances of each country, and questionnaire instruments, translated from the English original, that are as similar as possible, given the linguistic and cultural differences among the participating countries.

The ISSP database for the 1995 surveys comprises a total of 28 456 subjects from 23 countries. The countries' sample sizes, in the range 612–2089, are not related in any obvious way to their populations. Eighteen of the participating countries are from Europe, nine of them former communist-block countries or their parts. Four other countries are economically advanced (U.S.A., Canada, Japan and New Zealand), and the remaining country is the Philippines. Separate surveys were conducted in the former West Germany and German Democratic Republic, even though they were united several years earlier. To simplify the discourse, we refer to them as different countries. We treat Great Britain and Northern Ireland similarly because they are separate members of ISSP. Apart from Northern Ireland, Australia and Israel were two other members of ISSP in 1995 that did not conduct the 1995 survey.

The database contains 214 variables, but some of them, such as religion and political affiliation, have categories specific to each country. Further, some variables apply only to specific countries and some questionnaire items were not administered in all the countries. For languages spoken by the subject, there are several variables (first, second, ... language), but a monolingual subject has an entry only for the first variable; no response and 'not applicable' are confounded for the other variables. The variables can be classified as administrative, background and substantive. The latter are responses to the questions about the main theme of the survey, national identity. These 55 questions are organised in eight blocks.

We give details of MI for the block of six questions about subjects' attitudes to immigration. The response rate varies a great deal from country to country. Table 5.2 gives the relevant details for the block of questions about immigration. We use two summaries, the number of records that are incomplete (8132 out of $n = 28\,456$, that is, 28.6%), and the number of items missing (16 211 out of $6n$, that is, 9.5%). We classify the countries as historically immigration and emigration countries. The industrialised countries of northwestern Europe (including Austria), U.S.A., Canada and New Zealand belong to the former (type I in Table 5.2) and east European countries and Philippines belong to the latter (type E). East Germany, Italy, Ireland, Japan and Spain are classified as neither emigration nor immigration (type O), and are omitted from the comparisons discussed below.

Table 5.2. Countries involved in ISSP 1995, their sample sizes and the extent of missing data.

Country	Type	Sample size	Incomplete records	%	Missing items	%
Bulgaria	E	1105	579	52.4	1798	27.1
Czech Republic	E	1111	298	26.8	477	7.2
Hungary	E	1000	183	18.3	313	5.2
Latvia	E	1044	430	40.2	968	15.5
Philippines	E	1200	114	9.5	208	2.9
Poland	E	1598	822	51.4	1689	17.6
Russia	E	1585	852	53.8	2166	22.8
Slovakia	E	1388	454	32.7	845	10.1
Slovenia	E	1036	342	33.0	612	9.8
Austria	I	1007	233	23.1	379	6.3
Canada	I	1543	321	20.8	471	5.1
Great Britain	I	1058	210	19.8	398	6.3
the Netherlands	I	2089	412	19.7	758	6.0
New Zealand	I	1043	171	16.4	323	5.2
Norway	I	1527	400	26.2	710	7.7
Sweden	I	1296	352	27.2	590	7.6
U. S. A.	I	1367	382	27.9	784	9.6
West Germany	I	1282	374	29.2	721	9.4
East Germany	O	612	187	30.6	329	9.0
Ireland	O	994	142	14.3	194	3.3
Italy	O	1094	151	13.8	189	2.9
Japan	O	1406	427	34.0	750	10.0
Spain	O	1221	296	24.2	539	7.4
Total		28 456	8132	28.6	16 211	9.5

Notes: The country types are: E — historically emigration countries (Eastern Europe and Philippines), I — historically immigration countries (Western Europe, North America and New Zealand), and O — other countries.

The fraction of missing items is much smaller than the fraction of incomplete records, suggesting that many subjects skipped single questions. But this pattern varies from country to country. For example, Poland and Bulgaria have similarly high percentages of incomplete records but very different percentages of missing items. At the other extreme, Italy and Philippines have nearly identical (low) percentages of missing items, but very different percentages of incomplete records.

An obvious motive for not responding is the ethical and political sensitivity of the questions. It might be expected that subjects not wishing to respond to a particular question would refuse to respond to all similar questions (in the same block) or would abandon responding altogether. The corresponding response patterns are far from dominant, so this simple mechanism, associated with NMAR, is not prevalent. These and other plausible reactions to the questions are likely to differ from country to country; this suggests that imputations should be conducted separately for each country. This is advantageous also for practical implementation, as fewer records have to be handled at a time.

5.3.1 Imputation for 'national identity' items

Although theoretically preferable, simultaneous (proper) imputation for all the variables is not feasible. All the variables are categorical, some with many categories, and so it is not possible to define a joint distribution for them. Instead, we organise the imputations in stages, starting with socio-demographic background variables that tend to have few missing values, proceeding to income, trade-union and political-party affiliations, and concluding with the blocks of questions about national identity, for which conditioning on background is natural. To avoid near repetition, we discuss details only for West Germany and focus on one block of substantive questions.

At the first stage, plausible values are generated for sex, marital status (married, widowed, divorced, separated or never married) and 'cohabitation with a steady partner' (yes, no or not applicable). In the sample for West Germany, 49 subjects (3.8% out of 1282) have incomplete records on these three variables; eight records are empty, 29 have only marital status missing (pattern 101, or x?x), and the other twelve records belong to four of the five remaining patterns. Note that being married implies the response 'not applicable' to the question about cohabitation, so only 18 distinct response patterns are possible. As there are so few incomplete records, it suffices to fit a model to the complete records and, assuming MAR, use it for generating plausible values for the missing items.

At the second stage, plausible values are generated for education, an ordinal categorical variable with seven values, from 'none or still in education' to 'completed university education'. Only seven values are missing. The conditioning is on sex and marital status, and the latter variable is collapsed to two categories, whether married or not. There are so few missing values that generating plausible values by any naively justified process would seem to make little difference. Completion is highly desirable because data reduction in complex analyses with many variables would lead to smaller sample sizes, and there is no obvious value to be imputed for most missing items.

At the next stage, plausible values are generated for the variables inquiring about employment circumstances: employment status (12 missing values), employed in the private or public sector (38), whether self-employed (38) and whether having any supervisory role in employment (16). The conditioning is on sex, marital status (dichotomy) and education (dichotomy, whether possessing any tertiary education).

Table 5.3. Blocks of items on the subject of national identity in the 1995 ISSP and information on the response patterns for West Germany.

Block of items	Number of items	Complete records (%)	Missing values (%)
1. How close do you feel ...	5	586 (45.7)	1096 (17.1)
2. Move to improve conditions ...	5	1045 (81.5)	696 (10.9)
3. Important to be ...	7	1126 (87.8)	365 (4.1)
4. Nation – Country – Citizenship	6	945 (73.7)	607 (7.9)
5. Proud of ...	11	769 (60.0)	1521 (10.8)
6. Traditions vs. foreign countries	9	770 (60.1)	1030 (8.9)
7. Immigrants should (be) ...	6	908 (70.8)	721 (9.4)
8. Ethnicity & citizenship	3*	956 (74.6)	373 (9.7)
All items	52	186 (14.5)	6409 (9.6)

Note: * Block 8 comprises six questions, but only three were administered in West Germany.

The following stages generate plausible values for earnings (six ordered categories, 133 missing values), family income (seven ordered categories, 114 missing values), social class (seven categories, 24 missing values), trade union and party affiliation (39 and 62 missing values, respectively), religion and attendance of services and household size. None of the models is strongly predictive, so much of the variation in the plausible values is random, reflecting our failure to recover the missing values. With any single imputation, we would have to commit ourselves to one of the values for each missing item. If a single imputation were successful in recovering some of the missing values the model used or the underlying scheme could be adapted for MI by incorporating the (small) uncertainty about the missing values when generating sets of plausible values.

Information about missing items for the eight blocks of substantive questions is summarised in Table 5.3 for West Germany. In total, 618 values are missing for the background variables. Although it may be attractive to store the plausible values generated for them in a single file of 618 rows and $M+2$ columns (a column each to identify the subject and the variable, followed by M columns of plausible values), the national-identity items have many more missing values, and so the file of plausible values is no longer compact. The most convenient solution for a user is to have the M completed datasets. This is made more practical by defining plausible values only for the total scores for each block of items. The scale has to be reversed for some questions, to make the total score meaningful. These aggregate scores are sufficient for most secondary analyses. An exception is presented in Section 5.3.2.

By imputing for the total scores, the imputation task is greatly simplified. The completed datasets are much smaller, as the national-identity items are reduced to $8M$ columns of plausible totals. In an alternative arrangement, the plausible values for the missing background items are stored in one file and the plausible totals for the blocks of substantive items in another. As there are so many incomplete records for the blocks, the savings by storing the plausible totals for them are not substantial, and probably not worth the added complexity in the instructions for completing the dataset.

In the database, two codes for missing values are used: 'cannot choose' and similar (code 8) and 'refused to respond' (code 9). For simplicity, we do not distinguish between the two codes and consider a single model for missing values. A more principled approach, but also more complex, would distinguish between the two codes and define separate models for them.

The first block comprises five questions with a common lead-in passage

How close do you feel to your ... ?

neighbourhood (question 1), town or city, county, country and the continent (question 5). Each item is scored on the Likert scale (very close — 1, close — 2, neutral — 3, distant — 4 and very distant — 5). Only 586 subjects (46%) responded to all five items. One item is missing for 509 records (40%), with none of the five response patterns prevailing among them; this suggests that momentary distraction is a more likely cause of nonresponse than any reaction to the substance of the questions.

The second block of questions has a similar format, with the lead-in passage

If you could improve your living and working conditions, would you be willing to move to another ... ?

(neighbourhood, city or town, county, country, or continent). The block has 1045 (81.5%) complete records for West Germany, and the most common incomplete-response patterns are 00000 and 10000 with 59 and 37 records, respectively. Both the extent and the relative frequencies of the response patterns differ substantially from the first block. It is difficult to point to any specific cause of this, other than the location of the blocks.

The model for the missing block-level total scores assumes MAR and conditions on a selected set of background variables (sex, marital status and education, the latter two variables recoded to dichotomies) and the available scores for the questions of the block. The plausible values are generated separately for each response pattern, and the patterns are ordered partially from the almost complete pattern (only one item missing) to the empty pattern (all items missing).

For records with a single item missing, the total of the recorded scores is matched with the corresponding total for the complete records. The plausible total score is drawn from the total scores of the matched complete records, with an adjustment for the uncertainty about the distribution of the complete-data total scores.

For the records with two or more missing values, their totals on the available responses are matched with the corresponding totals of the records that have less nonresponse. For these 'donor' records, the complete-data total score is either defined (uniquely) or plausible values have been generated earlier. In the latter case, the ith set of plausible totals for the donor records is generated from the matching records. In the last step, plausible values for empty records are based on all the non-empty records, using their completely recorded or imputed total scores.

In a few instances, no donor could be found for a total score within the combination of the conditioning background variables. In such a case, the pool is expanded to include the neighbouring categories (with total score greater or smaller by one). This procedure for generating plausible values is not proper because the pools of donors overlap, and so the distributions from which plausible totals are drawn are not independent. We believe that the improperness involved is preferable to a single imputation procedure, as the procedure is relatively simple and requires only a modest programming effort. In any case, expanded pools of donors are required for very few recipients.

5.3.2 Attitudes to immigration

In this section, we describe an analysis of the block of questions about attitudes to immigration in ISSP 1995. We compare the historically emigration and immigration countries on the responses to the individual questionnaire items, and conduct a sensitivity analysis to assess how the conclusions of the analysis are altered with the departure of the assumed nonresponse mechanism from MAR.

We are concerned with six questionnaire items formulated as statements that directly relate to immigration issues:

1. Immigrants increase crime rates.
2. Immigrants are generally good for [*your country*]'s economy.
3. Immigrants take jobs away from people who were born in [*your country*].
4. Immigration makes [*your country*] more open to new ideas and cultures.
5. Number of immigrants to [*your country*] should ...
6. Refugees who have suffered political repression in their country should be allowed to stay in [*your country*].

The statements have the five response options of the Likert scale given in Table 5.4. The scoring scale for statements 1 and 3 is reversed, so that low scores indicate negative and high scores positive attitude to immigrants for each statement.

The response patterns are summarised in Table 5.5. More than half of the incomplete records have only one item missing. More detail is obtained by tabulating the $2^6 = 64$ response patterns. Every one of them is represented in

Table 5.4. The response options for the statements about attitudes to immigration.

Score	Statements 1–4 and 6	Statement 5
1	Disagree strongly	Be reduced a lot
2	Disagree	Be reduced a little
3	Neither agree nor disagree	Remain the same as it is
4	Agree	Be increased a little
5	Agree strongly	Be increased a lot

Table 5.5. Tabulation of the numbers of missing items.

	Number of items missing						
	0	1	2	3	4	5	6
Number of subjects	20 324	4446	1732	739	433	340	442
Percent	71.4	15.6	6.1	2.6	1.5	1.2	1.6

Table 5.6. Subjects with one nonresponse and subjects with one response.

	Number of subjects for statement No.					
	1	2	3	4	5	6
Sole nonresponse	335	600	247	781	1655	828
Sole response	148	52	11	55	8	66

the data, although the counts of subjects for quite a few of them are in single digits. In 4446 cases, only one statement is without response. Many more of these nonresponses are for the last three statements. Similarly, among the 340 cases with only one response, disproportionately many occur for the first statement. The counts are given in Table 5.6. They suggest that nonresponse may be informative.

As the statements are closely related, the recorded parts of the responses are good informants of the missing responses. When several responses are available the number of score patterns is very large, and so it is not practical to condition on the recorded scores. We collapse some of the response categories to avoid handling small within-cell counts. The imputations are carried out by hot deck, separately for each country, starting with records that have one missing item each, then dealing with records with two missing items, and so on, and concluding with imputations for empty records.

One item missing

Imputations are carried out separately for each response pattern (statement for which no response is recorded). The available quintets of scores have $5^5 = 3125$ possible patterns, so many of them are not represented among the complete records. The available scores are recoded to dichotomous variables that indicate whether the scores exceed the middle category 3. In this way, the number of response patterns is reduced to $2^5 = 32$. The categories defined by these patterns can be collapsed further by aggregating the smallest cells with their neighbours. The aggregation is carried out until each cell contains at least 50 records. Plausible values are drawn from the plausible multinomial distribution with values 1, ..., 5, implied by the aggregated score patterns among the complete records.

Two items missing

The response patterns for the four matching statements are collapsed to $2^4 = 16$ patterns, and aggregated further to have at least 100 records in each cell. The matching set of two statements has 25 distinct patterns. The plausible values are drawn from a plausible multinomial distribution with 25 categories.

Three items missing

The response patterns are collapsed by considering three categories, (1,2), (3,4) and 5, and are further collapsed until each cell has at least 120 records. The matching set is collapsed similarly to $3^3 = 27$ cells. A plausible cell for a missing triplet of items is drawn first, and the responses are then generated by drawing at random from the two alternative categories.

Four items missing

The 25 categories of the response patterns are left intact, and the matching responses are collapsed to $2^4 = 16$ categories.

Five or six items missing

When only one item is recorded the response patterns are left intact, and a draw is made from the pool of records with the same response on the available item. For empty records, the complete and completed records are used as a single pool of donors.

The imputations are 'recycled'; in imputations for records with k items missing, the matches are made on the records completed by imputations carried out earlier (for records with 1, ..., $k-1$ items missing). In replicate imputations, different pools of donors are used, contributing to the between-imputation variance.

The method of chained equations is a viable alternative to this approach. The neutral category 3 is the obvious default value for the initial imputation.

5.3.3 Sensitivity analysis

As the assumption of MAR is problematic, we explore departures from it and search for the 'critical' departure which no longer supports the original conclusion based on MAR. The NMAR models considered correspond to altering the plausible values generated under MAR in the following way. For a given probability p, an independent draw Δ is made from the binomial distribution $\mathcal{B}(p, 4)$ for each missing item. Suppose the estimated mean scores under MAR are higher for the emigration countries. The plausible values generated under MAR are reduced by Δ for each missing item in an emigration country and increased by Δ for each missing item in an immigration country. If the resulting value falls outside the range 1–5, it is truncated. MAR corresponds to $p = 0$ and the extreme NMAR to $p = 1$ when each missing item in an emigration country is replaced by 1 and each missing item in an immigration country by 5.

The analysis intended for the complete data is summarised in Figure 5.4. Each country is represented by a set of segments connecting the estimated deviations of the national mean scores from the overall means for the six statements. The mean scores are replaced by their deviations from the overall mean vector estimated for the following datasets or assumptions:

A. Complete records	(3.383, 3.202, 3.085, 2.748, 3.833, 2.693)
B. All available data	(3.389, 3.203, 3.089, 2.722, 3.860, 2.660)
C. MI, assuming MAR	(3.390, 3.202, 3.092, 2.754, 3.816, 2.677)
D. Extreme NMAR	(3.342, 3.157, 3.054, 2.672, 3.680, 2.636)

The segments for the emigration countries are plotted on the left- and for the immigration countries on the right-hand side of each panel. The panels A–D present the results for the analysis based on complete records, all available data (listwise deletion), with MI based on MAR, and for the extreme NMAR with 1 imputed for all missing items in the emigration countries and 5 for all missing items in the immigration countries. The panels A–C lead to the same conclusion, that emigration countries tend to have higher mean scores, but the conclusion from panel D is very different. The standard error of a typical estimator used in the diagram is about 0.03, so the differences observed are largely genuine, if the treatment of missing values is appropriate. Panel D corresponds to the adjustment of the plausible values by $\pm\mathcal{B}(p = 1, n = 4)$. As it is an extreme NMAR mechanism it can be ruled out as implausible. However, it would be difficult to come to a consensus about the largest plausible value of p.

Although the mean is a natural way of summarising the distribution of the responses for each statement, it is not the only choice. Alternatives attractive for some purposes focus on the balance between agreement and disagreement with the statement. The odds of agreement vs. disagreement is one such sum-

Figure 5.4. The estimated deviations of the within-country mean scores for the questionnaire items related to immigration.

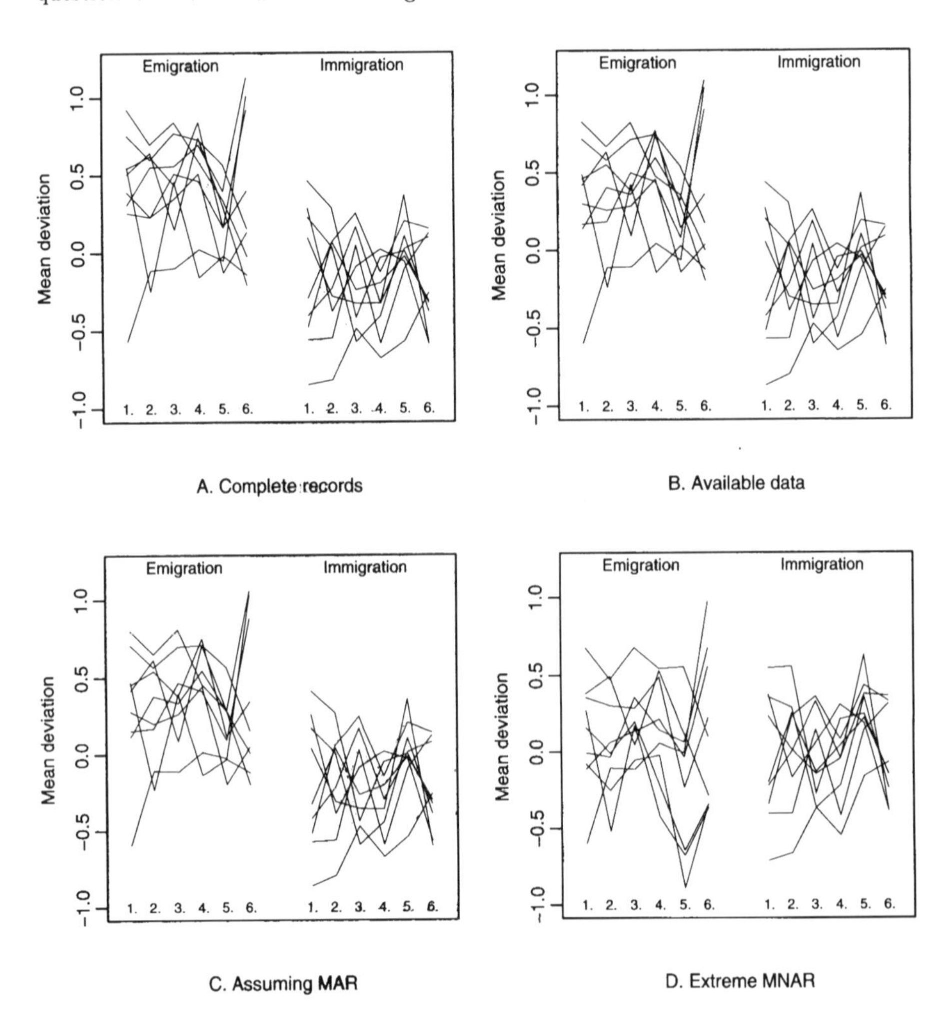

mary. It is defined as the ratio of the probabilities of agreement (response categories 4 and 5) and disagreement (categories 1 and 2). With this summary, no distinction is made between scores 4 and 5 on the one hand, and 1 and 2 on the other. A related summary is based on the odds of the extreme response categories 1 and 5. This corresponds to regarding the responses 2–4 as neutral and drawing no distinction among them.

An element of arbitrariness is involved in the choice of the summary, so establishing that its details do not have a strong impact on the inferences drawn is essential. Figure 5.5 presents the comparisons of the estimated odds

Figure 5.5. The estimated deviations of the within-country odds of the extreme responses to the six questionnaire items related to immigration.

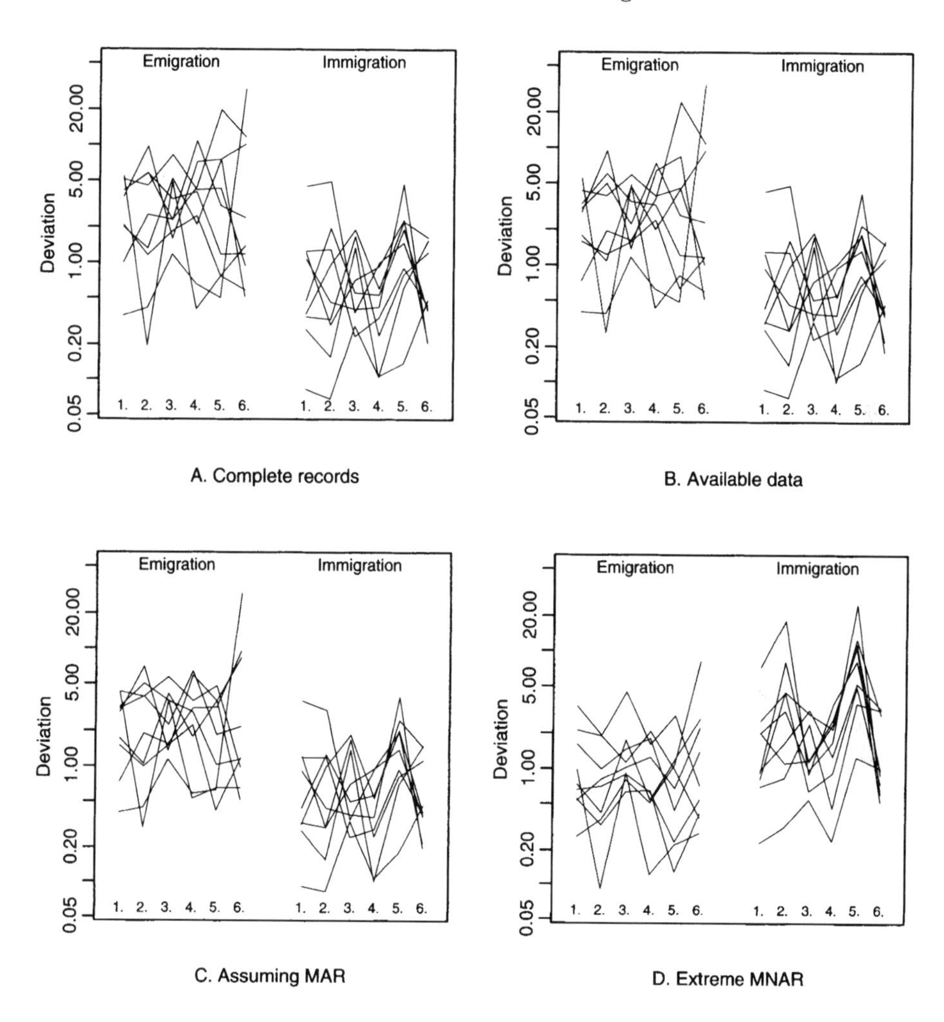

of the extreme categories for the emigration and immigration countries, using the same layout as in Figure 5.4. The vertical axis in each panel is on the log-scale, so that the observed vertical distances can be interpreted as differences in log-odds.

As in Figure 5.4, the extreme NMAR mechanism leads to a conclusion that contradicts the conclusion based on the MAR mechanism, and so it is essential to consider intermediate NMAR mechanisms. Ideally, the most extreme NMAR mechanism that is still plausible, say, defined by a (binomial) probability p^*, would be identified. If the conclusions based on the probabilities $0 < p < p^*$ do not differ appreciably, we can dismiss any concerns about NMAR; otherwise the assumed mechanism is an essential caveat of our analysis.

Note that unlike for deviations from the mean score in Figure 5.4, the complete-records and MI estimates of odds differ substantially for a few emigration countries for responses to statements 5 and 6. In these countries (Czech Republic, Slovenia and Latvia in particular), category 1 is very rare, so the plotted points are associated with large sampling variation in each analysis. However, the overall comparison of the two groups of countries is unaffected.

Instead of seeking a consensus about the probability p^*, we present the results for the entire range of values of p in Figure 5.6. For $p < 0.2$, the conclusions are not changed substantially; the odds in the emigration countries tend to be higher than in the immigration countries. For $0.2 < p < 0.6$, the odds are similar, and for $p > 0.6$, the immigration countries appear to have greater odds. Thus, the conclusions of the analysis are vulnerable to the assumption of MAR, and this should be addressed by qualitative assessment of the range of feasible departures from MAR, so that at least some of the extreme scenarios in Figure 5.6 could be ruled out.

In this example, the uncertainty due to sampling, reflected by the complete-data standard errors is but a small component of the overall uncertainty about some population quantities. Nonresponse poses a much greater threat to our confidence about the conclusions of the analysis. The database contains little information about the nature of the response mechanism, and so clues have to be sought elsewhere to narrow down the range of NMAR mechanisms that are feasible. This includes identifying variables that are suitable for conditioning. By including them in the model for nonresponse, the range of feasible departures from MAR would be reduced. But, in general, NMAR cannot be ruled out.

5.4 The Scottish House Condition Survey

The Scottish House Condition Survey (SHCS) is a survey of the residential housing stock in Scotland. It was conducted in 1991, 1996 and 2002. In this section, we describe a MI-based method that addresses the inconsistency of the surveyors engaged to assess the sampled dwellings in the 1996 survey. *Surveyor inconsistency* is defined as a disagreement of two surveyors' assessments of the same dwelling. It is related to misclassification, although the direct (ideal) assessment cannot be established, as it is not defined unambiguously.

The survey employs a stratified clustered sampling design based on the sampling frame obtained from the list of all residential addresses to which the Post Office delivers mail. The sample size in 1996 was around 16 000, and around 20 000 in 2002. The data collected from a sampled address comprises a 'social' and a 'physical' part. The social part inquires about the household composition, income of its adult members, intentions (e.g., to move in the

Figure 5.6. The estimated odds of the within-country extreme responses to the questionnaire items related to immigration under a range of NMAR assumptions.

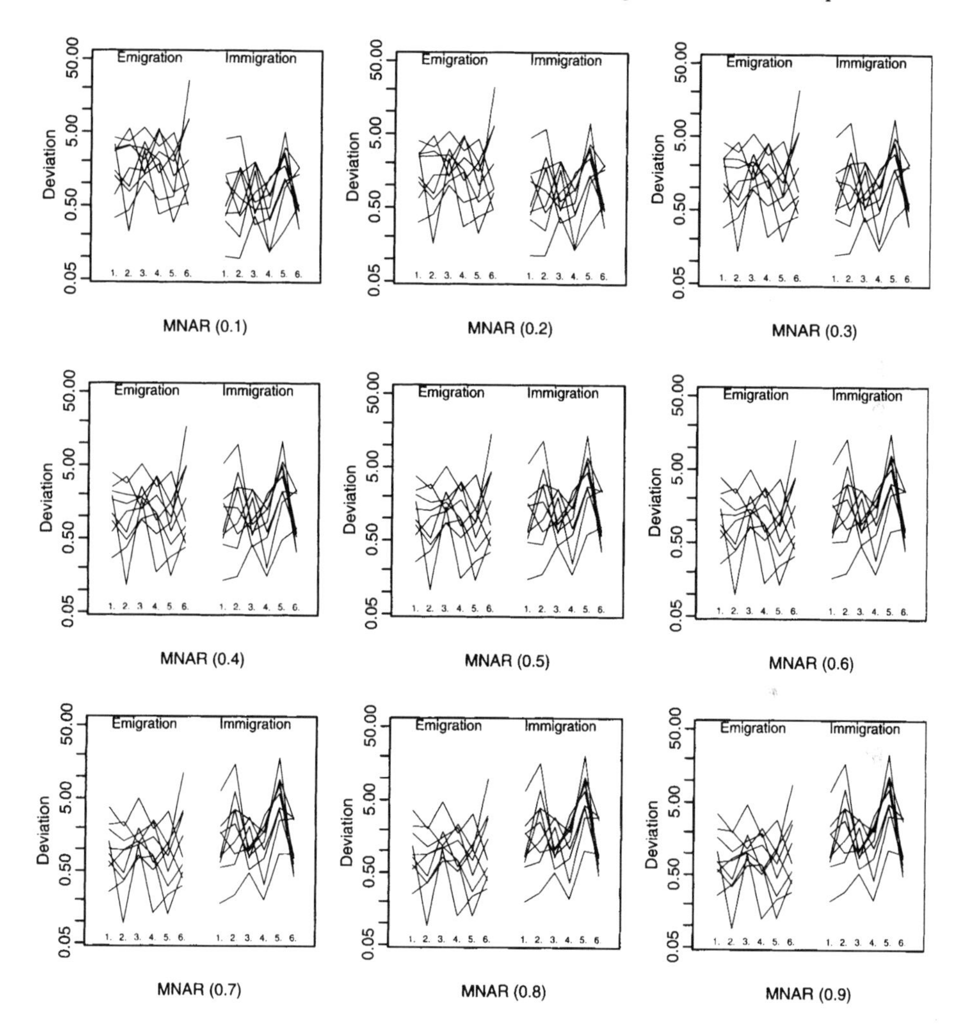

near future), and the like. In the physical part, the assigned surveyor assesses a large number of *elements*, such as dwelling type (seven categories), the extent of repairs required for an amenity (four percentage bands and a category for 'amenity missing'), and presence of central heating (none, partial, or full); most of the recorded variables are categorical; they are nominal, ordinal or have a partial ordering with one or a few categories outside the hierarchy (for example, 'not applicable'). Many elements are scored by the surveyors on the integer scale from 0 to 10 according to the level of disrepair. Zero stands for no repair required, and category k is interpreted that the element requires repairs which would cost about $10k$% of the replacement (full) price of the element. These assessments are combined into monetary values expressing the total cost of bringing the dwelling up to an established standard (*visible repair costs*, VRC) and maintaining that standard for the next ten years (*comprehensive repair costs*, CRC). These costs are calculated using extensive tables of typical costs that take into account the (area-dependent) cost of labour, economies of scale (applicable when a lot of repairs are required), existing maintenance contracts (e.g., for local-authority owned dwellings), and other factors.

As a form of quality control, a subsample of 545 surveyed dwellings was assessed second time. This 'sub-survey' intended to over-sample dwellings likely to be in poor condition — dwellings erected before 1945 and local-authority owned dwellings in particular. For each of these dwellings, two distinct surveyors were engaged. The pairs were not informed about one-another's identity, so that the assessments would be independent.

Despite careful selection of the surveyors, detailed instructions given to them, and training provided when applicable, the paired surveyors' assessments of a dwelling are not identical. Although differences in the assessments are quite rare for most of the assessed elements (the vast majority of assessments are zeros, indicating that no repair of the inspected element is required), the impact of the surveyor inconsistency on the overall assessment (VRC and CRC), aggregated over the many elements, is not trivial. By way of an illustration, suppose the survey comprises 20 elements and each element is assessed appropriately in 98% of the surveyed dwellings. Then, assuming that inappropriate assessments arise at random, the chance of a dwelling being assessed appropriately on all its elements is $0.98^{20} = 0.67$; one-third of the assessed dwellings will have at least one element assessed inappropriately. In the calculation of CRC, one 'error' may be (approximately) offset by another made on the same dwelling, while for another dwelling the errors are compounded. Surveyor inconsistency refers to the fact that another surveyor might have assessed an element of a dwelling differently.

As an example, Table 5.7 gives a cross-tabulation of the assessments of the element 'dwelling type'. The element has seven categories. Among them, we can recognise pairs of types that could easily be confused, such as semi-detached and terraced. We refer to such categories as *neighbours*. For ordinal categorical variables, the neighbours of a category are defined in the obvious way; the extreme categories (say, 0 and 10) have only one neighbour each (1 and 9, respectively), and the other categories have two neighbours each (for example, 3 and 5 are the neighbours of category 4).

From the collected data we cannot establish which assessments are appropriate and which are not. For the dwellings assessed twice, the assessment is very likely to be correct when the two surveyors agree, because the probability of both of them being incorrect, and making the same misjudgement, is very small. However, only about 3% of the dwellings were assessed twice.

The population quantities of interest are the means (and totals) and the distributions of VRC and CRC for the whole country, its regions and for

Table 5.7. Cross-tabulation of the element 'dwelling type' for the dwellings assessed twice in SHCS 1996.

	Category	DT	SM	TR	TN	4B	FL	TW
DT	Detached house	81	2	0	0	0	1	0
SM	Semi-detached house	2	88	8	0	0	0	0
TR	Terraced house	0	3	139	0	0	0	0
TN	Tenement	0	0	0	130	1	1	1
4B	Four in a block	0	0	0	4	60	6	0
FL	Flat converted bldg	0	0	0	1	1	8	0
TW	Tower/slab	0	0	0	2	0	0	6

various categories of dwellings (defined by ownership — owner-occupier, privately rented, local-authority owned; by dwelling type; and by age of property — built prior to 1919, in 1919–44, 1945–64 and after 1964). We are therefore concerned about the impact of surveyor inconsistency on the inferences about these population quantities.

We assume that each element of a dwelling has an *ideal assessment* (score), and regard any deviation from this (unknown) score as a misjudgement. The impact of surveyor inconsistency is governed by two factors: the distribution (frequency and extent) of misjudgements and the replacement cost of the elements. Some elements may be more difficult to judge, and so misjudgements of their assessments are more frequent, but the elements involve very disparate costs. For example, repairing some structural defects costs tens of thousands of pounds, whereas replacing the entrance door costs only hundreds of pounds. More expensive elements tend to be assessed with less inconsistency, although this association is far from perfect.

5.4.1 Missing information

We regard surveyor inconsistency as a source of data incompleteness. The data would be complete if the ideal (appropriate) score were available for every element. With MI, we generate sets of plausible scores and conduct the complete-data analysis for each set separately. The differences among these (completed-data) results represent the inflation of the sampling variance due to surveyor inconsistency. When the data are analysed as if they were complete (regarding the surveyors as consistent) the sampling variance is underestimated.

The first step of MI specifies a model for incompleteness. In our setting, the inconsistency is observed on a subsample of dwellings that were surveyed twice. For these dwellings, most of the assessments are in agreement and the majority of the remaining assessments differ by one point of the scale. This motivates the model in which two kinds of deviations from the ideal assessment take place:

- discrepancy — an assessment to a neighbour of the ideal score;
- gross error — a score assigned at random (without any regard for the state of the element).

The probabilities of these two kinds of deviations are denoted by p_d and p_g, respectively. A more complete notation includes the element as another subscript. Throughout, we assume that the probabilities are so small that the majority of assessments coincide with the ideal. In particular, $p_g \ll p_d \ll 1/K$, where K is the number of categories.

Suppose the ideal score for an element with an ordinal categorical assessment is 3. The probability that the recorded (realised) assessment is 2 is $p_d + p_g - p_d p_g$; this is approximately $p_d + p_g$, as both p_d and p_g are small. The probability that the recorded assessment is 4 is the same, but the probability of any other assessment is p_g because it can arise only as a result of a gross error. More generally, suppose category k has L_k neighbours. Then the probability of assessing a dwelling by the ideal category k is

$$\mathrm{P}(X = X^* \mid X^* = k) = 1 - L_k p_d - (K-1)p_g + (K-1)L_k p_d p_g \,. \tag{5.1}$$

(An element may be assigned to the neighbour of the ideal category also as a result of a gross error.) The product term $(K-1)L_k p_d p_g$ can be ignored because p_d and p_g are small.

More complex models can be defined by having different probabilities for each direction of misclassification (assigning higher or lower score), and by defining layers of neighbourhoods. For example, category 1 may be regarded as a 'distant' neighbour of category 3, with probability of misclassification p_{d_2} smaller than for the 'next-door' neighbour 2. As the number of categories is at most 11 (for integers 0–10), and the majority of assessments are zero, such complexity is not warranted.

We assume that misclassifications are independent across the dwellings and across elements within a dwelling. Dependence may arise among the assessments made by a surveyor whose misclassifications tend to be systematic. This is highly unlikely; most misclassifications can be ascribed to inexplicable deviations in the surveyor's judgements, many of them in borderline cases.

We generate plausible ideal scores by the following process. First, the probabilities p_d and p_g are estimated, separately for each element. The assumption of independent misclassifications for the elements is essential for this, so as to make the problem essentially univariate. The probabilities p_d and p_g define the process of misclassification. If the probabilities were known plausible ideal scores would be generated from the conditional distribution $\mathrm{P}(X^* \mid X)$ where, as in the standard notation, X^* denotes the (complete-data) ideal score and X the recorded score. This conditional distribution is derived by the Bayes theorem from $\mathrm{P}(X \mid X^*)$,

$$\mathrm{P}(X^* = k \mid X = h) = \frac{\mathrm{P}(X = h \mid X^* = k)\mathrm{P}(X^* = k)}{\sum_{k'} \mathrm{P}(X = h \mid X^* = k')\mathrm{P}(X^* = k')}\,, \tag{5.2}$$

where each conditional probability is given by (5.1), with p_d and p_g estimated.

5.4.2 Estimating the misclassification probabilities

The first step of MI, model fitting, involves estimating the probabilities p_d and p_g. Assume first that each pair of categories are neighbours and that all misjudgements are discrepancies. This is equivalent to the assumption that there are no discrepancies (or no neighbours) and every misjudgement is a gross error. Then the probability of a disagreement between two surveyors of a dwelling is

$$\begin{aligned} d &= 2(K-1)p_g\{1-(K-1)p_g\} + (K-1)(K-2)p_g^2 \\ &= 2(K-1)p_g - K(K-1)p_g^2\,. \end{aligned} \tag{5.3}$$

This is obtained by considering the two ways how a misjudgement can arise: either one surveyor makes the ideal assessment and the other one does not, or they make different non-ideal assessments. The probability d is estimated by the proportion of the twice-surveyed dwellings that involve disagreements. For example, for 'dwelling type', $\hat{d} = 33/545 = 0.0606$, obtained by adding up the off-diagonal entries in Table 5.7. From $\hat{d}$ we estimate p_g by moment matching, solving the quadratic equation

$$2(K-1)\hat{p}_g - K(K-1)\hat{p}_g^2 \;=\; \hat{d}\,.$$

The solution is

$$\begin{aligned} \hat{p}_g &= \frac{K-1-\sqrt{(K-1)^2 - \hat{d}K(K-1)}}{K(K-1)} \\ &= \frac{1}{K} - \frac{1}{K}\sqrt{1-\hat{d}\frac{K}{K-1}}\,; \end{aligned} \tag{5.4}$$

the other solution is discarded as it exceeds $\frac{1}{K}$. The sampling variance of $\hat{p}_g$ is approximated by the delta method (Taylor expansion). Denote first $c = \sqrt{1-dK/(K-1)}$; equation (5.4) implies that $c = 1 - Kp_g$. We have

$$\begin{aligned} \hat{p}_g &\doteq \frac{1-c}{K} + \frac{\hat{d}-d}{2c(K-1)} \\ &= p_g + \frac{\hat{d}-d}{2c(K-1)}\,, \end{aligned}$$

so the sampling variance is estimated by

$$\widehat{\text{var}}(\hat{p}_g) = \frac{\hat{d}(1-\hat{d})}{4n_2(K-1)^2(1-K\hat{p}_g)^2}, \tag{5.5}$$

where $n_2 = 545$ is the number of twice-surveyed dwellings. The quality of the approximations related to $\hat{p}_g$ and $\widehat{\text{var}}(\hat{p}_g)$ can be assessed straightforwardly by simulations that mimic the assumed process of misclassification. For a given set of n_2 ideal scores and probability p_g, n_2 pairs of assessments are generated, the proportion $\hat{d}$ evaluated and, based on it, the estimate $\hat{p}_g$. This process is replicated 10 000 times, with the same set of ideal values, resulting in a good approximation to the distribution of $\hat{p}_g$. This *empirical* variance is then compared with the *analytical* approximation in (5.5). A typical deviation for a range of examples tested was much smaller than 1%.

Next, suppose there are no gross errors. For a dwelling with ideal score k, the probability of a discrepancy is

$$\begin{aligned} d_k &= 2L_k p_d(1-L_k p_d) + L_k(L_k-1)p_d^2 \\ &= L_k p_d(2-L_k p_d - p_d), \end{aligned}$$

obtained similarly to (5.3). Let w_k be the probability of ideal score k among the twice-surveyed dwellings, and set $M_1 = \sum_k L_k w_k$ and $M_2 = \sum_k L_k^2 w_k$. The probability of a discrepancy is

$$\begin{aligned} d &= \sum_{k=1}^{K} L_k(2-L_k p_d - p_d)p_d w_k \\ &= 2M_1 p_d - (M_1+M_2)p_d^2 . \end{aligned}$$

Hence the moment-matching estimator of p_d is the solution of the quadratic equation

$$(M_1+M_2)p_d^2 - 2M_1 p_d + \hat{d} = 0,$$

which is

$$\hat{p}_d = \frac{M_1 - \sqrt{M_1^2 - \hat{d}(M_1+M_2)}}{M_1+M_2}. \tag{5.6}$$

The Taylor expansion for $\hat{p}_d$ around $\hat{d} = d$ yields the approximation

$$\hat{p}_d \doteq p_d + \frac{\hat{d}-d}{2\{M_1-(M_1+M_2)p_d\}},$$

which implies that

$$\text{var}(\hat{p}_d) \doteq \frac{\text{var}(\hat{d})}{4\{M_1-(M_1+M_2)p_d\}^2}.$$

When both discrepancies and gross errors are possible we estimate the probabilities p_d and p_g as follows. First we consider the cells of the cross-tabulation of the pairs of assessments for the non-neighbouring categories. Disregarding the small probability of different discrepancies committed by both surveyors in a pair, a dwelling can fall into such a cell only by a gross error in at least one of the assessments. We estimate the probability of gross error as in (5.6). The remaining off-diagonal cells contain the dwellings that were assessed with either a discrepancy or a gross error (or both), so we can estimate the total $p_+ = p_d - p_g$ or, more precisely, $p_+ = p_d + p_g - p_d p_g$, by (5.6) applied to the cells that correspond to pairs of neighbouring categories. From the estimators of p_+ and p_g, $\hat{p}_d$ is obtained as their difference. Independence of $\hat{p}_d$ and $\hat{p}_g$ implies that $\mathrm{var}(\hat{p}_d) \doteq \mathrm{var}(\hat{p}_+) - \mathrm{var}(\hat{p}_g)$. The approximation arises because the product $\hat{p}_d \hat{p}_g$ is ignored.

5.4.3 Generating plausible scores

Plausible scores for each element are drawn from their plausible distribution given by the probabilities in (5.2) evaluated for plausible values of p_d and p_g, drawn from their estimated joint sampling distribution. The denominator in (5.2) is more practically evaluated as the unconditional probability $\mathrm{P}(X = k)$. The estimators $\hat{p}_d$ and $\hat{p}_g$ are correlated, but $\hat{p}_g$ and $\hat{p}_+$ are not. It is therefore more practical to draw first plausible probabilities $\tilde{p}_g$ and $\tilde{p}_+$, and then set $\tilde{p}_d = \tilde{p}_+ - \tilde{p}_g$. One set of plausible scores for an element is generated with a fixed pair $(\tilde{p}_d, \tilde{p}_g)$. The sets of plausible scores are based on independent draws of $(\tilde{p}_d, \tilde{p}_g)$ from their estimated joint sampling distribution.

The sampling distributions for distinct elements are assumed to be mutually independent. This assumption is violated, for instance, when discrepancies or gross errors committed on one element are compensated on another element of the same dwelling. A realistic scenario arises when the surveyors may ascribe a particular sub-standard feature of a dwelling to different elements. Identifying such connections is very difficult, and implementing them in an MI procedure would be too complex, especially as such connections may span several elements and the associations among them are uneven. By assuming independence, we are likely to err on the side of greater variation in generating plausible values, so that our assessment of inconsistency is pessimistic, but honesty of our inferences is maintained.

Each surveyor's assessments may depart from the ideal scores in a systematic way. For instance, some surveyors may tend to err on the side of greater disrepair in general, or specifically for some types of elements, may prefer assessing higher scores for some elements at the expense of others, or may have different tendencies for the various types of dwellings. Such deviations are difficult to evaluate because each surveyor assesses a relatively small number of dwellings. Also, the assignment of surveyors to dwellings cannot be completely randomised, so that the level of scores awarded is partially confounded with the underlying level of disrepair. The method of generating plausible scores ignores these issues.

A precursor to most analyses is the calculation of the sets of plausible values of CRC and VRC. With the sets of plausible costs, each planned (complete-data) analysis is applied to every set of plausible scores and the results are averaged for each target, with an inflation for the sampling variance by the between-imputation term $(1 + 1/M)\hat{B}$. This term informs about the (undesirable) impact of surveyor inconsistency on the precision of the estimator.

A more detailed exploration of this impact aims to identify individual elements that make large contributions to it. To isolate the impact of the inconsistency for a single element, we compare the MI estimates of the sampling variances for a selected set of analyses under two conditions. Under condition A, plausible scores are used for each element and under condition B, the recorded scores are used for the selected element and the plausible scores for the other elements. In other words, in condition B we pretend that the selected element is assessed consistently. The (appropriate) sampling variance under condition A is greater than under B. The difference is a measure of the information lost because of inconsistent assessment of the selected element.

Carrying out such comparisons systematically is not practical; elements that either have a high probability of discrepancies and gross errors or are associated with high disrepair costs should be the first candidates for such an exploration. The exploration can be applied to a group of elements, by pretending in condition B that each element of the group is assessed consistently, but then the impact is not evaluated for either of the elements in the group. The purpose of such an evaluation may be to find areas in the training and instruction of the surveyors that have to be reviewed or emphasised.

For a routine analysis, $M = 5$ sets of plausible scores are sufficient, but for studying the impact of surveyor inconsistency on the precision, a larger M is necessary because the between-imputation variance B has to be estimated with greater precision.

5.5 Suggested reading. Software

The sections of this chapter are adapted from [164] (Section 5.1), [166] (Section 5.2), [159] (Section 5.3) and an unpublished report (Section 5.4), where further details can be found. `Splus`, [279] and R, [215], were used for all the computing. Although it requires more programming than software packages with modules designed for specific tasks, an advantage of this approach is the customisation for the specific problem and the integration of the functions for multiple imputation with the other data processing, statistical computing and graphical displays.

Software written by other parties can save a lot of programming effort and the analyst may benefit from the software author's expertise and experience that may be enhanced by feedback from other users. A suite of `Splus` functions based on [243] is available from the author's website at `www.stat.psu.edu`.

The functions cater for multiple imputation in multivariate normally distributed data (NORM), in multivariate categorical data (CAT), in data that contain both continuous (normally distributed) and categorical data (MIX) and in normally distributed panel and clustered data (PAN). The performance of these routines is improved by programming the computationally most demanding elements in Fortran.

`Solas`™ (`www.statsol.ie/solas`) is a software package dedicated to multiple imputation. It implements MI based on linear regression and propensity scoring, as well as several single-imputation methods such as LOCF and hot deck. It has a limited capacity for complete-data analyses, but the most commonly used methods are implemented as options. A script language enables programming and reliable replication of procedures as well as development of complex procedures.

`IVEware` (`www.isr.unich.edu/src/smp/ive`) comprises a collection of `SAS` macros for single and multiple imputation described in [218]. In the imputation, carried out for a variable at a time, various constraints can be implemented to conform with the a priori specified associations among the variables. The software has a limited selection of complete-data analyses, but they take account of the sampling design (sampling weights, clustering and stratification).

The software `MICE` (`web.inter.nl.net/users/S.van.Buuren/mi`) implements the method of chained equations. It caters for a wide range of models for nonresponse and complete-data methods. It is written in `Splus/R`, and allows users to supply their own programs (functions) for the steps of MI.

These software packages implement Bayesian methods, but this feature is not 'visible' to the analyst and has no impact on how they are used in complete-data analyses. The original development of MI, described in [233], is also formulated in a Bayesian framework. Thus, the model for nonresponse is specified with prior distributions for the unknown parameters and the plausible values are drawn from the (estimated) joint posterior distribution of the missing values given the observed data, including auxiliary information, and the posited models for nonresponse.

`SPSS` and `SAS` have procedures for some of the tasks in MI, for instance, for repeated imputation and averaging of the completed-data results. See [109] for a comprehensive review.

Reference [77] is a comprehensive text on modern Bayesian analysis. Drawing samples from conditional distribution by efficient routine is an important prerequisite for Bayesian computing. `BUGS` (`www.mrc-bsu.can.ac.uk/bugs` and [84]) is a popular software for Bayesian computing. Its core is an efficient implementation of the Markov chain Monte Carlo (MCMC) method. It is accompanied by modules for specific applications and for the convergence diagnostics in MCMC.

Part II

Small-area estimation

6

Introduction

Small is beautiful. Like my country.

Small-area statistics encompasses a wide variety of methods for making inferences about geographical and other sub-domains of the survey domain. An often quoted example is the estimation of the means of a variable in each district of a country. The sampling design of a typical national survey aims to ensure that inferences can be made with sufficient precision for the domain, and possibly for a few large sub-domains, such as the country's regions. Prescribing the sample sizes for each of several hundred *small areas* (districts) is rarely feasible. In an ideal arrangement, the subsample size within each district would be adequate for making the desired inferences with a prescribed precision. Such inferences would be based solely on the observed values of the variable in question (the *target* variable) in the district. In many settings, this would require an overall (national) sample size well beyond what can be afforded. This part of the book deals with methods for small-area estimation, which address this problem by drawing on information from outside the district, from the values of other variables in the district, and from outside the survey.

The key idea developed can be described as *exploiting similarity*. In its simplest form, with the task of estimating the district-level population mean of a variable recorded in the survey, we exploit the fact that the district-level means are similar. If the means were identical an efficient estimator of the national population mean would also be efficient for every district, because the two targets coincide. When the areas differ insubstantially, the national mean may still be competitive as an estimator for the district; it may be preferable to incur the bias arising from the difference between the district and the nation as a whole. When the national sample size is much greater than the subsample size for the area the bias may be richly compensated by a radical reduction of the sampling variance.

The first step in this approach is to establish how similar the districts are, or whether they are similar enough. This task is not straightforward when most districts are only sparsely represented in the survey. The sample means of the districts vary because so do the underlying quantities, the district-level subpopulation means, *and* because of the vagaries of the sampling process. The sample means would vary even if the subpopulation means were identical. We will summarise the district-level differences by the variance of the district-level subpopulation means, and estimate this summary as the variation of the district-level sample means that is in excess of the sampling variation. Variation is the opposite of similarity. Small variation (of districts) corresponds to great similarity.

Having estimated the level of similarity of the districts, we might decide whether to estimate the district-level subpopulation mean by the national or the district-level sample mean. This would not yield very good results. Given a certain level of similarity, the national mean may be quite efficient for a district with a small subsample size, but far less efficient than the sample mean for a district with a substantial subsample size. Thus, an obvious improvement is to use the national mean for the 'small' districts and the district-level subsample mean for the 'large' districts, with a suitable classification of the districts to small and large ones.

The next refinement abandons the inflexible dichotomy of district-level versus national sample mean. Instead of choosing one of them, the two means are combined (linearly) so as to estimate the district-level population mean as efficiently as possible. It is essential to allow the combination to be specific to each district. For a district that is not represented in the survey, we have no choice but to rely solely on the national mean. In contrast, for a district that is represented in the survey by a large sample size, it may be hard to improve on the district-level subsample mean; the national mean is (almost) redundant for estimation of the district's subpopulation mean.

This theme is developed further to take advantage of the similarity of variables (their area-level means), subpopulations, surveys and other data sources (registers and censuses in particular), and small changes from one time point (year) to another. We aim to satisfy the standard formulated in Part I — making the best use of the information in our possession, irrespective of its source or format.

The general method is related to a more traditional model-based approach in which we specify an hierarchical model that enables *borrowing strength* across the districts. This concept is related to exploiting similarity. The modelling approach is quite powerful, but its weakness is that the results it yields are contingent on the validity of the model. So, the methods offer more caveats than confidence when the model applied is found wanting in one aspect or another. And, even if no deficiency of the model is identified, the concern about the appropriateness of the model is not allayed because our model criticism may have been not thorough enough. We cannot afford to return to the subjects of the survey and ask them for more information if the model based on the data they have provided is inadequate. It is also desirable to bypass other model assumptions, such as normality. Failure to identify a suitable distribution for the data is not a good reason for not estimating the specified targets, or for estimating them without any input from the auxiliary information that has been found less than ideal.

Most large-scale (national) surveys are very expensive enterprises, requiring an extensive infrastructure involving business considerations (income from clients and secure long-term funding), public relations, questionnaire design, sampling design, information about the surveyed population, training and instruction of interviewers, coding and data management, and the like. Conducting a single survey is not as profitable, both from the economic and information points of view, because much of the infrastructure would be assembled for a single use; it could not be reused for a different survey without a substantial adaptation. Subcontractors who contribute to the infrastructure are keener to participate, and do so on more favourable terms, if their services are likely to be required regularly. Furthermore, the analysis of a survey in its isolation is often of limited value because the scales used, methods applied and conventions adopted may be unfamiliar to the clients and other survey users. The results from the analyses become more meaningful and easier to interpret when compared with the results from the same survey conducted in the recent past or from a similar survey conducted in a different population (country). Being a substantial enterprise, the survey entails a process of learning and continual improvement and gradual accumulation of experience. Next time, some of the operational glitches would be ironed out and difficulties resolved much more effectively. Higher quality is thus achieved, not necessarily with a greater effort or expenditure. In fact, some surveys have trials — small-scale rehearsals that aim to identify difficulties in the operation and deficiencies in the planning. Inferences may also be more efficient, even without any change in the sampling design and sample size, if the information collected in the past surveys can be effectively exploited for inferences about the current population.

In brief, it takes a few repeats before a survey approaches its full potential in terms of the quality of its operation, familiarity of all the parties with its procedures, analyses, conventions, reporting formats and scales used. As the clientele, and the public at large, get acquainted with the contribution of the survey to the overall information about the specific aspects of the society, economy, public services, environment, and the like, and find them relevant, asking for more detail is a natural reaction.

For example, the unemployment rate has been a familiar headline figure in the U.S. and European national media for several decades. Both laymen and experts have a relatively good understanding of the figures and how they reflect the state of the country's economy. There is a general agreement that unemployment in the UK in 2003, when there were fewer than one million unemployed (counted according to a specific definition), was a problem on a scale very different from the early 1980's when there were around three million unemployed, in a labour force of about 26.5 million, slightly smaller than in 2003 (around 28.5 million). The unemployment rate, around 3.25% in 2003, is probably a more familiar figure (compared with over 10% in the early 1980's). Comparisons with the UK's leading trading partners and competitors (U.S.A., Japan, Germany and France), both in the rates and in the changes of the rates over time, add further meaning and importance to the figures. They do so *today* because of a decades-long record of collecting related statistics, extensive research establishing their validity, and a high level of standardisation of the processes that yield the end-product — the estimate of the unemployment rate.

The national unemployment rate, or a similar economic indicator, is a rather simplified summary for the country. It hides the unequal unemployment rates in the regions and districts. The steady reduction in the rate of unemployment over several years may suggest that the rate, or its change, have been uniform across the country; the areas with the highest unemployment rate have remained as such, despite a reduction in the levels. But this need not be the case; the impact of the underlying processes may be uneven in the country's districts. In the today's environment, with insatiable appetite for information, it is a natural progression to ask for more detail:

What are the rates of unemployment in the country's districts?

Similar processes may be at play with other key social and economic indicators. As more and more surveys acquire a history of regular conduct, the procedures they employ are standardised and the dissemination of their products in both professional and lay communities becomes more effective, their profiles become more prominent, their data is more widely distributed and analysed, and the demand for more detailed analyses strengthens.

The analyses of the 'geographical' detail are referred to as small-area estimation. In this part, we develop methods for small-area estimation, formulate general principles underlying them, and then discuss applications of these principles outside the confines of the geographical detail; first in survey analysis, and then in Part III in statistical modelling in general.

6.1 Preliminaries

Suppose the domain of a survey, such as a country, comprises districts (small areas) $d = 1, \ldots, D$. The districts cover the whole country, but they do not overlap. The collection of these districts forms a *partition* of the country. It is also referred to as a *division* of the country. We say that one division, into districts, is *finer* than another, into regions, if each district is subsumed in a region and at least one region contains several districts. The converse of finer is *coarser*; in the quoted example, the division into regions is coarser than the division into districts.

The survey collects the values of a variable y on a sample of subjects drawn according to a specified sampling design that may have been informed by the division. For instance, the strata may be collections of (contiguous) districts, or the clusters may coincide with the districts. In other settings, the small areas may not be known to the survey designers, or the various parties may wish to estimate summaries for different partitions of the country.

The sampling design, together with the anticipated level of response, usually ensures that the key inferences for the country and its few large subdomains, such as regions, are sufficiently precise. We assume that similar arrangements for all the districts are not feasible; the districts differ in their population sizes, and some districts may even end up not being represented in the survey at all. (Each one of them might be represented in a replication of the survey.)

The vector of values of the variable of interest in the studied population is denoted by $\mathbf{Y}$. Let the survey data on this variable be $\mathbf{y}$, and let $\hat{\theta} = \hat{\theta}(\mathbf{y})$ be an estimator of the parameter of interest θ. In most practical settings, θ is the population total or mean of the variable, or the proportion of subjects with a specific set of values of the variable. The estimator $\hat{\theta}$ depends, apart from $\mathbf{y}$, also on the sampling design π. For district d, we define θ_d as the same summary as θ, but applied to the district; $\theta_d = \theta(\mathbf{Y}_d)$, where $\mathbf{Y}_d$ is the sub-vector of $\mathbf{Y}$ for the population in district d. The obvious way to derive an estimator of θ_d is to apply $\hat{\theta}$ on the variable that coincides with $\mathbf{y}$ in district d but vanishes outside d. This estimator is $\hat{\theta}_d = \hat{\theta}(I_d\mathbf{y})$, where I_d is the indicator of the district d: $I_d(j) = 1$ if subject j belongs to the district, and $I_d(j) = 0$ otherwise. Note that an adjustment for sample size has to be made when θ is a mean.

We assume that $\hat{\theta}$ is an unbiased estimator of θ for any population vector $\mathbf{Y}$, but do not assume that it has any specific form or that the values of $\mathbf{Y}$ satisfy some condition that would not be satisfied by its sub-vector $\mathbf{Y}_d$ for district d. Then $\hat{\theta}_d$ is unbiased for θ_d for any district d. We refer to $\hat{\theta}_d$ as a *direct* estimator derived from $\hat{\theta}$. When based, in effect, on a small sample of size n_d, the absence of bias is of little value. The large sampling variance $\mathrm{var}(\hat{\theta}_d)$ diminishes the usefulness of $\hat{\theta}_d$. The 'national' estimator $\hat{\theta}$, or its suitable adjustment for the population size, has a much smaller variance, but is biased for θ_d. No adjustment is necessary if θ is a mean or a proportion, and the adjustment for a total is by a reference to the mean.

If we knew that the country's districts are homogeneous (have identical values of θ_d or of its adjustment), $\hat{\theta}$ would have no competitor for estimating θ_d because it would be unbiased and have a small variance. If the districts are extremely heterogeneous (have vastly different values of θ_d), $\hat{\theta}$ conveys little information about θ_d because the differences $\theta_d - \theta$ are widely dispersed. If we estimated θ_d by $\hat{\theta}$ we would risk a large bias. For some districts we may be lucky, when $|\,\theta_d - \theta\,|$ is small, for others $\hat{\theta}$ would be very inefficient, burdened by the squared bias $(\theta_d - \theta)^2$.

In this discussion, the dispersion of the district-level quantities θ_d plays a central role. Since in many other contexts we measure dispersion by variance, we denote by σ_{B}^2 the finite-sample variance of the (unknown) district-level quantities θ_d:

$$\sigma_{\mathrm{B}}^2 = \frac{1}{N_2} \sum_{d=1}^{D} (\theta_d - \theta)^2 . \qquad (6.1)$$

Throughout, we will use the notation E, var and cov for expectation, variance and covariance, respectively, with reference to hypothetical replications of the sampling process. It will be useful to consider the same moments also for averaging over the districts. To avoid any confusion, we use the subscript $\mathcal{D}$ with E, var and cov to indicate the reference to the districts. Thus, (6.1) can be written compactly as

$$\sigma_{\mathrm{B}}^2 = \mathrm{var}_{\mathcal{D}}(\theta_{\mathcal{D}}) . \qquad (6.2)$$

The symbol $\mathcal{D}$ in the argument of θ indicates that the variance is applied to the districts' values of θ. Note that there is a slight inconsistency between (6.1) and (6.2). The sum of squares in the variance should be centred around $\mathrm{E}_{\mathcal{D}}(\theta_{\mathcal{D}})$, the mean of the district-level values of θ_d. This in general does not coincide with the national value θ. When $\theta = \theta(\mathbf{Y})$ is a linear function of $\mathbf{Y}$ and the districts have identical population sizes, θ and $\mathrm{E}_{\mathcal{D}}(\theta_{\mathcal{D}})$ coincide. But it is easy to construct realistic examples in which θ and $\mathrm{E}_{\mathcal{D}}(\theta_{\mathcal{D}})$ differ substantially. For illustration, suppose θ is a population mean and the values of θ_d are greater in a few districts that have subpopulation sizes much greater than the rest of the districts. Then $\theta > \mathrm{E}_{\mathcal{D}}(\theta_{\mathcal{D}})$ because more populous districts contribute to θ by more values than less populous districts, whereas in $\mathrm{E}_{\mathcal{D}}(\theta_{\mathcal{D}})$ each district is equally important, irrespective of its population size.

We will use the definition in (6.2) throughout. The 'variance' σ_{B}^2 in (6.1) is at least as large as its counterpart in (6.2). In several applications, we will estimate σ_{B}^2 and will prefer positive bias because the consequences of underestimating σ_{B}^2 will be more serious. One device for doing so will be estimating (6.1) without bias and using the estimate as a substitute for (6.2).

The mean squared error (MSE) of an estimator $\hat{\theta}$ aimed at the target θ is defined as

$$\mathrm{MSE}(\hat{\theta};\theta) = \mathrm{E}\left\{(\hat{\theta} - \theta)^2\right\} .$$

The argument θ in MSE is essential because $\hat{\theta}$ can be also used for estimating θ_d; clearly, $\mathrm{MSE}(\hat{\theta};\theta) \neq \mathrm{MSE}(\hat{\theta};\theta_d)$, unless $\theta_d = \theta$. The bias of an estimator $\hat{\theta}$ of θ is denoted by $\mathrm{B}(\hat{\theta};\theta)$. Just like for MSE, the argument θ is essential; we will omit it only when its identity is obvious from the context. We have

$$\mathrm{MSE}(\hat{\theta};\theta) = \mathrm{var}(\hat{\theta}) + \{\mathrm{B}(\hat{\theta};\theta)\}^2 . \qquad (6.3)$$

This implies that σ_{B}^2 in (6.1) exceeds its counterpart in (6.2) by the squared difference $\{\theta - \mathrm{E}_{\mathcal{D}}(\theta_{\mathcal{D}})\}^2$.

We regard MSE as the measure of efficiency. That is, we prefer estimators with smaller MSE. However, MSE is usually not known and has to be estimated; its value may depend on one or several parameters, sometimes even on the target itself. An estimator may be efficient for some values of the parameters but not for others. All this makes the search for the most efficient estimator challenging.

6.2 Choosing the estimator

So far, we have identified two candidates for estimating the summary θ_d for district d: the direct estimator $\hat{\theta}_d$ and the national estimator $\hat{\theta}$. Let their sampling variances be $v_d = \mathrm{var}(\hat{\theta}_d)$ and $v = \mathrm{var}(\hat{\theta})$. We assume that $v_d \gg v$; otherwise the direct estimator would be adequate, given a sampling design suitable for estimating θ. The (sampling) covariance of $\hat{\theta}$ and $\hat{\theta}_d$ is denoted by c_d; usually $c_d > 0$, as the subsample of subjects from district d contributes to both $\hat{\theta}_d$ and $\hat{\theta}$.

In this section, we discuss ways of selecting between the two estimators. The two methods described, although adhering to established approaches of model-based estimation, are poorly suited for small-area estimation, but it is important to discuss why that is so. For simplicity, we set aside the context of survey sampling, and consider the special case when θ is a population mean, so that our problem closely resembles the analysis of variance (ANOVA), with the D districts as the groups.

6.2.1 Uniform choice

If σ_B^2 is very small we should estimate each θ_d by $\hat{\theta}$. If σ_B^2 is very large $\hat{\theta}_d$ is preferred. What to do in intermediate situations when σ_B^2 is neither very small nor very large? The standard textbook treatment proposes to form the ANOVA table, and test the hypothesis that the groups are homogeneous $(\theta_1 = \ldots = \theta_D)$, that is, $\sigma_\mathrm{B}^2 = 0$, and then act upon the conclusion of the test.

If the null-hypothesis is rejected we use the direct estimator $\hat{\theta}_d$ for each district d. Otherwise we use the national estimator $\hat{\theta}$ for each district. Although this is a deeply ingrained practice in statistics, there is little good to say about it. First, $\hat{\theta}$ may be more efficient for θ_d even when $\sigma_\mathrm{B}^2 > 0$. Next, when the null-hypothesis is not rejected we have no evidence that $\sigma_\mathrm{B}^2 = 0$, so we should not act as if the null-hypothesis held true. Further, if the null-hypothesis is rejected we reach an impasse for districts that are not represented in the sample. But the direct estimators $\hat{\theta}_d$ for sparsely represented districts (small n_d) are also worthless. On the other hand, when the null-hypothesis is not rejected, the national estimator is imposed even on some districts with large subsample sizes, for which the direct estimator would have been adequate.

And finally, the decision made by hypothesis testing is not correct with certainty. This is an inherent limitation of the hypothesis testing as a method. Alternative methods for choosing between the two models may be superior (e.g., the Akaike information criterion, AIC), but they do not resolve the strategic mistake made — committing ourselves to the 'winner', $\hat{\theta}_d$ or $\hat{\theta}$, for every one of the D districts. The model selection is not sensitive to the subsequent use of the decision based on it.

With an inappropriate choice of $\hat{\theta}$ we risk bias and with an inappropriate choice of $\hat{\theta}_d$ we fail to take advantage of useful information from outside the district. We should weigh the potential gains and losses in achieving our objective of efficient estimation for every district; the hypothesis test, or more generally, model selection, is oblivious to this objective. This theme is developed fully in Chapter 11. For the time being, and with a specific reference to small-area estimation, we conclude that the solution by choosing an estimator (direct or national) is far from optimal.

6.2.2 Tailored choice

The alternative estimators have MSEs $\mathrm{var}(\hat{\theta}_d) = v_d$ and $\mathrm{MSE}(\hat{\theta}; \theta_d) = v + (\theta_d - \theta)^2$. With simple random sampling within the district, v_d is a decreasing function of the sample size n_d; $v_d = \sigma^2_{\mathrm{W}}/n_d$, where σ^2_{W} is the within-district variance. When v_d is very large (because n_d is very small), the advantage of the variance reduction, from v_d to v, may outweigh the bias $\theta_d - \theta$. When the variance reduction $v_d - v$ is more modest, incurring the bias may not be worth it. In other words, for districts with large enough n_d the direct estimator is sufficient, whereas for districts with small n_d we should resort to the national estimator. To implement this, we select a threshold sample size n_*, use $\hat{\theta}$ for each district that has sample size $n_d \le n_*$, and use $\hat{\theta}_d$ otherwise.

Ideally, $\hat{\theta}$ should be chosen when $\mathrm{MSE}(\hat{\theta}; \theta_d) < \mathrm{var}(\hat{\theta}_d)$, that is, when

$$v + (\theta_d - \theta)^2 \;<\; v_d \,.$$

We do not know the bias $\theta_d - \theta$ and, for most districts, we are unable to estimate it with any precision. We sacrifice a bit of the ideal of minimum-MSE estimation by replacing the squared bias $(\theta_d - \theta)^2$ with its district-level expectation σ^2_{B}. Thus, we choose $\hat{\theta}$ when $v_d > v + \sigma^2_{\mathrm{B}}$, and $\hat{\theta}_d$ otherwise. The threshold sample size is then

$$n_* \;=\; \frac{\sigma^2_{\mathrm{W}}}{v + \sigma^2_{\mathrm{B}}} \,.$$

Note that the variances σ^2_{W}, σ^2_{B} and v have to be estimated. However, they are quantities related to the survey domain, and so are estimated with much greater precision than any district-specific quantities, such as the squared bias $(\theta_d - \theta)^2$. On the one hand, it is not practical to assume that each district has a distinct value of σ^2_{W}; on the other hand, the assumption of a common value of σ^2_{W} may not be realistic. A suitable compromise may be the assumption that σ^2_{W} is constant within each of a small number of regions or groups of districts defined by their attributes (such as urbanity, population size or presence of a particular feature).

The MSE of $\hat{\theta}$ involves the squared deviation $(\theta_d - \theta)^2$, which is also the squared bias $\mathrm{B}^2(\hat{\theta}; \theta_d)$; the sampling variance v is usually of smaller order of magnitude. When $n_d > 0$, the bias $B_d = \mathrm{B}(\hat{\theta}; \theta_d) = \theta - \theta_d$ is estimated (without bias) by $\hat{B}_d = \hat{\theta} - \hat{\theta}_d$. However, $\hat{B}_d^2$ is biased for B_d^2. In fact,

$$\mathrm{E}(\hat{B}_d^2) = B_d^2 + v + v_d - 2c_d \,,$$

so the bias sought is $\mathrm{B}(\hat{B}_d^2;\, B_d^2) = v + v_d - 2c_d$. When $v_d \gg v$, this is approximately v_d. The unbiased estimator $\hat{B}_d^2 - \hat{v} - \hat{v}_d + 2\hat{c}_d$ (or $\hat{B}_d^2 - \hat{v}_d$, which is approximately unbiased) attains negative values with positive probability. If its values are truncated at zero, the unbiasedness is surrendered. However, unbiased estimators of v, σ_B^2 and σ_W^2 would not result in an unbiased (or efficient) estimator of the threshold n_*.

Estimation of σ_B^2 is dealt with in Section 6.4, after we further enhance its role as a key quantity in small-area estimation.

6.3 Composition

In the previous section, we considered two estimators, $\hat{\theta}_d$ and $\hat{\theta}$. The tailored choice, although somewhat more complex than the uniform choice, appears to be superior. For districts with sample sizes near the threshold n_*, we have a strange anomaly. If one or a few observations were removed or added to the subsample for such a district, the estimate might be changed radically because the many observations from outside the district would be either discarded or involved in estimating θ_d.

We resolve this anomaly by considering the linear combinations

$$\hat{\theta}_d^\mathrm{C} = (1 - b)\hat{\theta}_d + b\hat{\theta} \,, \tag{6.4}$$

in which we would choose, in ideal circumstances, the coefficient b so as to minimise $\mathrm{MSE}(\hat{\theta}_d^\mathrm{C};\, \theta_d)$. This could be accomplished if we knew v, v_d and c_d. We find the optimal coefficient b, as a function of these (co-)variances, and then make provisions for the practical setting in which only $\mathbf{y}$ and the district identification of the observations are available. Estimators constructed as linear (or, more precisely, convex) combinations of other estimators, as in (6.4), are called *composite* estimators.

We allow the coefficient b to be specific to the district. After all, the minimum MSE is bound to depend on v_d and c_d, which differ from district to district. To indicate that $\hat{\theta}_d^\mathrm{C}$ depends on b, we write $\hat{\theta}_d^\mathrm{C}(b)$. Later we will consider estimators of the optimal value of b, and so the argument of $\hat{\theta}_d^\mathrm{C}$ will be a random variable.

The MSE of $\hat{\theta}_d^\mathrm{C}(b)$ is

$$\mathrm{MSE}\left\{\hat{\theta}_d^\mathrm{C}(b); \theta_d\right\} = (1-b)^2 v_d + 2b(1-b)c_d + b^2(v + B_d^2)$$

$$= v_d - 2b(v_d - c_d) + b^2(v_d + v - 2c_d + B_d^2)$$
$$= R_{0,d} - 2bR_{1,d} + b^2 R_{2,d} \,. \tag{6.5}$$

This is a quadratic function with a positive quadratic coefficient, $R_{2,d} = v_d + v - 2c_d + B_d^2 = \mathrm{E}\{(\hat{\theta}_d - \hat{\theta})^2\}$, and so it has a unique minimum. The minimum is attained at

$$b_d^* = \frac{R_{1,d}}{R_{2,d}} = \frac{v_d - c_d}{v_d + v - 2c_d + B_d^2} \,, \tag{6.6}$$

and the minimum attained is

$$\begin{aligned} \mathrm{MSE}\left\{\hat{\theta}_d^{\mathrm{C}}(b_d^*)\right\} &= R_{0,d} - \frac{R_{1,d}^2}{R_{2,d}} = v_d - \frac{(v_d - c_d)^2}{v_d + v - 2c_d + B_d^2} \\ &= v + B_d^2 - \frac{(v + B_d^2 - c_d)^2}{v_d + v - 2c_d + B_d^2} \,. \end{aligned} \tag{6.7}$$

Two (artificial) examples of the MSE given by (6.5) are drawn in Figure 6.1. In the left-hand panel, MSE attains the minimum of 0.12 at $b^* = 0.35$ and in the right-hand panel, the minimum of 0.20 is attained at $b^* = 0.75$. In the left-hand panel, the direct estimator is more efficient than the national estimator; $\mathrm{MSE}(\hat{\theta}_d) = 0.24$ and $\mathrm{MSE}(\hat{\theta}) = 0.54$. In the right-hand panel, the direct estimator is less efficient; $\mathrm{MSE}(\hat{\theta}_d) = 0.76$ and $\mathrm{MSE}(\hat{\theta}) = 0.26$. In both cases, either estimator $\hat{\theta}_d$ and $\hat{\theta}$ can be improved by moving b, however slightly, from its extreme value, (0 for $\hat{\theta}_d$ and 1 for $\hat{\theta}$) toward $\frac{1}{2}$. This corresponds to combining $\hat{\theta}_d$ with $\hat{\theta}$ with a small weight assigned to $\hat{\theta}$ or $\hat{\theta}_d$.

Since $v_d > v$, necessarily $v_d > c_d$, and so $b_d^* > 0$. The variance v and covariance c_d are usually much smaller than v_d. Then

$$b_d^* \doteq \frac{v_d}{v_d + B_d^2} \,.$$

Thus $b_d^* < 1$, unless the squared bias, B_d^2, is negligible. Note that $B_d = 0$ when $\theta_d = \theta$; estimating θ_d by $\hat{\theta}_d^{\mathrm{C}}(1) = \hat{\theta}$ is then a sound proposition. For $b = 1$, we discard $\hat{\theta}_d$ completely. However, the data from district d still contributes to $\hat{\theta}$, although it is not any more important than the data from any other district. This contradicts any reasonable intuition when $n_d > 0$. When the district is not represented in the sample, $b = 1$ is a reasonable choice. This avoids the involvement of $\hat{\theta}_d$ which is not defined, or could formally be defined as having infinite variance.

If $b = 0$, we would rely on data from district d entirely; $\hat{\theta}_d^{\mathrm{C}}(0) = \hat{\theta}_d$. The composite estimator $\hat{\theta}_d^{\mathrm{C}}$ can be interpreted as a *shrinkage estimator*, as it moves all the direct estimators $\hat{\theta}_d$ toward the national estimator $\hat{\theta}$:

$$\hat{\theta}_d^{\mathrm{C}}(b_d^*) = \hat{\theta} + (1 - b_d^*)(\hat{\theta}_d - \hat{\theta}) \,.$$

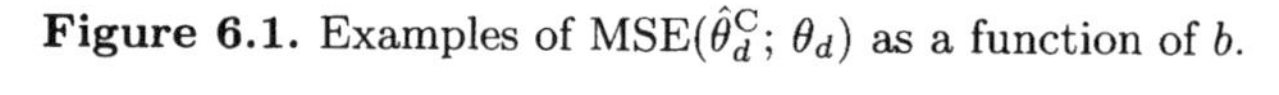

Figure 6.1. Examples of MSE$(\hat{\theta}_d^{\mathrm{C}};\,\theta_d)$ as a function of b.

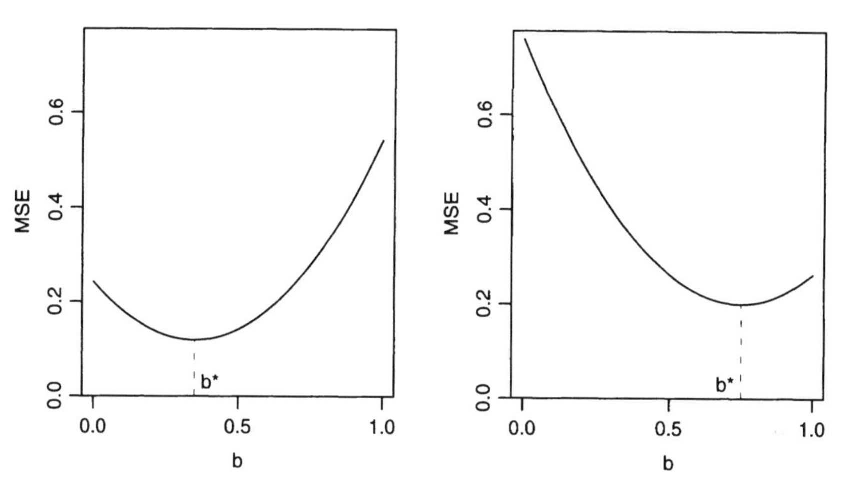

The shrinkage, controlled by the (shrinkage) coefficient b_d^*, is stronger for districts with greater v_d (typically, the districts with smaller subsample sizes n_d), which need more 'assistance' with estimation of their θ_d. The gain in precision (the reduction of MSE) of the composite estimator over the direct estimator is also an increasing function of v_d, if the covariance c_d can be ignored. This is the case not only for the differences $v_d - \mathrm{MSE}(\hat{\theta}_d^{\mathrm{C}}\,;\theta_d)$; see (6.7), but also for the ratios $v_d/\mathrm{MSE}(\hat{\theta}_d^{\mathrm{C}}\,;\theta_d)$. By construction, $\hat{\theta}_d^{\mathrm{C}}(b_d^*)$ would be more efficient than both $\hat{\theta}_d$ and $\hat{\theta}$ because these estimators are specific (extreme) choices in (6.4). This is also illustrated in Figure 6.1. By restricting our choice to $\hat{\theta}_d$ and $\hat{\theta}$, we set our eyes merely on matching the more efficient of them.

A formidable obstacle to realising the full potential of the composite estimator $\hat{\theta}_d^{\mathrm{C}}$ is that the quantities required for evaluating b_d^* are not known. The squared bias B_d^2 is particularly problematic because it involves our target θ_d. We resolve this problem by replacing B_d^2 with its expectation over the districts, $\sigma_{\mathrm{B}}^2 = \mathrm{E}_{\mathcal{D}}(B_{\mathcal{D}}^2)$. Introducing σ_{B}^2 does not solve all the problems; σ_{B}^2 also has to be estimated. However, it is estimated with much greater precision because it is a domain-related quantity — the entire sample $\mathbf{y}$ will contribute to its estimation. Estimation of σ_{B}^2 is dealt with in Section 6.4.

By replacing B_d^2 with σ_{B}^2, that is, by replacing b_d^* in (6.6) with

$$b_d = \frac{v_d - c_d}{v_d + v - 2c_d + \sigma_{\mathrm{B}}^2}\,, \tag{6.8}$$

we have reduced the standard to which we aspire. The minimum MSE given in (6.7) is not attained with $\hat{\theta}_d^{\mathrm{C}}(b_d)$, even in the unrealistic setting when σ_{B}^2 is known.

The coefficient b_d minimises the *expected* MSE (eMSE) of $\hat{\theta}_d^{\mathrm{C}}$; eMSE is defined as the district-level expectation of the MSE:

$$\mathrm{eMSE}(\hat{\theta}_d^{\mathrm{C}};\, \theta_d) \;=\; \mathrm{E}_{\mathcal{D}} \left\{ \mathrm{MSE}(\hat{\theta}_d^{\mathrm{C}};\, \theta_d) \right\} .$$

The minimum eMSE is

$$\mathrm{eMSE} \left\{ \hat{\theta}_d^{\mathrm{C}}(b_d);\, \theta_d \right\} \;=\; v_d - \frac{(v_d - c_d)^2}{v_d + v - 2c_d + \sigma_{\mathrm{B}}^2} \,; \qquad (6.9)$$

it is a decreasing function of σ_{B}^2. Thus, *on average*, similarity is conducive to improvement in the precision of the composite estimator over the direct estimator. Note that in the district-level expectation we regard v_d and c_d as fixed, and average only over θ_d. This is closely related to assuming that the subsample sizes n_d are fixed. In practice, they rarely are, but many other methods in survey analysis also condition on the sample size.

The expression $\mathrm{var}(\hat{\mu}_d - \hat{\mu}) \;=\; v_d + v - 2c_d$ in the formulae for b_d^* and b_d may at first sight be avoided by considering combinations of $\hat{\mu}_d$ and the estimator of the population mean for the country with district d removed. The attraction of this is that these two estimators are in most sampling designs independent. When independent, they can be combined more easily, as the coefficients in their composition are proportional to their precisions.

We show that this approach also yields the composite estimator $\hat{\theta}_d^{\mathrm{C}}$. Suppose $\hat{\mu}$ is a combination of $\hat{\mu}_d$,

$$\hat{\mu} \;=\; \frac{1}{u_+} \sum_{d'=1}^{D} u_{d'} \hat{\mu}_{d'} \,,$$

for some positive weights $u_{d'}$ with total $u_+ = u_1 + \cdots + u_D$, and define

$$\hat{\mu}_{-d} \;=\; \frac{1}{u_+ - u_d} \sum_{d' \neq d} u_{d'} \hat{\mu}_{d'} \,.$$

We can express the composition of $\hat{\mu}_d$ and $\hat{\mu}$ as

$$(1 - b_d)\hat{\mu}_d + b_d\hat{\mu} \;=\; \left\{ 1 - b_d \left(1 - \frac{u_d}{u_+} \right) \right\} \hat{\mu}_d + b_d\, \hat{\mu}_{-d} \left(1 - \frac{u_d}{u_+} \right) , \qquad (6.10)$$

so that it corresponds to composition of $\hat{\mu}_d$ and $\hat{\mu}_{-d}$ with shrinkage coefficient $b_d(1 - u_d/u_+)$.

The bias of $\hat{\mu}_{-d}$ in estimating μ_d is

$$\mathrm{B}(\hat{\mu}_{-d}\,;\mu_d) \;=\; \frac{u_+}{u_+ - u_d}(\mu - \mu_d)$$

and its sampling variance is

$$\mathrm{var}(\hat{\mu}_{-d}) \;=\; \frac{u_+^2 v - u_d^2 v_d}{(u_+ - u_d)^2} \,.$$

Hence, after taking the district-level expectation of $\mathrm{B}^2(\hat{\mu}_{-d}\,;\mu_d)$, the optimal combination of $\hat{\mu}_d$ and $\hat{\mu}_{-d}$ has the coefficient

$$\frac{v_d(u_+ - u_d)^2}{u_+^2(\sigma_\mathrm{B}^2 + v) + v_d\{(u_+ - u_d)^2 - u_d^2)\}} \,,$$

which coincides with the coefficient in (6.10). Thus, nothing is gained, either in terms of simplicity or improved estimation, by combining $\hat{\mu}_d$ with $\hat{\mu}_{-d}$ instead of combining $\hat{\mu}_d$ with $\hat{\mu}$. Using $\hat{\mu}_{-d}$ is perhaps less natural as it is not an estimator that could itself be used for any purpose. As an aside, $\hat{\mu}_{-d}$ is encountered in jackknife estimation [285].

Example 1

We illustrate the differences between MSE and eMSE on an artificial example of a country with 40 districts. The national mean of the target variable is 10.0, the district-level variance is $\sigma_\mathrm{B}^2 = 1$ and the within-district variance is $\sigma_\mathrm{W}^2 = 7$. In practice, these three quantities would not be known. The first two columns of Table 6.1 give the sample sizes and population means of the districts. The next two columns give the shrinkage coefficients — minimising the MSE and eMSE, respectively, followed by the corresponding values of MSE or eMSE. The right-most column gives the MSEs based on the composition (shrinkage) that minimises eMSE.

Recall that minimising MSE is our 'real' aim and minimising eMSE is a 'similar' aim that is easier to achieve because the coefficient b_d does not involve the district-level mean μ_d. The shrinkage coefficients that minimise MSE and eMSE differ substantially for many districts. The extreme is district 16, for which $b_{16}^* = 0.94$ and $b_{16} = 0.32$. The former suggests that we can rely on the national mean $\hat{\mu}$, whereas the latter makes us put much more faith in $\hat{\mu}_{16}$. The cause of this discrepancy is that μ_{16} is very close to the national mean $\mu = 10$. Effectively, $\hat{\mu}$ is unbiased for μ_{16}, and has a much smaller sampling variance than $\hat{\mu}_{16}$. If estimation of μ_{16} were not informed that μ_{16} is so close to μ, we would trust $\hat{\mu}_{16}$ more, responding to the concern about the possible bias of $\hat{\mu}$. $\mathrm{MSE}\{\hat{\mu}_{16}^\mathrm{C}(b_{16}^*)\,;\mu_{16}\}$ is extremely small, exceeding $\mathrm{var}(\hat{\mu})$ only slightly. In contrast, $\mathrm{var}(\hat{\mu}_{16})$ is $7/14 = 0.50$. The minimum eMSE for district 16 is 0.34, an overstatement of the MSE when b_{16} (which minimises eMSE) is used.

The results for MSE and eMSE nearly coincide for district 17. The reason for the close agreement is that the district mean, 11.01, happens to be close to $\mu + \sigma_\mathrm{B}$; it is in the same distance from the national mean as is, in effect, assumed by eMSE.

The differences between b_d^* and b_d are greatest for districts with μ_d close to μ. The differences between MSE and eMSE tend to be greater for districts

Table 6.1. Small-area estimation for a country with 40 districts. An artificial example.

District No.	Sample size	Mean	b_d^* (MSE)	b_d (eMSE)	MSE (with b_d^*)	eMSE (with b_d)	MSE (with b_d)
1	23	9.45	0.48	0.22	0.17	0.24	0.21
2	10	11.75	0.18	0.40	0.57	0.42	0.76
3	8	11.06	0.43	0.46	0.50	0.48	0.50
4	6	11.27	0.42	0.53	0.69	0.55	0.73
5	8	9.67	0.88	0.46	0.12	0.48	0.29
6	19	10.52	0.56	0.26	0.17	0.28	0.23
7	14	9.28	0.48	0.32	0.27	0.34	0.29
8	6	9.37	0.74	0.53	0.31	0.55	0.38
9	5	10.69	0.74	0.58	0.38	0.60	0.42
10	16	11.79	0.12	0.29	0.39	0.31	0.51
11	11	8.42	0.20	0.38	0.51	0.40	0.62
12	11	10.52	0.69	0.38	0.21	0.40	0.29
13	5	9.39	0.78	0.58	0.32	0.60	0.39
14	20	12.71	0.04	0.25	0.34	0.27	0.66
15	6	9.36	0.73	0.53	0.32	0.55	0.39
16	14	10.15	0.94	0.32	0.04	0.34	0.24
17	10	11.01	0.40	0.40	0.43	0.42	0.43
18	21	11.60	0.11	0.24	0.30	0.26	0.35
19	9	9.63	0.84	0.43	0.14	0.45	0.29
20	11	8.14	0.15	0.38	0.54	0.40	0.76
21	5	9.51	0.84	0.58	0.23	0.60	0.35
22	21	10.22	0.85	0.24	0.06	0.26	0.20
23	7	9.97	0.99	0.49	0.03	0.51	0.27
24	12	11.39	0.23	0.36	0.45	0.38	0.50
25	16	9.73	0.83	0.29	0.09	0.31	0.23
26	6	10.45	0.84	0.53	0.20	0.55	0.33
27	5	10.69	0.74	0.58	0.37	0.60	0.42
28	24	12.76	0.04	0.22	0.28	0.23	0.54
29	9	10.26	0.91	0.43	0.09	0.45	0.28
30	16	10.71	0.45	0.29	0.25	0.31	0.27
31	12	11.31	0.25	0.36	0.44	0.38	0.47
32	11	11.34	0.26	0.38	0.48	0.40	0.51
33	10	8.04	0.15	0.40	0.60	0.42	0.89
34	20	12.58	0.05	0.25	0.33	0.27	0.62
35	11	10.24	0.90	0.38	0.07	0.40	0.26
36	8	9.80	0.95	0.46	0.06	0.48	0.28
37	24	10.84	0.26	0.22	0.21	0.23	0.22
38	8	9.82	0.95	0.46	0.06	0.48	0.27
39	8	9.72	0.91	0.46	0.09	0.48	0.28
40	7	8.39	0.28	0.49	0.73	0.51	0.90

Figure 6.2. MSEs and eMSEs of the composite estimators of the mean for a set of 40 districts. Computer generated example. The optimum shrinkage for each district is indicated by a black disk, for MSE (panel A) and eMSE (panel B).

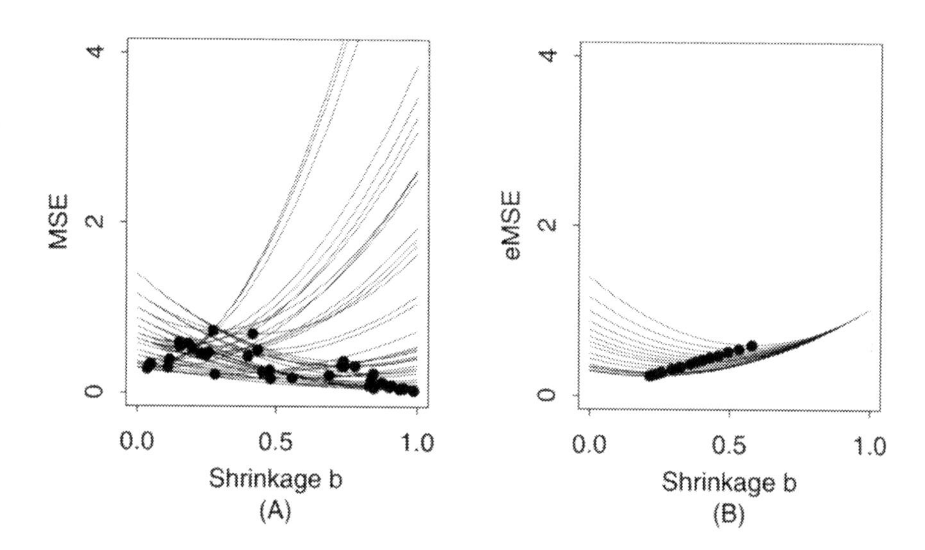

with smaller sample sizes n_d. For districts with greater n_d, the within-district information prevails, when minimising both MSE and eMSE, although the impact of the squared bias $(\mu_d - \mu)^2$ does not disappear altogether.

Figure 6.2 contains the plots of the MSEs and eMSEs, as functions of the shrinkage coefficient b, for the $D = 40$ district-level compositions. The optimal shrinkage is marked by a black disk for every district. A pattern is difficult to discern among the MSE curves or values of b_d^* in the left-hand panel because the values are affected by both sample size n_d and the squared bias $(\mu_d - \mu)^2$. In contrast, the eMSEs are aligned in an orderly fashion and the optimal shrinkage coefficients b_d decrease with the sample size n_d (increase with v_d). Although the minimum MSE is attained for high values of the shrinkage coefficient for several districts, the risk of high MSE is much smaller when less shrinkage takes place.

6.3.1 Combining the district-level means

As an alternative to combining the direct and national estimators, the direct estimators for all the districts may be combined. The quantity θ_d for district d is estimated using the direct estimator $\hat{\theta}_d$ and its counterparts $\hat{\theta}_{d'}$ for the other districts by

$$\hat{\theta}_d^{\mathrm{C}} = b_d \hat{\theta}_d + \sum_{d' \neq d} b_{d'} \hat{\theta}_{d'} ,$$

where $b_1 + \cdots + b_D = 1$. For brevity, we denote $\mathbf{b} = (b_1, \ldots, b_D)^\top$.

The notation b_d is not complete because the subscript of b should indicate not only the 'contributing' district d' but also the target district d; $b_{d',d}$. A district contributes to the estimation of different districts with different weights; in general, $b_{d',d_1} \neq b_{d',d_2}$ and $b_{d',d} \neq b_{d,d'}$. We omit the second index throughout, as the target district will always be d. Assuming that the sampling is independent across the districts, MSE of $\hat{\theta}_d^{\mathrm{C}}$ is

$$\mathrm{MSE}\left\{\hat{\theta}_d^{\mathrm{C}}(\mathbf{b});\, \theta_d\right\} = b_d^2 v_d + \sum_{d' \neq d} b_{d'}^2 \left\{v_{d'} + (\theta_{d'} - \theta_d)^2\right\} . \tag{6.11}$$

Since the squared differences $(\theta_{d'} - \theta_d)^2$ are estimated with poor precision, we replace them by their common expectation σ_{B}^2, yielding

$$\mathrm{eMSE}\left\{\hat{\theta}_d^{\mathrm{C}}(\mathbf{b});\, \theta_d\right\} = \sum_{d'=1}^{D} b_{d'}^2 v_{d'} + \sigma_{\mathrm{B}}^2 \sum_{d' \neq d} b_{d'}^2 .$$

As a function of the coefficients $\mathbf{b}$, subject to the constraint $\mathbf{b}^\top \mathbf{1} = 1$, $\mathrm{eMSE}\{\hat{\theta}_d^{\mathrm{C}}(\mathbf{b});\, \theta_d\}$ is minimised by finding the roots of its first-order partial differentials with respect to $b_{d'}$. ($\mathbf{1}$ stands for the vector of ones of length implied by the context, or indicated by its subscript.) For $d' \neq d$, we have

$$\frac{1}{2} \frac{\partial \mathrm{eMSE}}{\partial b_{d'}} = -b_d v_d + b_{d'}(v_{d'} + \sigma_{\mathrm{B}}^2) . \tag{6.12}$$

Here we have set $b_d = 1 - \sum_{d' \neq d} b_{d'}$, to avoid the constraint $\mathbf{b}^\top \mathbf{1} = 1$. The constraint could also be dealt with by the method of Lagrange multipliers. The partial differentials of eMSE vanish when

$$\frac{1 - b_d}{b_d} = v_d \sum_{d' \neq d} \frac{1}{v_{d'} + \sigma_{\mathrm{B}}^2} .$$

Hence, the optimal coefficients are $b_d^* = 1/U_+$ and, for $d' \neq d$,

$$b_{d'}^* = \frac{1}{U_+} \frac{v_d}{v_{d'} + \sigma_{\mathrm{B}}^2} , \tag{6.13}$$

where

$$U_+ = \frac{1}{b_d^*} = 1 + v_d \sum_{d' \neq d} \frac{1}{v_{d'} + \sigma_{\mathrm{B}}^2} .$$

The eMSE attained with the coefficients $b_{d'}^*$ is

$$\mathrm{eMSE}\left\{\hat{\theta}_d^{\mathrm{C}}(\mathbf{b}^*);\, \theta_d\right\} = \frac{v_d}{U_+} ,$$

so that U_+ is the quotient of improvement in precision over the direct estimator $\hat{\theta}_d$. It is a decreasing function of σ_B^2.

This approach appears at first to be unattractive because many coefficients have to be evaluated. However, the greater flexibility in combining the direct estimators $\hat{\theta}_d$ leads to an estimator with smaller eMSE than the composite estimator $\hat{\theta}_d^C$. That is the case when σ_B^2 is known. A drawback encountered later is that, unlike $\hat{\theta}_d^C$ given by (6.4), this estimator does not have useful generalisations. But its properties have not yet been explored thoroughly even in some simple settings.

6.3.2 Suboptimal composition

We refer to $\hat{\theta}_d^C(b_d^*)$ and $\hat{\theta}_d^C(b_d)$ that minimise the MSE or eMSE, respectively, as *ideal composite* estimators. We have to resign ourselves to using 'incorrect' (in practice, estimated) values of b_d^*. We explore therefore the consequences of using a coefficient $b_\dagger$ different from b_d^*, and discuss estimation of the quantities involved in b_d^*.

If we substitute a coefficient $b_\dagger$ instead of b_d^* in $\hat{\theta}_d^C$, we obtain an estimator less efficient than $\hat{\theta}_d^C(b_d^*)$. Perhaps $\hat{\theta}_d^C(b_\dagger)$ would still be satisfactory if it was more efficient than both original estimators $\hat{\theta}_d$ and $\hat{\theta}$. We compare $\hat{\theta}_d^C(b_\dagger)$ with them. The MSE of $\hat{\theta}_d^C(b_\dagger)$ is

$$\begin{aligned} \mathrm{MSE}\left\{\hat{\theta}_d^C(b_\dagger);\, \theta_d\right\} &= R_{0,d} - 2b_\dagger R_{1,d} + b_\dagger^2 R_{2,d} \\ &= R_{0,d} - b_\dagger(2b_d^* - b_\dagger) R_{2,d}\,; \qquad (6.14) \end{aligned}$$

$R_{0,d}$, $R_{1,d}$ and $R_{2,d}$ are defined in (6.5). Therefore, $\hat{\theta}_d^C(b_\dagger)$ is more efficient than $\hat{\theta}_d$ when $b_\dagger(2b_d^* - b_\dagger)$ is positive, that is, when $b_\dagger < 2b_d^*$. As $b_\dagger < 1$, this condition is relevant only when $b_d^* < \frac{1}{2}$. The MSE in (6.14) is smaller than $v + B_d^2 = R_0 - 2R_1 + R_2$ when

$$2(1 - b_\dagger)R_1 - (1 - b_\dagger^2)R_2 > 0\,,$$

that is, when $b_\dagger > 2b_d^* - 1$. This inequality is relevant only when $b_d^* > \frac{1}{2}$. In summary, $\hat{\theta}_d^C(b_\dagger)$ is more efficient than both $\hat{\theta}_d$ and $\hat{\theta}$ when

$$2b_d^* - 1 < b_\dagger < 2b_d^*\,.$$

The width of this interval, in which $b_\dagger$ has to lie, is 1.0. This might seem to allow us a considerable margin of error in guessing or estimating b_d^*; however, only part of the interval $(2b_d^* - 1,\, 2b_d^*)$ is contained in $(0, 1)$, and it is a narrow interval when b_d^* is close to zero or unity.

Figure 6.3 illustrates that there is nothing unexpected about this outcome. As a quadratic function of b, MSE is symmetric around its minimum b^*, its

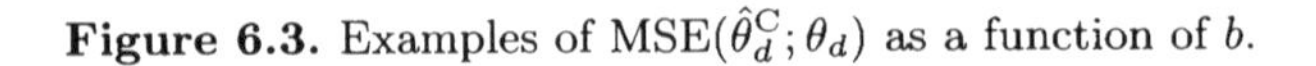

Figure 6.3. Examples of $\text{MSE}(\hat{\theta}_d^{\text{C}}; \theta_d)$ as a function of b.

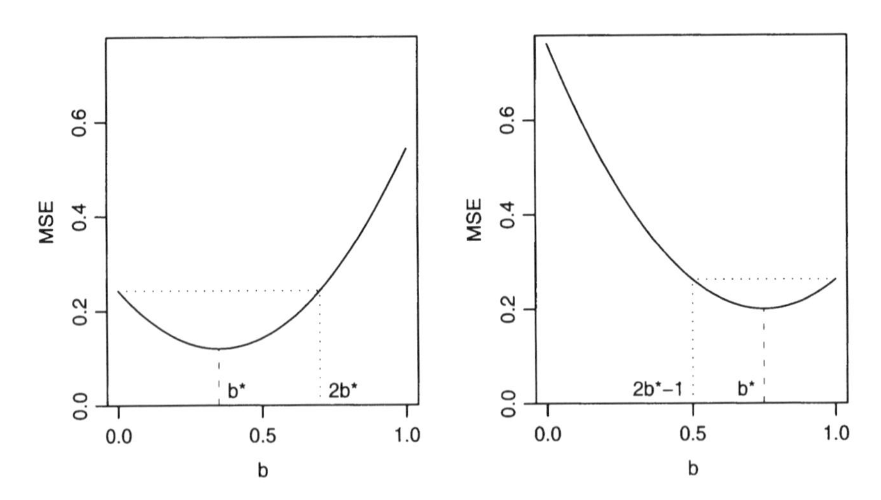

value is smaller than $\text{MSE}\{\hat{\theta}_d^{\text{C}}(0)\}$ in the range $(0, 2b^*)$ (relevant in the left-hand panel), and smaller than $\text{MSE}\{\hat{\theta}_d^{\text{C}}(1)\}$ in the range $(2b^* - 1, 1)$ (relevant in the right-hand panel).

In conclusion, the advantage of $\hat{\theta}_d^{\text{C}}$ over $\hat{\theta}_d$ and $\hat{\theta}$ is most vulnerable when the optimal shrinkage is either almost total ($b_d^* = 1$) or none ($b_d^* = 0$). These cases correspond respectively to very small and very large sample sizes n_d, but also to very small and very large district-level variances σ_{B}^2.

6.4 Estimating the district-level variance

In the previous section, we derived small-area estimators with minimum eMSE. The minimum eMSE could be attained only if we knew the district-level variance σ_{B}^2. As second best, we use an estimate of σ_{B}^2 in its place. In this section, we derive simple estimators of σ_{B}^2, assess the losses in precision due to not knowing σ_{B}^2 and explore how the impact of the uncertainty about σ_{B}^2 can be reduced.

An estimator of σ_{B}^2 is based on moment matching. We form a weighted sum of squares of the direct estimators, S, evaluate its expectation, and estimate σ_{B}^2 by equating S to it. We deviate from the usual moment matching by averaging not only over the replications, as is the standard, but also over the districts. The method can be interpreted as separating the two sources of variation: due to estimation and because of the between-district differences.

Let

$$S = \sum_{d=1}^{D} w_d (\hat{\theta}_d - \hat{\theta})^2 ,$$

for a set of weights (positive numbers) w_d. The expectation of S is

$$\mathrm{E}(S) = \sum_{d=1}^{D} w_d \left\{ v_d + v - 2c_d + (\theta_d - \theta)^2 \right\} ,$$

and taking expectation over the districts amounts to replacing the squared district-level deviations $(\theta_d - \theta)^2$ with their district-level expectation σ_{B}^2:

$$\mathrm{E}_{\mathcal{D}} \left\{ \mathrm{E}(S) \right\} = \sum_{d=1}^{D} w_d (v_d - 2c_d) + w_+ (\sigma_{\mathrm{B}}^2 + v) ,$$

where $w_+ = w_1 + \cdots + w_D$. Hence the moment-matching estimator

$$\hat{\sigma}_{\mathrm{B}}^2 = \frac{1}{w_+} \left\{ S - \sum_{d=1}^{D} w_d (v_d - 2c_d) \right\} - v . \qquad (6.15)$$

Usually v_d is much greater than v and c_d and little efficiency is lost by assuming that v and c_d vanish. Then

$$\hat{\sigma}_{\mathrm{B}}^2 = \frac{1}{w+} \left(S - \sum_{d=1}^{D} w_d v_d \right) .$$

This indicates that σ_{B}^2 is estimated from S by adjusting for the sampling variation of the direct estimators $\hat{\theta}_d$.

A practical choice for the weights are the subsample sizes n_d. They yield the estimator

$$\hat{\sigma}_{\mathrm{B}}^2 = \frac{1}{n} \left(S - \sum_{d=1}^{D} n_d v_d \right) , \qquad (6.16)$$

which simplifies further when v_d are inversely proportional to n_d, as when $v_d = \sigma_{\mathrm{W}}^2 / n_d$. The added advantage of the weights $w_d = n_d$ in this case is that the sampling variances v_d do not have to be estimated, since $n_d v_d = \sigma_{\mathrm{W}}^2$.

6.4.1 The sampling variance of $\hat{\theta}_d$

Composite estimators $\hat{\theta}_d^{\mathrm{C}}$ require the sampling variances v_d of the direct estimators $\hat{\theta}_d$. As there are many districts, we should be concerned that the errors in estimating the numerous v_d may inflate the eMSE, by contributing to both bias and sampling variance of $\hat{\sigma}_{\mathrm{B}}^2$, and with it to a loss of precision in estimating θ_d by $\hat{\theta}_d^{\mathrm{C}} = \hat{\theta}_d^{\mathrm{C}}(\hat{b}_d)$, using an estimator $\hat{b}_d$ of either b_d^* or b_d.

The estimators $\hat{\sigma}_{\mathrm{B}}^2$ in (6.15) and (6.16) are linear functions of the v_d, so we have to focus only on the sampling variation of the $\hat{v}_d$. Districts with larger sample sizes tend to have smaller sampling variances of $\hat{\theta}_d$ but their variances v_d contribute to $\hat{\sigma}_{\mathrm{B}}^2$ with greater weight, n_d/n in (6.16). So, the poorly estimated variances v_d are 'sheltered' under small coefficients in (6.16). In fact, we can define the weights w_d in such a way as to reduce the impact of uncertainty about v_d. Assigning larger weights for districts with larger subsample sizes is an obvious prescription, although there is still a myriad of choices for how fast the weight w_d should increase with the subsample size n_d. Also, we should pay attention to the representation of the districts in (6.16).

There may be consistent differences in the sampling variances, due to differential within-district variation. For example, the larger districts may be more variable (have greater within-district variances σ_W^2). If we assume a common within-district variance σ_W^2 but pool the within-district estimated variances, the sampling variances v_d may be underestimated for the large and overestimated for the small districts. With sample-size dependent weights assigned to the districts' values of v_d (or $\hat{v}_d$), σ_B^2 is estimated with bias. Assigning equal weights w_d is not a good solution for this problem because then the total $(w_1\hat{v}_1 + \cdots + w_D\hat{v}_D)/w_+$ is too variable.

Nevertheless, it is necessary to pool the within-district variance estimates when the variances are estimated with low precision in most districts. However, the variance could be pooled over suitable subsets of the districts, defined either by an attribute, such as urbanity (urban districts tend to be more populous and more heterogeneous), or by classifying the districts according to their population into a few categories.

The covariances c_d

For estimators $\hat{\theta}_d$ and $\hat{\theta}$ that are linear in $\mathbf{y}$, the covariances c_d are estimated straightforwardly, especially when $\hat{\theta}$ is a linear combination of the $\hat{\theta}_d$. When $\hat{\theta} = (u_1\hat{\theta}_1 + \cdots + u_D\hat{\theta}_D)/u_+$ and the direct estimators $\hat{\theta}_d$ are mutually independent,

$$c_d = \operatorname{cov}(\hat{\theta}_d, \hat{\theta}) = \frac{u_d}{u_+} v_d < v_d .$$

Thus, the covariance c_d is a substantial fraction of v_d for no more than a few districts d that have large weights u_d. Such districts would also have large sample sizes, and so v_d would be small, as would be c_d. Composition for such districts is not particularly effective, but the direct estimator is quite efficient.

District-level means and simple random sampling

By way of an example, consider a survey with a simple random sampling design from an effectively infinite population. Suppose the district-level means θ_d of a continuous variable y are of interest and the districts have a common within-district variance σ_W^2. The direct and national estimators are the sample means over the district-subsample and the sample, respectively. Their respective sampling variances are $v_d = \sigma_W^2/n_d$ and $v = \sigma_W^2/n$, and the covariance of the two estimators is $c_d = \sigma_W^2/n$. Hence, $v_d + v - 2c_d = v_d - c_d = \sigma_W^2(1/n_d - 1/n)$. The within-district variance σ_W^2 is estimated as

$$\hat{\sigma}_{\mathrm{W}}^2 = \frac{1}{n-D} \sum_{d=1}^{D} \sum_{j=1}^{n_d} (y_{jd} - \hat{\theta}_d)^2$$

(assuming that each district is represented in the sample). The district-level variance estimate, based on S with $w_d = n_d$, is

$$\begin{aligned} \hat{\sigma}_{\mathrm{B}}^2 &= \frac{1}{n} \left\{ S - \hat{\sigma}_{\mathrm{W}}^2 \sum_{d=1}^{D} n_d \left(\frac{1}{n_d} - \frac{2}{n} \right) \right\} - \frac{\hat{\sigma}_{\mathrm{W}}^2}{n} \\ &= \frac{S - (D-1)\hat{\sigma}_{\mathrm{W}}^2}{n} . \end{aligned}$$

The covariances c_d contribute to this expression by $-2/n$ in the first line. If they are ignored, $D - 1$ in the second line is replaced by D. This change is inconsequential when there are many districts D.

Denote the variance ratio $\omega = \sigma_{\mathrm{B}}^2/\sigma_{\mathrm{W}}^2$, and its (naive) estimator by $\hat{\omega}$. The shrinkage coefficient b_d that minimises $\mathrm{eMSE}(\hat{\theta}_d^{\mathrm{C}})$ is estimated by

$$\hat{b}_d = \frac{g_j}{g_j + \hat{\omega}} ,$$

where $g_j = 1/n_d - 1/n$; see (6.8). Ignoring the uncertainty about σ_{W}^2 and ω, the eMSE of $\hat{\theta}_d^{\mathrm{C}}(\hat{b}_d)$ is estimated by

$$\widehat{\mathrm{eMSE}} \left\{ \hat{\theta}_d^{\mathrm{C}}(\hat{b}_d) \right\} = \hat{\sigma}_{\mathrm{W}}^2 \left(\frac{1}{n_d} - \frac{g_j}{1 + \hat{\omega}/g_j} \right) .$$

This estimator is downward biased because the uncertanty about ω is bound to inflate the sampling variance of $\hat{\theta}_d^{\mathrm{C}}$. The uncertainty about σ_{W}^2 is minor in comparison.

If we consider the mean of the district-level means $\theta^* = \mathrm{E}_{\mathcal{D}}(\theta_{\mathcal{D}})$ instead of the national mean θ, $\hat{\theta}$ is replaced by

$$\hat{\theta}^* = \frac{1}{D} \sum_{d=1}^{D} \hat{\theta}_d .$$

If each district is represented in the sample,

$$(v^* =) \quad \mathrm{var}(\hat{\theta}^*) = \frac{1}{D^2} \sum_{d=1}^{D} v_d .$$

As soon as one district is not represented in the sample, $v^* = +\infty$. This is a serious weakness of $\hat{\theta}^*$.

Binary data

For binary data y_{jd} (say positive, coded as 1, and negative as 0), there is only one meaningful parameter to estimate, the proportion (rate or percentage) of positive outcomes. Another peculiarity of binary data is that the sampling variance of the estimated rate $\hat{\theta}_d$ is related to the rate itself. With simple random sampling with replacement within districts,

$$\operatorname{var}(\hat{\theta}_d) = \frac{1}{n_d}\theta_d(1-\theta_d),$$

so that we can regard $\theta_d(1-\theta_d)$ as the within-district variance, akin to σ_{W}^2. The association of the proportion (mean) with the sampling variance has several implications. First, the error committed in estimating θ_d is duplicated when estimating $v_d = \operatorname{var}(\hat{\theta}_d)$ naively by $\hat{\theta}_d(1-\hat{\theta}_d)/n_d$. Since v_d is a non-linear function of θ_d, its naive estimator is biased even when $\hat{\theta}_d$ is not biased for θ_d. It may be preferable to estimate each v_d by using $\hat{\theta}$ instead of $\hat{\theta}_d$. By $\hat{\theta}(1-\hat{\theta})/n_d$, v_d may be estimated with much smaller sampling variance, especially when θ_d is close to zero or unity. And we reach full circle if we consider composition — combining $\hat{\theta}_d(1-\hat{\theta}_d)/n_d$ and $\hat{\theta}(1-\hat{\theta})/n_d$ according to their (estimated) precisions in estimating v_d. The barrier to effective solution by this route is that, as before, we require the value of the district-level variance σ_{B}^2 (or its estimate).

However, for proportions distant from zero and unity, the sampling variance is a flat function of θ_d, so a substantial error in estimating θ_d converts to a minute error in estimating v_d. In contrast, for proportions close to zero or unity, the sampling variance is well approximated by a linear function of θ_d; θ_d at zero and $1-\theta_d$ at unity. In these cases, the problem is more acute.

A practical proposition is to evaluate $\hat{\theta}_d^{\mathrm{C}}$ with naively estimated v_d, but then to re-estimate v_d based on the composite estimator $\hat{\theta}_d^{\mathrm{C}}$ and repeat the composite estimation. This is a compromise between using the naive estimators of v_d and the 'stable' estimators based on the national estimator $\hat{\theta}$.

Similar comments apply to estimation with variables that can be regarded as outcomes from other single-parameter families of distributions. A notable example is the Poisson distribution for counts, for which the mean and variance coincide. We caution that count data may have distributions very different from the Poisson. The association of the mean and variance is relied on heavily, so the consequences of a departure from it should be carefully weighed.

6.4.2 The impact of uncertainty about σ_{B}^2

The orthodox reaction to not knowing σ_{B}^2 is to estimate it efficiently — as precisely as possible, and substitute the estimate for the parameter in b_d. However natural this approach may appear, it fails to take into account how the estimate $\hat{\sigma}_{\mathrm{B}}^2$ is used. For instance, the consequences of the estimate being greater than the target, $\hat{\sigma}_{\mathrm{B}}^2 = \sigma_{\mathrm{B}}^2 + \Delta$, may be much less serious than the converse, $\hat{\sigma}_{\mathrm{B}}^2 = \sigma_{\mathrm{B}}^2 - \Delta$, for *any* positive Δ. The eMSEs with the 'incorrectly' substituted values of $\sigma_{\mathrm{B}}^2 \pm \Delta$ instead of σ_{B}^2, that is, with $b_d = R_{1,d}/(R_{2,d} \pm \Delta)$ in (6.5), are

$$r_{\pm} = R_0 - \frac{R_1^2(R_2 \pm 2\Delta)}{(R_2 \pm \Delta)^2};$$

(we drop the district-index d). The difference of the two eMSEs is

$$r_- - r_+ = \frac{4\Delta^3 R_1^2}{(R_2 + \Delta)^2(R_2 - \Delta)^2} > 0\,.$$

Thus, it is preferable to err on the side of greater σ_{B}^2, irrespective of the values of v, v_d and c_d, which are involved in R_0, R_1 and R_2.

Figure 6.4 illustrates this on an example. The curve drawn in solid in panel A is the eMSE as a function of the coefficient b for a district; it is based on the setting $v_d = 1$, $v = c_d = 0.1$ and $\sigma_{\mathrm{B}}^2 = 0.25$, so that the minimum of eMSE is attained at $b^* = 0.78$, and the value attained is 0.296. The dashed lines are the eMSE's evaluated for σ_{B}^2 set (incorrectly) to 0.4 and 0.1, erring by 0.15 in both cases. With these two values of σ_{B}^2, the shrinkage coefficients $b^+ = 0.69$ and $b^- = 0.90$ are obtained. Based on the respective values of σ_{B}^2, we obtain the eMSEs of 0.377 and 0.190. The eMSEs based on the correct value of $\sigma_{\mathrm{B}}^2 = 0.25$, but 'incorrect' shrinkage coefficients b^+ and b^- are 0.305 and 0.312, respectively. Thus, with smaller σ_{B}^2 we obtain a poorer estimator, but the solution will indicate to the contrary (eMSE $= 0.190$). By overestimating σ_{B}^2, the eMSE will be overestimated, so the precision of $\hat{\theta}_d^{\mathrm{C}}$ is assessed with honesty.

Panel B illustrates what happens when the error is multiplicative. The same values of v_d, c_d, v and σ_{B}^2 are used, but the errors committed with regard to σ_{B}^2 are multiplicative; the shrinkage coefficient b^+ is based on the 1.5-multiple and b^- on two-thirds of σ_{B}^2. Now, underestimation of σ_{B}^2 is preferable (eMSE of 0.300 against 0.302). Note that the differences in eMSE are quite small with what might be regarded as substantial errors, in both the additive and the multiplicative case. The errors in assessing the precision of the estimators are much greater, though.

A similar conclusion is drawn if we give priority to improving on the direct estimator $\hat{\theta}_d$. $\mathrm{MSE}\{\hat{\theta}_d^{\mathrm{C}}(b);\, \theta_d\}$ is a quadratic function of b, with local maxima at $b = 0$ and $b = 1$, so sufficiently small values of b will yield an improvement over the direct estimator $\hat{\theta}_d$; improvement is achieved when $b < 2b_d^*$. As b_d^* is a decreasing function of σ_{B}^2, smaller b corresponds to greater value of $\hat{\sigma}_{\mathrm{B}}^2$. Therefore, by erring on the side of greater σ_{B}^2, we keep unchanged or increase the number of districts for which $\hat{\theta}_d^{\mathrm{C}}(b_d^\dagger)$ with $b_d^\dagger$ based on $\hat{\sigma}_{\mathrm{B}}^2$ is more efficient than $\hat{\theta}_d$. In other words, composite estimation of θ_d is conservative if we overestimate σ_{B}^2. The moment-matching estimator in (6.15) suggests that

Figure 6.4. The consequences of an error in the guess or estimate of σ_B^2. Additive and multiplicative errors.

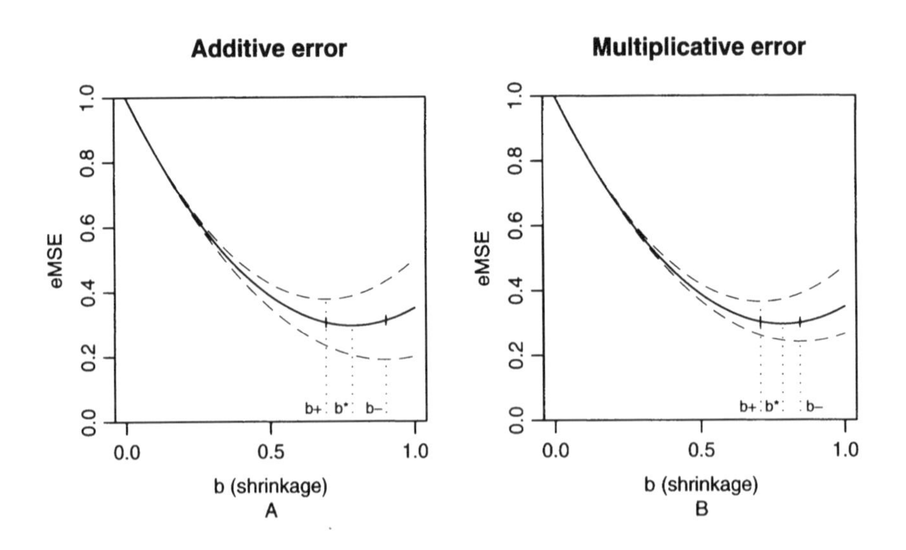

overestimation of σ_B^2 is achieved by underestimating the sampling variances v_d. Conservatism should, however, be applied in moderation — if the shrinkage coefficients b_d are set very small, we improve the estimation for almost every district, but the improvement is minute for every one of them.

We can interpret the switch from minimising MSE to minimising eMSE as 'estimation' of the squared bias $B_d = (\mu_d - \mu)^2$ by the district-level variance σ_B^2, or its estimator. We could explore whether this estimation can be improved. An interesting approach is to reuse the idea of composition by combining $(\hat{\mu}_d - \hat{\mu})^2$ and $\hat{\sigma}_B^2$, aiming to estimate $(\mu_d - \mu)^2$ efficiently. When there are many districts D this will have the effect of assigning to $(\hat{\mu}_d - \hat{\mu})^2$ weight increasing with n_d, from zero when $n_d = 0$ to full weight when n_d is a substantial fraction of n. This shrinkage is somewhat more complex to work out because both $(\hat{\mu}_d - \hat{\mu})^2$ and $\hat{\sigma}_B^2$ are biased for $(\mu_d - \mu)^2$ and their MSEs depend on the quantities that we aim to estimate.

Exceptional districts

The location and other characteristics of the districts may be an important factor in the district-level variation. For example, a few districts may be known to be exceptional; without them the districts are much more homogeneous. Or the country's regions may differ a great deal, but the districts within the regions are much more homogeneous. In these settings, it is preferable to consider each region, or the country without the exceptional districts, as a separate domain. Smaller district-level variance is preferable, see (6.9), as greater gains in precision are then realised. However, with a smaller dataset, the district-level variance is estimated with less precision, although, for a fixed sample size, a smaller variance is estimated with greater precision than a greater variance.

6.5 Spatial similarity

In the previous section, we recognised two sources of variation: *sampling variation*, described by the sampling variances $v_d = \mathrm{var}(\hat{\theta}_d)$ (and the independence of the estimators $\hat{\theta}_d$), and *district-level variation*, which we assume to be such that $\mathrm{var}_{\mathcal{D}}(\theta_d - \theta_{d'} \,|\, \theta_d) = \sigma_{\mathrm{B}}^2$, a constant. Note that without conditioning on $\hat{\theta}_d$, $\mathrm{var}_{\mathcal{D}}(\theta_d - \theta_{d'}) = 2\sigma_{\mathrm{B}}^2$.

Assumptions about both sources of variation may have to be loosened. For example, the sampling in distinct small areas may be dependent. An extreme case of dependence is that only one of a pair of districts is sampled. This may occur when districts, or units containing districts, are sampled systematically. But even in stratified clustered sampling, when a small set number of clusters is sampled without replacement from a stratum, the inclusion of one cluster is negatively associated with the inclusion of another cluster. Such associations can be incorporated in the evaluation of MSE in (6.11) by including the $b_{d_1} b_{d_2}$-multiples of the sampling covariances for all pairs of districts d_1 and d_2.

District d' for which the sampling is dependent on the sampling for district d is called a *sampling neighbour* of district d. Most of the $\frac{1}{2}D(D-1)$ covariances that would appear in (6.11) vanish, and in the partial differentials in (6.12), only the sampling neighbours of district d appear. In practice, it is difficult to sort out the 'neighbourhoods', especially when the number of districts is large, and the associations involved are not very strong; so, they are ignored altogether.

Another intuitively appealing model for the district-level variation is that neighbouring districts (that is, districts that have a common border) are more similar than districts further apart. Suppose d_1 and d_2 are neighbouring districts. If being neighbours implies more similarity than for the districts country-wide, then

$$\mathrm{var}_{\mathcal{D}}(\theta_{\mathcal{D}} \,|\, \theta_d \,; \mathrm{neighbour}) \;=\; \sigma_{\mathrm{B}}^2 \rho$$

for some $\rho < 1$. The variation of the means of the neighbours of a district is smaller than the variation among the districts in general. A typical district has only a few neighbours, so it is practical to consider ρ as a 'national' quantity, defined by pooling over the neighbourhoods of all the districts. Such neighbour-similarity can be represented by the ratio of the conditional and unconditional district-level variances:

$$\rho = \frac{\mathrm{var}_{\mathcal{D}}(\theta_{\mathcal{D}} \,|\, \theta_d \,; \mathrm{neighbour})}{\sigma_{\mathrm{B}}^2} \,. \tag{6.17}$$

We relate ρ to the (constant) correlation of the pairs of neighbouring districts. Suppose the values of θ_d for any two neighbouring districts d_1 and d_2 are related by the model

$$\theta_{d_2} = \varrho\theta_{d_1} + \varepsilon_{d_1,d_2}\,, \tag{6.18}$$

where ε_{d_1,d_2} are mutually independent and independent of all θ_d. The definition of σ_{B}^2 implies that $\mathrm{var}(\varepsilon_d) = (1-\varrho^2)\sigma_{\mathrm{B}}^2$, and so $\mathrm{var}_{\mathcal{D}}(\theta_{\mathcal{D}}\,|\,\mathrm{neighbour}) = \mathrm{var}(\varepsilon_{d_1,d_2}) = (1-\varrho^2)\sigma_{\mathrm{B}}^2$. Thus, ρ in (6.17) can be equated with $1-\varrho^2$. Suppose next that district d_3 is a neighbour of district d_2, but is not a neighbour of d_1. Then

$$\theta_{d_3} = \varrho^2\theta_{d_1} + \varrho\varepsilon_{d_2,d_3} + \varepsilon_{d_1,d_2}\,,$$

and so $\mathrm{var}_{\mathcal{D}}(\theta_{\mathcal{D}}\,|\,\mathrm{neighbour's\ neighbour}) = (1-\varrho^4)\sigma_{\mathrm{B}}^2$.

We can define the distance Δ_{d_1,d_2} between districts d_1 and d_2 as the smallest number of borders that have to be crossed on the way from one district to the other. For this definition, we have to assume that each district is contiguous; that it does not have separated parts (enclaves). Thus, each district is in zero distance from itself, in unit distance from its neighbours, and so on.

For settings with $\varrho \neq 0$, we can talk about *spatial similarity*, and the squared correlation ϱ^2 can be regarded as its measure. It is obvious that efficient estimation of θ_d should draw on the information in its neighbours more than on the information in more distant districts. As in Section 6.3.1, we consider linear combinations of the direct estimators

$$\hat{\theta}_d^{\mathrm{C}}(\mathbf{b}) = \sum_{d'=1}^{D} b_{d'}\hat{\theta}_{d'}\,,$$

evaluate their eMSEs, and choose the vector of coefficients $\mathbf{b}$ that yields the minimum $\mathrm{eMSE}\{\hat{\theta}_d^{\mathrm{C}}(\mathbf{b})\}$. The solution $\mathbf{b}^*$ depends on d.

To evaluate $\mathrm{eMSE}\{\hat{\theta}_d^{\mathrm{C}}(\mathbf{b})\}$, we have to express $\mathrm{var}_{\mathcal{D}}(\theta_{\mathcal{D}}\,|\,\mathrm{neighbour})$ in terms of ϱ and σ_{B}^2. For the model considered in (6.18), these conditional variances depend on the pairwise distances Δ_{d_1,d_2}; $\mathrm{var}_{\mathcal{D}}(\theta_{\mathcal{D}}\,|\,\theta_d) = (1-\varrho^{2\Delta_{\mathcal{D},d}})$. Since it is discrete, we may classify the districts by the distance, and write

$$\hat{\theta}_d^{\mathrm{C}}(\mathbf{b}) = b_d\hat{\theta}_d + \sum_{\Delta=1}^{\Delta_{\max}} \sum_{\{d';\Delta(d',d)=\Delta\}} b_d'\hat{\theta}_{d'}\,,$$

and for the eMSE,

$$\mathrm{eMSE}\{\hat{\theta}_d^{\mathrm{C}}(\mathbf{b})\} = b_d^2 v_d + \sum_{\Delta=1}^{\Delta_{\max}} \sum_{\{d';\,\Delta(d',d)=\Delta\}} {b_{d'}}^2\left\{v_{d'} + \sigma_{\mathrm{B}}^2(1-\varrho^{2\Delta})\right\}.$$

Minimising this expression as a function of $\mathbf{b} = (b_1,\ldots,b_D)^\top$, subject to the constraint that $\mathbf{b}^\top\mathbf{1} = 1$, yields

$$\frac{b_{d'}}{b_d} = \frac{v_d}{v_{d'} + \sigma_{\mathrm{B}}^2\left(1-\varrho^{2\Delta_{d',d}}\right)}$$

and

$$b_d^* = \frac{1}{v_d U_+}$$

$$b_{d'}^* = \frac{1}{U_+} \frac{1}{v_{d'} + \sigma_B^2 (1 - \varrho^{2\Delta_{d',d}})}, \qquad (6.19)$$

where $U_+ = \sum_{d'=1}^{D} \{v_{d'} + \sigma_B^2 (1 - \varrho^{2\Delta_{d',d}})\}$. Note that the equation for b_d^* does not have to be quoted separately, as $\Delta_{d,d} = 0$.

For $\varrho = 0$, (6.19) reverts to (6.13). For $\varrho \neq 0$, the coefficient $b_{d'}$ is boosted for districts neighbouring on district d; the denominator $v_{d'} + \sigma_B^2(1 - \varrho^{2\Delta})$ is smaller for $\Delta = 1$ than for greater distances.

Flexibility is further enhanced by defining the variances $\mathrm{var}_{\mathcal{D}}(\theta_{\mathcal{D}} \mid \theta_d)$ as functions of the distance $\Delta_{\mathcal{D},d}$, without a reference to a model. The distance can be defined in a different way, not necessarily as an integer (a discrete variable). The definition of the distance can be bypassed altogether, by specifying the conditional variances $\mathrm{var}_{\mathcal{D}}(\theta_{\mathcal{D}} \mid \theta_d)$ directly, as a $D \times D$ symmetric array with zero diagonal.

Does the distance matter?

This is a question about the nature of similarity. Whereas some phenomena are transported contiguously, from one district to its neighbours, many others do not respect any administrative or even national boundaries, or rather respect some other boundaries for which we have a limited understanding and they defy any concise description. Thus, an epidemic may spread from one city or airport to another, affecting the small towns and rural districts with delay and much less profoundly, or from one farm, to another in a considerable distance mediated more strongly by business associations than physical proximity. Physical proximity is distorted by the communication infrastructure. For example, in passenger rail transport, express railway stations are connected by fast and frequent services, whereas travelling between the local stations on the same line is much slower and less convenient. Airlines connect major cities, with relatively little regard for distance because accessing airports and dealing with the security and other formalities at the airport takes up a substantial part of the overall travel time. Information spread electronically has even less respect for distance or administrative boundaries.

6.6 Suggested reading

A number of approaches to small-area estimation are reviewed by [213] and [214]. Shrinkage estimators for a collection of means (e.g., for small areas) were proposed by [273] and were put on a theoretical basis by [55], [56] and [57]. They draw on the celebrated finding of [264] and [115] that, when estimating more than four means, each of them can be estimated more efficiently than by the corresponding sample means. These ideas are applied by [67] to a U.S. Federal Program for distributing funds to localities in the U.S.A., based on their (estimated) mean income. References [88] and [60] are their important precursors.

Reference [52] describes a study that evaluates the performance of several small-area estimators intended for the Canadian Labour Force Survey. A similar goal is pursued by [62], in the context of the Italian Labour Force Survey.

The populations of administrative units are in many countries determined by adjusting the census figures by extrapolation to the current date. The imperfect coverage of the U.S. Decennial Census (Census undercount) has generated a great deal of controversy spanning constitutional, legal and statistical issues. These include adjustment of the population (and subpopulation) figures for small areas, such as U.S. counties. References [248] and [286] propose solutions of this problem. See [257] for a UK perspective on a related problem.

6.7 Exercises

1. Suppose an island country comprises of only two regions called Inland and Coastal. The population of the Coastal region is ten times greater. A survey with a stratified sampling design is conducted in which the values of a continuous target variable are recorded for a simple random sample of $10n$ subjects from the Coastal and for an independent simple random sample of n subjects from the Inland region. Discuss the merits of estimating the population mean of this variable for the Inland region by a, the sample mean for the Inland region; b, the sample mean for the Coastal region; c, the national sample mean; d, the combination of the two subsample means with weights 10/11 (for Inland) and 1/11 (for Coastal). (For simplicity, assume that the two within-region variances are identical.) e, the national mean, if the test of the hypothesis that the two regions have identical means is not rejected, and by the sample mean for the Inland region otherwise.
2. Find in the literature, or on the Internet, the unemployment rates, median house prices, or some other socio-economic summaries in your country and region for a sequence of recent years (quarters, months, or the like), and compare the trends of the two sequences. Search for the details of the sources of this information (surveys or registers) and, if applicable, for the estimators applied.
3. Apply the uniform and tailored choice methods to the data in Example 1 and Table 6.1.

   Hint: Use the parameter values given in the introduction to the example.
4. Simulate a set of direct and composite estimators for a country with 200 districts. Generate first their population means and sample sizes, from

suitable distributions (e.g., gamma and Poisson, respectively). Either assume that each district has the same variance, or generate the within-district variances by drawing them from a distribution, or setting them to one of a small number of positive values. Draw a sample mean for each district (assume normality, independence of the within-district subsamples and simple random sampling design in each district). Compare the direct and composite estimates by counting the number of districts for which either estimate is closer to the target (the district's population mean). Repeat the steps of drawing a sample mean for each district and applying the direct and composite estimates. For one generated dataset, compare the results using the district-nation covariances c_d estimated or set to zero. Repeat the simulation exercise and compare the ideal composition (based on known variance of the district-level means) with the composition based on the estimated between-district variance. Estimate (from simulations) the distribution of the estimator $\hat{\sigma}^2_{\mathrm{B}}$. Match the distribution with a χ^2 distribution. Why has the matched distribution fewer degrees of freedom than the number of districts D?

5. On a simulated or real example, study the difference between composite estimators $\hat{\theta}^{\mathrm{C}}_d$ based on the naive estimator of b_d in (6.8) and its approximation with c_d and v set to zero. Draw suitable graphs to show that the approximation is problematic only for the areas with the largest representation in the sample.
6. With a dataset used in the previous example, apply for each district the composite estimators $\hat{\theta}^{\mathrm{C}}_d(\hat{b}_d)$, $\hat{\theta}^{\mathrm{C}}_d(0.9\hat{b}_d)$ and $\hat{\theta}^{\mathrm{C}}_d(0.8\hat{b}_d)$. Compare the three sets of estimates with their targets. Define and evaluate summaries of the deviations $\hat{\theta}^{\mathrm{C}}_d - \theta_d$ that reflect the estimation errors of an estimator type. Hint: Consider $\sum_d(\hat{\theta}^{\mathrm{C}}_d - \theta_d)^2$.
7. Show that the ratios $v_d/\mathrm{MSE}(\hat{\theta}^{\mathrm{C}}_d;\,\theta_d)$ and $v_d/\mathrm{eMSE}(\hat{\theta}^{\mathrm{C}}_d;\,\theta_d)$ are decreasing functions of v_d. (Ignore the value of c_d or assume that $c_d = v$.) Plot these ratios as functions of v_d for a setting of your choice, without ignoring c_d.
8. Consider the problem of estimating district-level means of income (of members of the labour force, or of households) or unemployment rate. How would you define suitable distances between pairs of districts (in your country)? For your (or a selected) district, tabulate the totals of the subsample sizes of the areas for each distance. Assuming that only a handful of the districts are your neighbours and most of the districts are distant, assess the difference between composition that takes distance into account and one that ignores it.

7

Models for small areas

Models are an important conduit to understanding phenomena that we study. A good model captures the principal features of the complex phenomenon and ignores the secondary features. The behaviour of the model, deduced theoretically or observed in simulations, is then assumed to be similar to the behaviour of the studied phenomenon. In the context of population surveys, the interest is in the values of variables on the members of a population. Inferences are desired about (population) summaries of these variables; measures of association, such as a correlation or a regression coefficient can be regarded as model-related multivariate summaries, involving several variables. The models we consider describe the phenomena in terms of systematic (consistent) and random (inexplicable) features.

The systematic features are present in every replication of the study, whereas the random features are not predictable (replicable). In a model building exercise, we consider the most important features of the studied population, the variables of interest, and of the process of data collection (sampling and, if applicable, nonresponse and measurement), and match them as closely as we can to a class of models. For small-area estimation, the key feature is the presence of the districts, and the understanding (prior information) that they have similar but not identical means or other subpopulation summaries.

7.1 Analysis of variance

Models for small areas (districts) have to capture two sources of variation: within districts and among them. The obvious starting point for estimating the district-level means μ_d is the model

$$y_{jd} = \mu_d + \varepsilon_{jd} , \tag{7.1}$$

acknowledging that the districts have different means μ_d and that the values of y for the units within each district vary around this mean. The nature of the variation can be specified by the distributions of the within-district deviations ε_{jd} and the district-level means μ_d. For the within-district deviations, we may specify a distribution common to all the districts, different distributions for each district (district-specific distributions) or common distributions for subsets of districts. A common distribution is the simplest choice, but it may not be appropriate. District-specific distributions allow much more flexibility, but may be impractical when many districts are sparsely represented in the sample.

Commonly, a class of distributions, such as normal, is assumed for the deviations ε_{jd}. The purpose of such an assumption is to justify the application of estimation procedures that are efficient when the assumption is appropriate. Expediency is an important factor in this — assumptions that lead to simple estimation procedures are greatly preferred. That is why the normal distribution is the first candidate, and is used unless there is strong evidence against it. A secondary factor is that models with normality assumptions are much better understood; the well established link to linear algebra is particularly valuable.

Without any assumption about the district-level means μ_d, (7.1) is a model for the one-way *analysis of variance* (ANOVA). With its standard treatment, it yields the direct estimator $\hat{\mu}_d$ or the national estimator $\hat{\mu}$ for each district d, depending on whether we conclude that the district-level means are identical or not. We have discredited this approach in Section 6.2. The development of composition in Section 6.3 suggests that we should reexamine the standard application of ANOVA even in settings other than small areas. This we do in Section 11.4.

In Section 6.3, we identified the district-level variance σ_B^2 as the key quantity for finding a composite estimator that is superior to both the direct and national estimators. The obvious way of introducing this variance in the ANOVA model is by assuming a distribution for the district-level means. Expediency suggests that it should be normal, $\mathcal{N}(\mu, \sigma_B^2)$, unless there is a compelling reason for another choice. Note that this is a district-level distribution; $\sigma_B^2 = \mathrm{var}_{\mathcal{D}}(\mu_{\mathcal{D}})$.

The ANOVA model with an assumption about the distribution of the means μ_d is called *random-effect* ANOVA (rANOVA). We can express (7.1) equivalently as

$$y_{jd} = \mu + \delta_d + \varepsilon_{jd}, \tag{7.2}$$

and declare that δ_d is a random sample from $\mathcal{N}(0, \sigma_B^2)$. Since both δ_d and ε_{jd} are random variables, we can regard them on equal footing as subject- and district-level deviations, so that μ and the variances σ_B^2 and σ_W^2 define the model completely. Summarising the D district-level means μ_d by their mean μ and variance σ_B^2 is very useful — instead of D 'degrees of freedom' we use only two parameters. However, this does not absolve us from estimating each district-level mean μ_d. Even if the three 'global' parameters, μ, σ_B^2 and σ_W^2, are known, we still cannot separate δ_d from the ε_{jd}, $j = 1, \ldots, n_j$, so as to estimate $\mu_d = \mu + \delta_d$.

In rANOVA, μ_d is a random variable, so we estimate its realisation by its conditional expectation. If both δ_d and ε_{jd} are normally distributed (and mutually independent), the conditional distribution of δ_d given the data $\mathbf{y}$ and the global parameters is

$$(\delta_d \,|\, \mathbf{y};\, \mu, \sigma_{\mathrm{W}}^2, \sigma_{\mathrm{B}}^2) \sim \mathcal{N}\left\{ (\hat{\mu}_d - \mu)\frac{n_d \omega}{1 + n_d \omega}, \, \frac{\sigma_{\mathrm{B}}^2}{1 + n_d \omega} \right\}, \tag{7.3}$$

where $\omega = \sigma_{\mathrm{B}}^2 / \sigma_{\mathrm{W}}^2$ is the variance ratio. Hence the estimator

$$\begin{aligned} \tilde{\mu}_d &= \hat{\mu} + (\hat{\mu}_d - \hat{\mu})\frac{n_d \hat{\omega}}{1 + n_d \hat{\omega}} \\ &= \hat{\mu}_d \frac{n_d \omega}{1 + n_d \omega} + \hat{\mu}\frac{1}{1 + n_d \omega}\,. \end{aligned} \tag{7.4}$$

This coincides with the estimator $\hat{\theta}_d^{\mathrm{C}}$ derived in Section 6.3, if we ignore the covariance c_d and variance v in (6.8), and set $v_d = \sigma_{\mathrm{W}}^2 / n_d$. In (7.3), we ignore the uncertainty about μ, whereas in (6.8) we do not. However, in neither case have we taken into account that the variance ratio ω is estimated.

The composite estimator seems to be preferable. We have made fewer assumptions in deriving it, yet we obtain, at least for small districts (when $c_d \doteq 0$), the same estimator as when normality is assumed. The assumption of normality seems to be redundant. Conceivably, we might obtain estimators more efficient than $\tilde{\mu}_d$ in (7.4) when another distributional assumption is adopted. But if the assumption is not appropriate we may be back to square one or even worse. Besides, the composite estimator $\hat{\theta}_d^{\mathrm{C}}$ is more versatile because it can be applied to quantities other than means (or proportions), and the sampling design can be incorporated in the direct and national estimators with no additional difficulties brought on by small-area estimation. Incorporating sampling weights in models such as ANOVA and rANOVA is straightforward (all the statistics used are replaced by their weighted versions), but not all the results extend to the models with weights.

The difference between ANOVA and rANOVA deserves a close examination. As we replicate the survey in the ANOVA setting, the same district-level means μ_d are realised (if the district is represented in the sample). In contrast, the replication implied by rANOVA would draw μ_d for each district d at random; any given district would have a different mean in every replication. In this aspect, the assumption of random δ_d is not correct; in the intended replications, each μ_d should be held constant. But with the corresponding model, (fixed-effect) ANOVA, we get no further than the direct estimator. This paradox is explained in Chapter 11 where we show that the established ANOVA (maximum likelihood) estimator is inefficient. The assumption of randomness of the district-level deviations is merely a device that enables a more natural application of a general principle that should be employed, or at least considered, universally.

We outline this principle in brief, in the context of one-way ANOVA. The obvious estimator of the district-level mean is $\hat{\mu}_d = (y_{1d} + \cdots + y_{n_d d})/n_d$. It is unbiased and its sampling variance is $\sigma^2_{\mathrm{W}}/n_d$. If the district-level means were identical, $\mu_1 = \ldots = \mu_D$, the overall sample mean $\hat{\mu} = (n_1\hat{\mu}_1 + \cdots + n_D\hat{\mu}_D)/n$ would be much more efficient for every district: $\mathrm{E}(\hat{\mu}) = \mu \equiv \mu_d$, and $\mathrm{var}(\hat{\mu}) = \sigma^2_{\mathrm{W}}/n$ is much smaller than $\mathrm{var}(\hat{\mu}_d)$. Since the gain in efficiency, from $\sigma^2_{\mathrm{W}}/n_d$ to σ^2_{W}/n would be quite dramatic for most districts (those with $n_d \ll n$), we can afford to incur some bias in estimating μ_d by $\hat{\mu}$, even when the districts do not have identical means. Finally, instead of arbitrating between $\hat{\mu}_d$ and $\hat{\mu}$ as estimators of μ_d, we should search for their convex combination that minimises the MSE. The composite estimator aims to do just that, although we developed it in Section 6.3 without a reference to any models.

7.2 Auxiliary information

The precision of a direct estimator of a district-level quantity θ_d is limited by the sample size n_d and the district-level variance $\sigma^2_{\mathrm{B}} = \mathrm{var}_D(\theta_D)$. Neither the sample size nor σ^2_{B} can be altered; n_d because it has been realised and σ^2_{B} because it is a characteristic of the population (a population quantity). Although the districts differ, often substantially, some of their variation may be accounted for by an association with one or several variables, either observed in the same survey or with its values available from other sources.

For example, the mean income may be higher on average in urban than rural districts. This information could be exploited by analysing rural and urban districts separately. We then estimate θ_d more efficiently if the district-level variance is smaller for both urban and rural districts than it is for the whole country. On the one hand, the estimate of the district-level variance is based on less data for both urban and rural districts, so it may be less precise. On the other hand, smaller variances tend to be estimated with higher precision (holding the sample size fixed), so the district-level variance is estimated not necessarily with less precision for a subpopulation than for the entire population.

Income is associated with educational level and age. It is plausible that such an association is present even at the district level — the districts have different mean incomes, but the within-district associations of income with educational level and age are much more similar. If by an adjustment for educational level and age the district-level mean incomes did become more similar, we could gain efficiency by estimating first the adjusted mean income for the district, and then correcting it for the deviations of the educational and age profiles from the national average.

An appropriate model for such an approach has to combine regression and ANOVA. This leads to models for analysis of covariance (ANCOVA) and their versions with random effects (rANCOVA). The latter class is generally referred to as two-level (a special case of *multilevel*) or *random coefficient* models. For a single covariate x recorded for every subject in the sample, we consider the rANCOVA model

$$y_{jd} = \beta_0 + \beta_1 x_{jd} + \delta_d + \varepsilon_{jd} \,, \tag{7.5}$$

with mutually independent random terms δ_d and ε_{jd}, with zero means and respective variances σ_{B}^2 and σ_{W}^2. Commonly, normality of these random terms is assumed. This, together with linearity, $\mathrm{E}(y) = \beta_0 + \beta_1 x$, and homoscedasticity, $\mathrm{var}(y \,|\, \delta_d) = \sigma_{\mathrm{W}}^2 = \mathrm{const}$, make the model in (7.5) rather restrictive. Either of these three conditions can be promoted by a transformation of x (and y), although promoting one condition may be at the expense of the other two.

The model in (7.5) implies a simple regression, $y = \beta_0 + \beta_1 x + \varepsilon$, in an average (typical) district in which $\delta_d = 0$. Within the districts, y is related to x, with parallel regressions; the within-district regressions share the same slope β_1, but differ in their intercepts $\beta_0 + \delta_d$. This model is also referred to as random-intercept model. If the model is too restrictive, the regressions can be 'let loose' by introducing district-specific deviations of the slope on x:

$$y_{jd} = \beta_0 + \beta_1 x_{jd} + \delta_{0,d} + \delta_{1,d} x_{jd} + \varepsilon_{jd} \,, \tag{7.6}$$

where $(\delta_{0,d}\,, \delta_{1,d})^\top$ have a bivariate normal distribution with mean $(0,0)^\top$ and variance matrix $\mathbf{\Sigma}$. The districts have regressions

$$\mathrm{E}(y_{jd} \,|\, \delta_{0,d}\,, \delta_{1,d}) = \beta_0 + \delta_{0,d} + (\beta_1 + \delta_{1,d}) x_{jd} \,,$$

each with residual variance σ_{W}^2. It is too restrictive to assume that the covariance in $\mathbf{\Sigma}$ vanishes. In fact, the covariance (or the correlation) in $\mathbf{\Sigma}$ indicates the pattern of variation of the regressions and it controls the value x^* at which the regressions attain their minimum variance. Let $\Sigma_h = \mathrm{var}_{\mathcal{D}}(\delta_{h,\mathcal{D}})$, $h = 0, 1$, and $\Sigma_{01} = \mathrm{cov}_{\mathcal{D}}(\delta_{0,\mathcal{D}}\,, \delta_{1,\mathcal{D}})$ be the elements of $\mathbf{\Sigma}$. Then the variance of the within-district regressions at a point x is

$$\begin{pmatrix} 1 \\ x \end{pmatrix}^\top \mathbf{\Sigma} \begin{pmatrix} 1 \\ x \end{pmatrix} = \Sigma_0 + 2\Sigma_{01} x + \Sigma_1 x^2 \,.$$

The minimum of this variance, $\Sigma_0 - \Sigma_{01}^2/\Sigma_1$, is attained for $x^* = -\Sigma_{01}/\Sigma_1$. Thus, when $\mathbf{\Sigma}$ is singular all the regressions cross at the point $(x^*, \beta_0 + \beta_1 x^*)$, unless $\Sigma_1 = 0$, in which case the regressions are parallel and $\mathrm{var}(y) = \sigma_{\mathrm{W}}^2 + \Sigma_0$ is constant. Identical regressions correspond to $\mathbf{\Sigma} = \mathbf{0}$.

Figure 7.1 gives examples of sets of varying regressions. In each panel, the intercepts and slopes have unit variances, and their correlation is given in the subtitle. In panel A, the intercepts and slopes are uncorrelated; there $x^* = 0$. In panel F, the intercepts and slopes are strongly negatively correlated; their lines cross in a narrow band around $x = 1$. When the intercepts and slopes

Figure 7.1. Sets of random regressions. Computer generated examples.

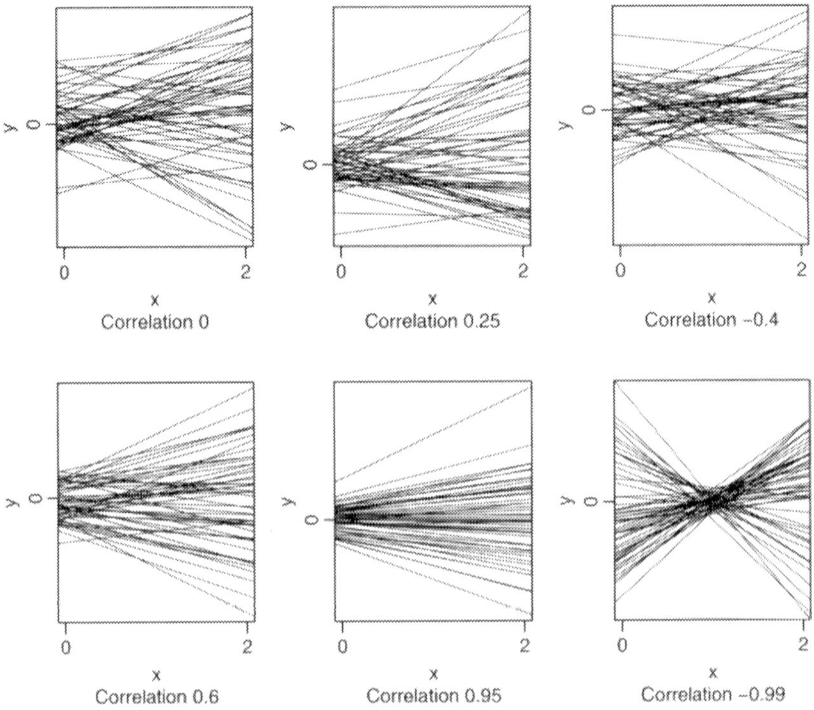

Correlation 0

Correlation 0.25

Correlation −0.4

Correlation 0.6

Correlation 0.95

Correlation −0.99

are strongly positively correlated, the regression lines intersect near a negative value of x, as in panel E.

If we move the origin of x, by a transformation $x^\dagger = x - c$, the pattern of the lines is not altered, but the 'window' is moved, from $(0, 2)$ in the panels in Figure 7.1 to $(c, 2+c)$. The covariance Σ_{01} and the variance of the intercepts, Σ_0, are also changed. The variance matrix for the model with $x^\dagger$ is

$$\mathbf{\Sigma}^\dagger = \begin{pmatrix} 1 & c \\ 0 & 1 \end{pmatrix} \mathbf{\Sigma} \begin{pmatrix} 1 & c \\ 0 & 1 \end{pmatrix}^\top .$$

Therefore, if we could conceivably use $x^\dagger$ instead of x as a covariate, we cannot assume that the covariance Σ_{01} vanishes or attains any specific value.

7.2.1 Several covariates

With several covariates, we specify the general two-level regression model as

$$\mathbf{y}_d = \mathbf{X}_d \boldsymbol{\beta} + \mathbf{X}_d \boldsymbol{\delta}_d + \boldsymbol{\varepsilon}_d , \tag{7.7}$$

where $\varepsilon_d \sim \mathcal{N}(\mathbf{0}_{n_d}, \sigma_W^2 \mathbf{I}_{n_d})$ and $\boldsymbol{\delta}_d \sim \mathcal{N}(\mathbf{0}_p, \boldsymbol{\Sigma})$, independently. ($\mathbf{0}$ is the vector of zeros of length indicated by its subscript and $\mathbf{I}$ is used similarly for the identity matrix.) The model parameters are $\boldsymbol{\beta}$ (a $p \times 1$ vector), the residual variance σ_W^2, and the $(p \times p)$ district-level variance matrix $\boldsymbol{\Sigma}$. This variance matrix has $\frac{1}{2}p(p+1)$ unique parameters and they characterise the pattern of the within-district regressions $\mathrm{E}(\mathbf{y}_d \,|\, \boldsymbol{\delta}_d) = \mathbf{X}_d(\boldsymbol{\beta} + \boldsymbol{\delta}_d)$:

$$\mathrm{var}_{\mathcal{D}} \left\{ \mathrm{E}(\mathbf{y}_d \,|\, \delta_{\mathcal{D}}\,;\, \mathbf{X}_d) \right\} \;=\; \mathbf{X}_d \boldsymbol{\Sigma} \mathbf{X}_d^{\top} \,.$$

The model in (7.7) can be paired up with the ANCOVA model which differs from it only by the assumptions about $\boldsymbol{\delta}_d$. In ANCOVA, the $\boldsymbol{\delta}_d$ are (fixed) parameters and the differences among the slopes in (7.7) are represented by the slope-by-district interactions. When there are many districts (groups) d the district-level variation is described by the $\frac{1}{2}p(p+1)$ (co-)variance parameters in rANCOVA more parsimoniously than by the $D(p-1)$ interaction parameters in the ANCOVA model.

Just as in ANCOVA we prefer models with fewer sets of interactions, in (7.7) we can also restrict the pattern of district-level variation. This is done by assuming that certain variances in $\boldsymbol{\Sigma}$ vanish. With each variance that is set to zero, all the covariances in the same row and column of $\boldsymbol{\Sigma}$ are also constrained to zero. If all the regression slopes are constrained in this way, only the intercepts vary,

$$\mathbf{y}_d \;=\; \mathbf{X}_d \boldsymbol{\beta} + \delta_{0,d} + \varepsilon_d \,; \tag{7.8}$$

now the regression lines are parallel and $\boldsymbol{\Sigma}$ contains only one parameter, the intercept variance.

As an alternative to the notation in (7.7) with the constraints on $\boldsymbol{\Sigma}$, we can write

$$\mathbf{y}_d \;=\; \mathbf{X}_d \boldsymbol{\beta} + \mathbf{Z}_d \boldsymbol{\gamma}_d + \varepsilon_d \,, \tag{7.9}$$

where $\mathbf{Z}_d$ is formed by the columns of $\mathbf{X}_d$ for which the within-district regressions vary (the corresponding variances in $\boldsymbol{\Sigma}$ are positive). The number of variables in each $\mathbf{Z}_d$ is denoted by r. The variables in $\mathbf{Z}$ are said to be *associated with variation*. For example, in (7.8), only the intercept is associated with variation; $\mathbf{Z} = \mathbf{1}$ and $r = 1$. The p variables in $\mathbf{X}$ are said to form the *regression part* and those in $\mathbf{Z}$ (associated with district-level variation) the *district-level variation part* of the model. The regression and variation parts are also referred to as the respective fixed and random parts of the model.

The analogy between ANCOVA and two-level models suggests a general strategy for selecting variables into the variation part. The regression part can be equated to the main effects and the variation part to the interactions in ANCOVA. First, the variation part should not contain any variables not included in the regression part — interactions in ANCOVA are not meaningful without the associated main effects. Second, we should be more selective about including variables in the variation than in the regression part — the model should have fewer sets of interactions than it has main effects. And finally, it is more appropriate to include a variable in the variation part when it is important in the regression part — it is more meaningful to consider interactions for variables that have substantial main effects. Variables that have values constant within each district, or are defined for districts, should not be included in the variation part because the within-district slopes on these variables are not identified. Variables that vary much less within districts than among districts should not be included in the variation part either, because their within-district slopes are poorly identified.

These rules imitate the conventions universally adopted in ANCOVA. In rANCOVA, they may be broken; such models may be meaningful, but the interpretation in terms of varying regressions is no longer applicable. For example, a district-level variable z may be included in the variation part, but its role is solely to model variance heterogeneity, the dependence of the variance $\mathrm{var}(y)$ on z.

Subject- and district-level models

The two-level model has an alternative formulation in terms of a subject- and a district-level model. Let $\mathbf{X} = \left(\mathbf{X}^{(1)}, \mathbf{X}^{(2)}\right)$ be the partitioning of the covariates (columns of $\mathbf{X}$) to variables defined for subjects and districts, respectively. The variation part is selected from the variables in $\mathbf{X}^{(1)}$.

We can formulate separate regression models for subjects and districts:

$$
\begin{aligned}
\mathbf{y}_d &= \mathbf{X}_d^{(1)} \boldsymbol{\beta}_d^{(1)} + \boldsymbol{\varepsilon}_d \\
\boldsymbol{\beta}_d^{(1)} &= \boldsymbol{\beta}^{(2)} \mathbf{x}_d^{(2)\top} + \boldsymbol{\gamma}_d \,,
\end{aligned}
\tag{7.10}
$$

where $\boldsymbol{\beta}^{(2)}$ is a matrix of parameters and $\mathbf{x}_d^{(2)}$ a row of $\mathbf{X}_d^{(2)}$. (The rows of $\mathbf{X}_d^{(2)}$ are identical for the subjects in district d.) The equation for $\boldsymbol{\beta}_d^{(1)}$ is a (multivariate) model for the (within-district) regression coefficients. Note that with the variables in $\mathbf{X}^{(2)}$ their interactions with $\mathbf{X}^{(1)}$ are also included in the model:

$$
\mathbf{y}_d = \mathbf{X}_d^{(1)} \boldsymbol{\beta}^{(2)} \mathbf{x}_d^{(2)\top} + \mathbf{X}_d^{(1)} \boldsymbol{\gamma}_d + \boldsymbol{\varepsilon}_d \,;
$$

compare with (7.9). Unless several parameters in $\boldsymbol{\beta}^{(2)}$ are constrained to zero, the interactions are absent only when the model for $\boldsymbol{\beta}_d^{(1)}$ is univariate, that is, when $\mathbf{X}_d^{(1)} = \mathbf{1}$ and a district-level model is specified only for the intercept.

The model formulation by (7.10) suggests that the effective sample size for certain parameters is n (σ_{W}^2 and the components of $\boldsymbol{\beta}_d^{(1)}$ that are constant across the districts), while for others (the parameters in $\boldsymbol{\beta}^{(2)}$ and $\boldsymbol{\Sigma}$) it is only D. District-level variables $\mathbf{X}^{(2)}$ can reduce only the district-level variation. Some subject-level variables vary not only within but also across districts; so, even if defined for subjects, they may contribute to reducing the district-level variation.

The district-level model in (7.10) may contain variables that are aggregates, such as the district-level means of some subject-level variables. The means, or other summaries, should be for the population, not the sample. The sample means are correlated with the subject-level variables, and their use raises some issues related to measurement errors in covariates.

7.2.2 Two-level models and small-area estimation

The variables in $\mathbf{X}$, used in the regression for the target variable $\mathbf{y}$, are called *auxiliary*. Their purpose, and the purpose of the models in which they are involved, is to contribute to small-area estimation, that is, to enable estimation of district-level population quantities with greater efficiency than if their values were not available. Having defined a rich class of models by (7.7) or (7.9), we have to choose a suitable model on which to base our inferences — to estimate the district-level means. Although in Chapter 11 we question the appropriateness of this general approach, we adhere here to this long-honoured convention.

We may start with a general model and search for terms in its regression and variation parts that are redundant — the quality of the model fit is reduced insubstantially by excluding them from the model. This may be accomplished in several steps, excluding variables one-by-one and reviewing the model fit at every step. Since the iterative procedures for fitting these models are more complex for more extensive variation parts, it is practical to start with a relatively simple model and look for variables that improve the model fit when included (first) in the regression and (then) in the variation part of the model. As an alternative, we may start with an extensive regression part and a trivial variation part (parallel district-level regressions), and proceed by reducing the regression and expanding the variation part, without breaking the ANCOVA-motivated convention that the variation part is subsumed in the regression part. (No interactions should be retained without both of their main effects.) For the selected model, the mean for a small area is estimated by the multivariate version of (7.3):

$$\hat{\bar{y}}_d = \overline{\mathbf{x}}_d\hat{\boldsymbol{\beta}} + \overline{\mathbf{z}}_d\hat{\boldsymbol{\gamma}}_d ,$$

where $\overline{\mathbf{x}}_d$ and $\overline{\mathbf{z}}_d$ are the within-district sample means of the covariates $\mathbf{x}$ and $\mathbf{z}$, $\hat{\boldsymbol{\beta}}$ is the estimate of $\boldsymbol{\beta}$ obtained by fitting the model in (7.9) and

$$\hat{\boldsymbol{\gamma}}_d = \mathrm{E}(\boldsymbol{\gamma}_d \,|\, \mathbf{y}) = \hat{\boldsymbol{\Omega}}\left(\mathbf{I}_r + \mathbf{Z}_d^\top\mathbf{Z}_d\hat{\boldsymbol{\Omega}}\right)^{-1}\mathbf{Z}_d^\top(\mathbf{y}_d - \mathbf{X}_d\hat{\boldsymbol{\beta}}) ;$$

$\hat{\boldsymbol{\Omega}}$ is the estimate of the scaled variance matrix $\sigma_{\mathrm{W}}^{-2}\boldsymbol{\Gamma}$ and $\boldsymbol{\Gamma} = \mathrm{var}(\boldsymbol{\gamma}_d)$. Details of the estimation procedure are given in the next section.

7.3 Computational procedures

Maximum likelihood (ML) is the traditional workhorse for models for which there are no intuitively derived estimation procedures. Many estimators derived by other methods are either ML or closely related to ML. In brief, ML has little competition in the field of efficient estimation. Its application is supported by powerful results about *asymptotic* efficiency — good properties for large samples, although what constitutes a large enough sample is often difficult to establish. Apart from the large enough sample size, another important caveat is that the properties of ML estimators refer to 'when the model applies'. In practice, we make an effort to identify *an* appropriate model, a parsimonious model that is not contradicted by the data, and then proceed regarding it as *the* model. Chapter 11 discusses this and related issues in greater depth.

The likelihood is defined as the joint density of the observations, regarded as a function of the parameters:

$$L(\boldsymbol{\theta}; \mathbf{y}, \mathbf{X}) \;=\; f(\mathbf{y}; \boldsymbol{\theta}, \mathbf{X}) \,.$$

That is, the roles of the data (argument of the density function f) and parameters (argument of the likelihood L) are interchanged. ML is defined as the global maximum of L, that is, as the vector of parameters for which the joint density *would be* the highest. Throughout, we work with the log-likelihood, $l = \log(L)$, because its maximisation is easier.

For the model in (7.9), with the usual assumptions of normality and independence of the random terms γ and ε, the log-likelihood is

$$l \;=\; -\frac{1}{2}\left\{ n\log(2\pi) + \sum_{d=1}^{D} \log(\det \mathbf{V}_d) + \sum_{d=1}^{D} \mathbf{e}_d^\top \mathbf{V}_d^{-1} \mathbf{e}_d \right\} , \qquad (7.11)$$

where $\mathbf{V}_d \;=\; \mathrm{var}(\mathbf{y}_d)$ is the variance matrix of the observations in district d and $\mathbf{e}_d \;=\; \mathbf{y}_d - \mathbf{X}_d\boldsymbol{\beta}$ is the vector of residuals for observations in district d. The summations in (7.11) can be dispensed with by defining $\mathbf{X}$ as the matrix constructed by vertically stacking $\mathbf{X}_d$, $d = 1, \ldots, D$, conforming with $\mathbf{y} = (\mathbf{y}_1^\top, \ldots, \mathbf{y}_D^\top)^\top$, defining $\mathbf{e} = \mathbf{y} - \mathbf{X}\boldsymbol{\beta}$ and denoting $\mathbf{V} = \mathrm{var}(\mathbf{y})$. $\mathbf{V}$ is the block-diagonal matrix composed of blocks $\mathbf{V}_d$. Then

$$l \;=\; -\frac{1}{2}\left\{ n\log(2\pi) + \log(\det \mathbf{V}) + \mathbf{e}^\top \mathbf{V}^{-1} \mathbf{e} \right\} \,.$$

Also, $\mathbf{X}^\top \mathbf{V}^{-1} \mathbf{X} = \sum_d \mathbf{X}_d^\top \mathbf{V}_d^{-1} \mathbf{X}_d$, and similarly for any other quadratic form in $\mathbf{V}^{-1}$. The model in (7.9) implies that

$$\mathbf{V}_d \;=\; \sigma_{\mathrm{W}}^2 \mathbf{I}_{n_d} + \mathbf{Z}_d \boldsymbol{\Sigma} \mathbf{Z}_d^\top \,.$$

A one-to-one reparametrisation of $(\sigma_{\mathrm{W}}^2, \boldsymbol{\Sigma})$ does not alter the model fit (the ML solution). It is advantageous to work with the scaled (relative) variance matrix $\mathbf{\Omega} = \sigma_{\mathrm{W}}^{-2}\mathbf{\Sigma}$ and with the matrices $\mathbf{W}_d = \sigma_{\mathrm{W}}^{-2}\mathbf{V}_d = \mathbf{I}_{n_d} + \mathbf{Z}_d\mathbf{\Omega}\mathbf{Z}_d^{\top}$ and $\mathbf{W} = \sigma_{\mathrm{W}}^{-2}\mathbf{V}$ which, with $\mathbf{\Omega}$, do not involve σ_{W}^2. The log-likelihood (7.11) can be expressed as

$$l = -\frac{1}{2}\left\{n\log(2\pi\sigma_{\mathrm{W}}^2) + \log(\det\mathbf{W}) + \frac{1}{\sigma_{\mathrm{W}}^2}\mathbf{e}^{\top}\mathbf{W}^{-1}\mathbf{e}\right\}. \tag{7.12}$$

Its maximum is found as the root of the vector of the first-order partial differentials of l. For $\boldsymbol{\beta}$, we have

$$\frac{\partial l}{\partial \boldsymbol{\beta}} = \frac{1}{\sigma_{\mathrm{W}}^2}\mathbf{X}^{\top}\mathbf{W}^{-1}\mathbf{e},$$

and its root is the weighted least squares (WLS) estimator

$$\hat{\boldsymbol{\beta}} = \left(\mathbf{X}^{\top}\hat{\mathbf{W}}^{-1}\mathbf{X}\right)^{-1}\mathbf{X}^{\top}\hat{\mathbf{W}}^{-1}\mathbf{y}. \tag{7.13}$$

Note that (7.13) depends on the estimate of $\mathbf{\Omega}$, involved in $\hat{\mathbf{W}}$. The partial differential of l with respect to σ_{W}^2 is

$$\frac{\partial l}{\partial \sigma_{\mathrm{W}}^2} = -\frac{1}{2}\left(\frac{n}{\sigma_{\mathrm{W}}^2} - \frac{1}{\sigma_{\mathrm{W}}^4}\mathbf{e}^{\top}\mathbf{W}^{-1}\mathbf{e}\right);$$

hence

$$\hat{\sigma}_{\mathrm{W}}^2 = \frac{1}{n}\hat{\mathbf{e}}^{\top}\hat{\mathbf{W}}^{-1}\hat{\mathbf{e}}. \tag{7.14}$$

This simple expression is obtained owing to the $\mathbf{\Omega}$-parametrisation.

For evaluating a quadratic form $\mathbf{u}_1^{\top}\mathbf{W}^{-1}\mathbf{u}_2$ for an arbitrary pair of vectors $\mathbf{u}_1$ and $\mathbf{u}_2$ of length n each, neither $\mathbf{W}$ nor its inverse $\mathbf{W}^{-1}$ have to be formed. Their blocks $\mathbf{W}_d$ and $\mathbf{W}_d^{-1}$ do not have to be formed either, as we show in Section 7.3.2.

Finally, for ω, an element of $\mathbf{\Omega}$, we have

$$\frac{\partial l}{\partial \omega} = -\frac{1}{2}\sum_{d=1}^{D}\mathrm{tr}\left(\mathbf{W}_d^{-1}\mathbf{Z}_d\frac{\partial\mathbf{\Omega}}{\partial\omega}\mathbf{Z}_d^{\top}\right)$$
$$+\frac{1}{2\sigma_{\mathrm{W}}^2}\sum_{d=1}^{D}\mathbf{e}_d^{\top}\mathbf{W}_d^{-1}\mathbf{Z}_d\frac{\partial\mathbf{\Omega}}{\partial\omega}\mathbf{Z}_d^{\top}\mathbf{W}_d^{-1}\mathbf{e}_d. \tag{7.15}$$

The partial differential $\partial\mathbf{\Omega}/\partial\omega$ is a matrix of the same dimensions as $\mathbf{\Omega}$. If ω is a variance $\partial\mathbf{\Omega}/\partial\omega$ is a matrix containing zeros in every element except for the location of ω, where there is a unity. If ω is a covariance $\partial\mathbf{\Omega}/\partial\omega$ contains zeros everywhere except for unities at the two locations to which ω refers. In principle, any parametrisation for $\mathbf{\Omega}$ can be used; some options are discussed in Section 7.3.2. All the terms in (7.15) can be evaluated from $\mathbf{Z}_d^{\top}\mathbf{W}_d^{-1}\mathbf{Z}_d$ and $\mathbf{e}_d^{\top}\mathbf{W}_d^{-1}\mathbf{Z}_d$, $d = 1, \ldots, D$, as the totals of products of their elements.

The root of (7.15) cannot be found analytically. The Newton-Raphson algorithm is a general method for locating the extremes of analytical functions. It proceeds by iterations of the formula

$$\hat{\boldsymbol{\theta}}_{\mathrm{new}} = \hat{\boldsymbol{\theta}}_{\mathrm{old}} + \boldsymbol{\mathcal{H}}^{-1}(\hat{\boldsymbol{\theta}}_{\mathrm{old}})\, \mathbf{s}(\hat{\boldsymbol{\theta}}_{\mathrm{old}})\,, \tag{7.16}$$

where $\mathbf{s}(\boldsymbol{\theta})$ is the vector of first-order partial differentials of l and $-\boldsymbol{\mathcal{H}}(\boldsymbol{\theta})$ the matrix of its second-order partial differentials with respect to $\boldsymbol{\theta}$. The vector $\mathbf{s}$ is called the *score* vector and $-\boldsymbol{\mathcal{H}}$ the *Hessian* matrix. A more rigorous notation is $\boldsymbol{\mathcal{H}}_{\boldsymbol{\theta}}(\hat{\boldsymbol{\theta}})$, indicating that the partial differentials are with respect to $\boldsymbol{\theta}$ and are evaluated at $\boldsymbol{\theta} = \hat{\boldsymbol{\theta}}$. When no ambiguity arises or the arguments are immaterial, one or both arguments are dropped.

The second-order partial differential with respect to any two parameters in $\boldsymbol{\Omega}$ is

$$\begin{aligned}
\frac{\partial^2 l}{\partial \omega_1\, \partial \omega_2} &= \frac{1}{2} \sum_{d=1}^{D} \mathrm{tr} \left(\mathbf{Z}_d^{\top} \mathbf{W}_d^{-1} \mathbf{Z}_d \frac{\partial \boldsymbol{\Omega}}{\partial \omega_1} \mathbf{Z}_d^{\top} \mathbf{W}_d^{-1} \mathbf{Z}_d \frac{\partial \boldsymbol{\Omega}}{\partial \omega_2} \right) \\
&\quad - \frac{1}{\sigma_{\mathrm{W}}^2} \sum_{d=1}^{D} \mathbf{e}_d^{\top} \mathbf{W}_d^{-1} \mathbf{Z}_d \frac{\partial \boldsymbol{\Omega}}{\partial \omega_1} \mathbf{Z}_d^{\top} \mathbf{W}_d^{-1} \mathbf{Z}_d \frac{\partial \boldsymbol{\Omega}}{\partial \omega_2} \mathbf{Z}_d^{\top} \mathbf{W}_d^{-1} \mathbf{e}_d \\
&\quad - \frac{1}{2} \sum_{d=1}^{D} \mathrm{tr} \left(\mathbf{Z}_d^{\top} \mathbf{W}_d^{-1} \mathbf{Z}_d \frac{\partial^2 \boldsymbol{\Omega}}{\partial \omega_1\, \partial \omega_2} \right) \\
&\quad + \frac{1}{2\sigma_{\mathrm{W}}^2} \sum_{d=1}^{D} \mathbf{e}_d^{\top} \mathbf{W}_d^{-1} \mathbf{Z}_d \frac{\partial^2 \boldsymbol{\Omega}}{\partial \omega_1\, \partial \omega_2} \mathbf{Z}_d^{\top} \mathbf{W}_d^{-1} \mathbf{e}_d \,.
\end{aligned} \tag{7.17}$$

This is a formidable expression, although it simplifies somewhat when $\boldsymbol{\Omega}$ is a linear function of both ω_1 and ω_2 (for example, when ω_1 and ω_2 are variances or covariances in $\boldsymbol{\Omega}$); then the last two terms, involving $\partial^2 \boldsymbol{\Omega} / (\partial \omega_1\, \partial \omega_2)$, vanish. But the entire expression is composed of cross-products of the elements of $\mathbf{Z}_d^{\top} \mathbf{W}_d^{-1} \mathbf{Z}_d$ and $\mathbf{Z}_d^{\top} \mathbf{W}_d^{-1} \mathbf{e}_d$, so its evaluation is not any more complex than for the other expressions required for maximising l.

The negative of the Hessian,

$$\boldsymbol{\mathcal{H}}_{\boldsymbol{\theta}} = -\frac{\partial^2 l}{\partial \boldsymbol{\theta}\, \partial \boldsymbol{\theta}^{\top}}\,,$$

where $\boldsymbol{\theta}$ is a vector of all the parameters involved in l, is also called the *observed information matrix*. As $\boldsymbol{\mathcal{H}}$ is defined for a parameter vector, it is altered by reparametrisation. $\boldsymbol{\mathcal{H}}$ is defined for the entire vector of parameters in the two-level model, comprising $\boldsymbol{\beta}$, σ_{W}^2 and $\boldsymbol{\omega}$, the vector of all the independent elements of $\boldsymbol{\Omega}$. The off-diagonal elements of $\boldsymbol{\mathcal{H}}$ that involve σ_{W}^2 and an element of $\boldsymbol{\omega}$ or $\boldsymbol{\beta}$ are of no importance, although they do not vanish.

The expectation of $\boldsymbol{\mathcal{H}}$ is called the *expected information matrix* and is denoted by $\boldsymbol{\mathcal{I}}$; $\boldsymbol{\mathcal{I}} = \mathrm{E}(\boldsymbol{\mathcal{H}})$. The theoretical importance of $\boldsymbol{\mathcal{I}}$ is that, under certain regularity conditions, its inverse is the *asymptotic* sampling variance matrix of the ML estimator;

$$a\mathrm{var}(\hat{\boldsymbol{\theta}}) = \{\mathcal{I}(\boldsymbol{\theta})\}^{-1} .$$

In practice, the qualifier 'asymptotic' (a in $a$var) is ignored. In large-scale surveys, this is appropriate for *some* parameters. Another important qualification is that $\mathcal{I}$ depends on unknown parameters, sometimes even on the target of estimation. So, we can at best *estimate* $\mathcal{I}$, by $\hat{\mathcal{I}}$. Having done so, caution is called for in estimating $\mathcal{I}^{-1}$ by $\hat{\mathcal{I}}^{-1}$. Conventionally, the square roots of the diagonal entries of $\hat{\mathcal{I}}^{-1}$ are quoted as the *standard errors.* We should bear in mind that they are *estimated* and they are problematic because of the string of non-linear operations (including matrix inversion) and naive estimation involved in their evaluation. The problems are most acute when the matrix $\hat{\mathcal{I}}$ is ill-conditioned.

Further imprecision in working with $\hat{\mathcal{I}}$ may occur when we invert its submatrix corresponding to the parameters of interest, instead of the whole matrix. With two-level models, this is not a problem for the separate sets of parameters $\boldsymbol{\beta}$ (regression), σ^2_{W} (within-district variation) and $\boldsymbol{\omega}$ (district-level variation), because $\mathcal{I}$ is block-diagonal, with its blocks corresponding to these sets of parameters. For example,

$$-\mathrm{E}\left(\frac{\partial^2 l}{\partial\boldsymbol{\beta}\,\partial\boldsymbol{\omega}}\right) = \mathbf{X}^\top\frac{\partial\mathbf{W}^{-1}}{\partial\boldsymbol{\omega}}\mathrm{E}(\mathbf{e}) = \mathbf{0} .$$

Furthermore, if the uncertainty about $\boldsymbol{\Omega}$ is ignored, $\mathrm{var}(\hat{\boldsymbol{\beta}}) = \mathcal{I}_{\boldsymbol{\beta}}^{-1}$ without a reference to asymptotics. This is derived from (7.13) directly:

$$\begin{aligned} &\mathrm{var}\left\{\left(\mathbf{X}^\top\mathbf{W}^{-1}\mathbf{X}\right)^{-1}\mathbf{X}^\top\mathbf{W}^{-1}\mathbf{y}\right\} \\ &= \sigma^2_{\mathrm{W}}\left(\mathbf{X}^\top\mathbf{W}^{-1}\mathbf{X}\right)^{-1}\mathbf{X}^\top\mathbf{W}^{-1}\mathbf{X}\left(\mathbf{X}^\top\mathbf{W}^{-1}\mathbf{X}\right)^{-1} \\ &= \sigma^2_{\mathrm{W}}\left(\mathbf{X}^\top\mathbf{W}^{-1}\mathbf{X}\right)^{-1} , \end{aligned}$$

assuming that $\boldsymbol{\Omega}$ and σ^2_{W} are known. Therefore, the quoted standard errors for $\hat{\boldsymbol{\beta}}$, derived from

$$\hat{\mathcal{I}}_{\boldsymbol{\beta}} = \hat{\sigma}^{-2}_{\mathrm{W}}\mathbf{X}^\top\hat{\mathbf{W}}^{-1}\mathbf{X} ,$$

are not tainted by any asymptotic dependence of $\hat{\boldsymbol{\beta}}$ and $\hat{\boldsymbol{\Omega}}$. The residual variance σ^2_{W} is usually estimated with high precision, and so the elements of $\mathcal{I}$ that involve σ^2_{W} are of no concern.

The reference to asymptotics is contentious for the parameters in $\boldsymbol{\Omega}$ because their sample size is more appropriately characterised by the number of districts, and even that may be an overstatement. To see this, suppose that the variance σ^2_{W} and the deviations γ_d, $d = 1, \ldots, D$, are known. Then the scaled variance matrix $\boldsymbol{\Omega}$ is estimated by scaling the sample variance matrix of γ_d, centred around $\mathbf{0}$, so it is distributed according to the scaled multivariate χ^2 (Wishart) distribution with D degrees of freedom. When the γ_d are not known each element of $\boldsymbol{\Omega}$ is bound to be estimated with less precision or, after matching to a χ^2 distribution, with fewer degrees of freedom than D.

The importance of $\hat{\mathcal{I}}$ for computations is that it is a more stable approximation to or estimator of $\mathcal{H}$. For maximising the log-likelihood, it is advantageous to replace $\hat{\mathcal{H}}$ by $\hat{\mathcal{I}}$; this induces some stability in the iterations, but also in many settings (including ours), the expression for $\mathcal{I}$ is simpler and easier to evaluate than for $\mathcal{H}$. The Newton-Raphson with this adaptation is called the Fisher scoring algorithm.

As $\mathcal{H}_{\boldsymbol{\beta}} = -\sigma_{\mathrm{W}}^{-2}\mathbf{X}^\top\mathbf{W}^{-1}\mathbf{X}$ does not depend on $\mathbf{y}$, $\mathcal{I}_{\boldsymbol{\beta}} = \mathcal{H}_{\boldsymbol{\beta}}$. For a pair of parameters involved in $\boldsymbol{\Omega}$, the expectation of (7.17) reduces to

$$-\mathrm{E}\left(\frac{\partial^2 l}{\partial\omega_1\,\partial\omega_2}\right) = \frac{1}{2}\sum_{d=1}^{D}\mathrm{tr}\left(\mathbf{Z}_d^\top\mathbf{W}_d^{-1}\mathbf{Z}_d\,\frac{\partial\boldsymbol{\Omega}}{\partial\omega_1}\,\mathbf{Z}_d^\top\mathbf{W}_d^{-1}\mathbf{Z}_d\,\frac{\partial\boldsymbol{\Omega}}{\partial\omega_2}\right). \qquad (7.18)$$

7.3.1 Restricted maximum likelihood

An apparent deficiency of ML is that its estimators of the variances are biased. For example, the denominator in (7.14) is n, whereas intuition and an analogy with ordinary least squares (OLS) suggest that it should be $n - p$. In fact, the ML estimator of the residual variance in the ordinary regression model also has the denominator n, whereas the denominator $n - p$ would yield an unbiased estimator of σ^2. The p degrees of freedom are lost because the p regression parameters in $\boldsymbol{\beta}$ are not known; ML procedures are oblivious to this fact. If $\boldsymbol{\beta}$ were known $\hat{\sigma}_{\mathrm{W}}^2$ in (7.14) would be unbiased.

A conceptual remedy for this deficiency of ML is to maximise the likelihood of the so-called 'error' contrasts of the outcomes ([204] and [94]). These contrasts $\mathbf{y}^*$ are a linear transformation of the outcomes $\mathbf{y}$ that is orthogonal and complementary to the regression design space spanned by $\mathbf{X}$. The transformation is not unique, but yields the same likelihood function, apart from a constant factor that is irrelevant for likelihood maximisation. A practical choice for the transformation is the projection $\mathbf{y}^* = \left\{\mathbf{I} - \mathbf{X}\left(\mathbf{X}^\top\mathbf{X}\right)^{-1}\mathbf{X}^\top\right\}\mathbf{y}$, and the resulting log-likelihood is

$$l_{\mathrm{R}} = l + \frac{1}{2}\log\left\{\det\left(\mathbf{X}^\top\mathbf{V}^{-1}\mathbf{X}\right)\right\}. \qquad (7.19)$$

This (log-)likelihood is called *restricted*, as opposed to the *full* (log-)likelihood in (7.11). The qualifiers 'full' and 'restricted', or ML and REML, are also used for the estimators obtained by maximising the respective likelihoods. They are not meant to indicate any superiority of l over l_{R}.

Since l_{R} is an adjustment of the original ('full') likelihood, it can be maximised by suitably adapting the Newton-Raphson or Fisher scoring algorithm for maximising l. First, since the adjustment $\log\left\{\det\left(\mathbf{X}^\top\mathbf{V}^{-1}\mathbf{X}\right)\right\}$ in (7.19) does not involve $\boldsymbol{\beta}$, the WLS estimator in (7.13) is unchanged, except for a change in $\hat{\mathbf{W}}$ stemming from an altered estimator of $\boldsymbol{\Omega}$. Next, as

$$\det\left(\mathbf{X}^\top\mathbf{V}^{-1}\mathbf{X}\right) = \left(\sigma_{\mathrm{W}}^2\right)^p \det\left(\mathbf{X}^\top\mathbf{W}^{-1}\mathbf{X}\right)$$

and $\mathbf{W} = \sigma_{\mathrm{W}}^{-2}\mathbf{V}$ depends only on $\boldsymbol{\Omega}$,

$$\frac{\partial l_{\mathrm{R}}}{\partial \sigma_{\mathrm{W}}^2} = \frac{\partial l}{\partial \sigma_{\mathrm{W}}^2} + \frac{p}{2\sigma_{\mathrm{W}}^2}\,.$$

Hence the REML estimator is $\hat{\sigma}_{\mathrm{W}}^2 = \hat{\mathbf{e}}^\top\hat{\mathbf{W}}^{-1}\hat{\mathbf{e}}/(n-p)$; the denominator is adjusted for the regression degrees of freedom.

The adjustment for estimating $\boldsymbol{\Omega}$ is somewhat more difficult to derive, but is still straightforward to implement. The first-order partial differential with respect to an element of $\boldsymbol{\Omega}$ is

$$\frac{\partial l_{\mathrm{R}}}{\partial \omega} = \frac{\partial l}{\partial \omega} - \frac{1}{2\sigma_{\mathrm{W}}^2}\mathrm{tr}\left\{\left(\mathbf{X}^\top\mathbf{W}^{-1}\mathbf{X}\right)^{-1}\sum_{d=1}^{D}\left(\mathbf{X}_d^\top\mathbf{W}_d^{-1}\mathbf{Z}_d\,\frac{\partial\boldsymbol{\Omega}}{\partial\omega}\,\mathbf{Z}_d^\top\mathbf{W}_d^{-1}\mathbf{X}_d\right)\right\}. \tag{7.20}$$

To evaluate this expression we need, apart from $\partial l/\partial\omega$, the quadratic forms $\mathbf{X}_d^\top\mathbf{W}_d^{-1}\mathbf{Z}_d$; their total is $\mathbf{X}^\top\mathbf{W}^{-1}\mathbf{Z}$.

The second-order partial differentials are rather formidable expressions in the general case, and are usually not evaluated. Details are given in the Appendix. Maximisation of l_{R} can proceed with $\mathrm{E}\{-\partial^2 l/(\partial\omega_1\,\partial\omega_2)\}$ instead of its counterpart with l_{R}, ignoring the adjustment given by (7.33).

Data for small-area estimation usually contain several (tens of) thousands of records, so the REML adjustment for σ_{W}^2 is unimportant. The adjustment for $\boldsymbol{\Omega}$ is a different matter altogether, because the effective sample size for it is at most D. In fact, it would be D if each district were represented by so many subjects that each deviation γ_d would be (almost) known. In practice, the effective sample size (number of degrees of freedom) is much smaller. So, a small adjustment can make a lot of difference. The loss of p degrees of freedom for σ_{W}^2 is unimportant, but a similar loss for $\boldsymbol{\Sigma}_{\mathrm{B}}$ or $\boldsymbol{\Omega}$ (from D to $D-p$) has a much greater impact. The response should not be an attempt to recover the loss (that is futile), but to understand the optimistic nature of the verdict proferred by the results of a 'full' ML analysis.

REML is concerned with reducing bias. This does not necessarily promote efficiency. Both bias and efficiency are fragile properties — they are lost by non-linear transformations. To illustrate this, suppose the variance of a normally distributed variable is estimated from a random sample $y_1, \ldots, y_n$ without bias by $\hat{\sigma}^2 = \sum_i (y_i - \overline{y})^2/(n-1)$, where $\overline{y}$ is the sample mean of the y_i. The $(n-1)/\sigma^2$-multiple of $\hat{\sigma}^2$ has χ^2_{n-1} distribution; $\mathrm{var}(\hat{\sigma}^2) = 2\sigma^4/(n-1)$. However,

$$\mathrm{MSE}\left(\frac{n-1}{n+1}\hat{\sigma}^2\right) = \frac{2\sigma^4}{n+1}\,.$$

Therefore, the denominator $n+1$ yields a more efficient estimator of σ^2. Further, $1/\hat{\sigma}^2$ is biased. It becomes unbiased if the denominator is set to $n-3$. But neither of these estimators is efficient; the optimal denominator is $(n-1)^2/(n-3)+2(n-3)/(n-5)$. The proof is left for an exercise.

7.3.2 Implementing ML and REML

When some of the sample sizes n_d are substantial, the computation of the various quadratic forms $\mathbf{u}_1^\top \mathbf{W}^{-1}\mathbf{u}_2$ is greatly speeded up by exploiting the specific form of $\mathbf{W}_d$, $\mathbf{W}_d = \mathbf{I}_{n_d} + \mathbf{Z}_d \boldsymbol{\Omega} \mathbf{Z}_d^\top$. It is easy to show that

$$\begin{aligned} \mathbf{W}_d^{-1} &= \mathbf{I}_{n_d} - \mathbf{Z}_d \boldsymbol{\Omega} \mathbf{G}_d^{-1} \mathbf{Z}_d^\top \\ \det\left(\mathbf{W}_d\right) &= \left(\sigma_{\mathrm{W}}^2\right)^{n_d} \det\left(\mathbf{G}_d\right) , \end{aligned} \tag{7.21}$$

where $\mathbf{G}_d = \mathbf{I}_r + \mathbf{Z}_d^\top \mathbf{Z}_d \boldsymbol{\Omega}$ are $r \times r$ matrices. With these expressions, we avoid the inversion and evaluation of the determinants of any sizeable matrices, irrespective of the sample sizes n_d. For example,

$$\mathbf{X}^\top \mathbf{W}^{-1} \mathbf{X} = \mathbf{X}^\top \mathbf{X} - \sum_{d=1}^{D} \mathbf{X}_d^\top \mathbf{Z}_d \, \boldsymbol{\Omega} \mathbf{G}_d^{-1} \, \mathbf{Z}_d^\top \mathbf{X}_d .$$

Further,

$$\hat{\mathbf{e}}^\top \mathbf{W}^{-1} \hat{\mathbf{e}} = \mathbf{y}^\top \mathbf{W}^{-1} \mathbf{y} - 2\mathbf{y}^\top \mathbf{W}^{-1} \mathbf{X} \hat{\boldsymbol{\beta}} + \hat{\boldsymbol{\beta}}^\top \mathbf{X}^\top \mathbf{W}^{-1} \mathbf{X} \hat{\boldsymbol{\beta}} ,$$

so we do not have to evaluate the vector of residuals $\hat{\mathbf{e}}$. Of course, when $n_d \leq r$ it is more practical to form the matrix $\mathbf{W}_d$ and invert it directly. The quadratic forms in (7.15), (7.17) and (7.20) involve $\mathbf{Z}$. These expressions can be reduced by using the identity

$$\begin{aligned} \mathbf{Z}_d^\top \mathbf{W}_d^{-1} \mathbf{u} &= \mathbf{Z}_d^\top \mathbf{u} - \mathbf{Z}_d^\top \mathbf{Z}_d \, \boldsymbol{\Omega} \mathbf{G}_d^{-1} \, \mathbf{Z}_d^\top \mathbf{u} \\ &= \mathbf{G}_d^{-1} \mathbf{Z}_d^\top \mathbf{u} \end{aligned} \tag{7.22}$$

for any vector $\mathbf{u}$ of length n_d.

In summary, the Fisher scoring algorithm requires the following statistics (data summaries):

- the sample matrix of cross-products $(\mathbf{X}, \mathbf{y})^\top (\mathbf{X}, \mathbf{y})$;
- the within-cluster matrices of cross-products $(\mathbf{X}_d, \mathbf{y}_d)^\top \mathbf{Z}_d$.

After calculating these before the first iteration, the Fisher scoring iterations involve no operations with subject-level data. An efficient organisation of the calculations is summarised by the following scheme:

1. Data input.
2. Calculate $(\mathbf{X}, \mathbf{y})^\top (\mathbf{X}, \mathbf{y})$ and $(\mathbf{X}_d, \mathbf{y}_d)^\top \mathbf{Z}_d$, $d = 1, \ldots, D$.

3. Fit OLS and define the initial solution. See Section 7.3.3.
4. Apply iterations until convergence. Each iteration comprises the following steps:
   a) Calculate $\mathbf{G}_d^{-1}$ and $\boldsymbol{\Omega}\mathbf{G}_d^{-1}$.
   b) Calculate $\mathbf{G}_d^{-1}\mathbf{Z}_d^{\top}(\mathbf{X}_d\,,\,\mathbf{y}_d)$.
   c) Calculate

$$(\mathbf{X},\,\mathbf{y})^{\top}\mathbf{W}^{-1}(\mathbf{X},\,\mathbf{y}) = (\mathbf{X},\,\mathbf{y})^{\top}(\mathbf{X},\,\mathbf{y}) - \sum_{d=1}^{D}(\mathbf{X}_d\,,\,\mathbf{y}_d)^{\top}\mathbf{Z}_d\,\boldsymbol{\Omega}\mathbf{G}_d^{-1}\,\mathbf{Z}_d^{\top}(\mathbf{X}_d\,,\,\mathbf{y}_d)\,.$$

   d) Update $\hat{\boldsymbol{\beta}}$ and $\hat{\sigma}_{\mathrm{W}}^2$. Evaluate the (restricted) log-likelihood.
   e) Calculate the various cross-products $(\mathbf{Z}_d\,,\,\hat{\mathbf{e}}_d)^{\top}\mathbf{W}_d^{-1}\mathbf{Z}_d$ required for updating $\hat{\boldsymbol{\Omega}}$.
   f) Update $\hat{\boldsymbol{\Omega}}$. Check positive definiteness of $\hat{\boldsymbol{\Omega}}$ and convergence.
5. Collect the results in a suitable object or array. Add displays related to model diagnostics and to the specific purpose of the analysis (such as small-area estimation).

7.3.3 Computational issues

This section discusses issues common to all iterative model fitting algorithms. They apply equally to ML and REML estimation.

Initial solution

All iterative algorithms require an initial solution, to be used in the first iteration. For the regression parameters, the OLS fit is an obvious choice, although the fit to the model with the same regression part but a different variation part ($\mathbf{Z}$) can also be used, when available from a previous model fit to the same dataset. The residual variance from the OLS fit usually exceeds the estimate $\hat{\sigma}_{\mathrm{W}}^2$ fitted to the two-level model, especially when the between-cluster variation is substantial. So, a substantial fraction of the OLS estimate of the residual variance can be used as the initial estimate of σ_{W}^2. In random-intercept models (when $\mathbf{Z} = \mathbf{1}$), the complementary fraction is a suitable initial solution for ω. For example, the OLS estimate $\hat{\sigma}^2$ can be split so that $0.9\hat{\sigma}^2$ and 0.1 are the respective initial estimates of σ_{W}^2 and ω.

When the variation part contains one or several variables, so that a matrix $\boldsymbol{\Omega}$ is estimated, the starting solution can be set to a diagonal matrix $\hat{\boldsymbol{\Omega}}$. For any reasonable model, the slopes can be expected not to vary wildly, so the ordinary regression slope can be used as a guide. Suppose the estimate of the slope on a variable involved in $\boldsymbol{\Omega}$ is substantial, say, equal to $\hat{\beta} > 0$. Then by setting the variance to $\hat{\beta}^2/4$ we are guessing that the slope is negative in only a small fraction of the clusters. In general, it is better to start with inflated variances in $\hat{\mathbf{\Omega}}$, although the speed of convergence should not depend strongly on the initial solution. If it does, it is a sign of instability in the solution, which can best be resolved by simplifying the model, especially its variation part $\mathbf{Z}$.

Alternatively, the variances in $\hat{\mathbf{\Omega}}$ can be set by simple moment matching applied to the cross-products $\hat{\mathbf{e}}_d^\top \mathbf{Z}_d$, or the variances can be set as guesses based on the OLS fit, assuming that the standard deviation of the slopes is of the same order of magnitude as the slope itself. This approach is not substantially superior; its main advantage is that $\hat{\mathbf{\Omega}}$ is initially set automatically, without the analyst's improvisation.

Convergence criteria

The iterations can be stopped when the log-likelihood or the estimates are changed by successive iterations only slightly, or when the score vector is close to $\mathbf{0}$. And these three criteria can be combined, for example, by insisting that either the maximum or the total of the norms of the updating corrections and of the score vector, and the absolute difference of the log-likelihoods in consecutive iterations is smaller than a prescribed value, such as 10^{-5}. An adjustment can be made for the number of parameters; the norm can be scaled to avoid handicapping problems with many parameters.

The convergence properties of the Fisher scoring algorithm are quite robust with respect to the starting solution, especially for models with few variables in the variation part. Usually one or two iterations make up for a poorly set initial solution.

Non-negative definiteness of $\hat{\mathbf{\Omega}}$

The Fisher scoring and Newton-Raphson algorithms do not intrinsically produce estimates of $\hat{\mathbf{\Omega}}$ (or $\hat{\mathbf{\Sigma}}$) that are non-negative definite. Special arrangements have to be made to force this. It does not suffice to force the variances to be non-negative and the correlations in $\hat{\mathbf{\Omega}}$ to be within the range $[-1, 1]$ at every iteration. A simple counterexample is provided by the matrix

$$\begin{pmatrix} 1.0 & 0.7 & -0.8 \\ 0.7 & 1.0 & 0.3 \\ -0.8 & 0.3 & 1.0 \end{pmatrix} .$$

Even though each off-diagonal element in it is within the range $(-1, 1)$, it is not a variance (or correlation) matrix because its eigenvalues are 1.9, 1.3 and -0.2.

The log-likelihood l in (7.12) is well defined as an analytical function beyond the space of non-negative definite matrices $\mathbf{\Omega}$; it suffices that all the matrices $\mathbf{G}_d = \mathbf{I} + \mathbf{Z}_d^\top \mathbf{Z}_d \mathbf{\Omega}$ are positive definite. Thus, we could search for a solution in this extended parameter space, and upon convergence project the solution back to the original parameter space. This can be done by replacing all the negative eigenvalues λ_k in the eigenvalue decomposition $\hat{\boldsymbol{\Omega}} = \sum_k \lambda_k \boldsymbol{\xi}_k \boldsymbol{\xi}_k^\top$ with zeros. Although sufficient for most practical purposes, the resulting solution is neither ML nor REML.

A solution that works in most cases halves the updating vector $\boldsymbol{\Delta} = \hat{\boldsymbol{\mathcal{H}}}^{-1}\hat{\mathbf{s}}$ whenever the new solution is not positive definite. The halving may have to be repeated several times and in several iterations. Since the initial solution is positive definite, halving, repeated sufficiently many times, leads to a positive definite matrix $\hat{\boldsymbol{\Omega}}$. At the same time, the solution can get arbitrarily close to a singular matrix. A problem with this approach is that if an intermediate solution happens to end up very close to a non-negative definite matrix (close to the boundary of the parameter space, the solution will not move from there, even if, conceivably, it might have got to a better fit through the outside of the parameter space proper.

Variances can be forced to be non-negative by estimating their square roots — the standard deviations. This is not a comprehensive solution because it does not 'restrain' the covariances. Moreover, if an intermediate estimate of a standard deviation is zero, it will not be altered by updating. To show this, suppose σ is the standard deviation, $\mathbf{H}$ the row of the observed information matrix corresponding to σ^2 and $s = \partial l/\partial \sigma^2$. By switching from σ^2 to σ, s is replaced by $2\sigma s$ and $\mathbf{H}$ by $2\sigma\mathbf{H}$, except for $-\mathcal{H}$, the (σ^2, σ^2) diagonal element of $-\boldsymbol{\mathcal{H}}$, which is changed to $-2\sigma\mathcal{H} - 2s$. Thus, for $\sigma = 0$, $\boldsymbol{\mathcal{H}}$ is block-diagonal with a block corresponding to σ and the first-order partial differential (the score) with respect to σ is zero. Therefore $\hat{\sigma} = 0$ is not changed by updating. This is a problem because an intermediate estimate of a variance may vanish merely because its initial estimate has been set too small.

A comprehensive solution estimates a decomposition of $\boldsymbol{\Omega}$, such as the Cholesky decomposition $\boldsymbol{\Omega} = \mathbf{L}^\top\mathbf{L}$ for an upper-diagonal matrix $\mathbf{L}$. All the partial differentials are adjusted according to the chain rule for differentiation:

$$\frac{\partial \boldsymbol{\Omega}}{\partial \omega} = \left(\frac{\partial \mathbf{L}}{\partial \omega}\right)^\top \mathbf{L} + \mathbf{L}^\top \frac{\partial \mathbf{L}}{\partial \omega} .$$

Singularity of the Hessian $-\boldsymbol{\mathcal{H}}$ may be reached at an iteration. The consequent indeterminacy of $\hat{\mathbf{L}}$ can be resolved only by deleting one of its rows. For a $r \times r$ matrix $\boldsymbol{\Omega}$, deletion of the bottom row of $\hat{\mathbf{L}}$ is equivalent to constraining the (r, r) element of $\mathbf{L}$ to zero. If singularity occurs again, the next deletion, of row $r - 1$, corresponds to two additional constraints on the elements of $\mathbf{L}$, and so on. The result of k deletions is an estimated matrix $\hat{\boldsymbol{\Omega}}$ of rank $r - k$. The rank of $\hat{\boldsymbol{\Omega}}$ should not be confused with the rank of $\boldsymbol{\Omega}$.

Slow convergence

More complex models, and models with more complex variation part $\mathbf{Z}$ in particular, tend to require more iterations. Slow convergence is a sure sign that there are too many parameters in the model. It is useful to monitor the convergence and identify the parameters that hold up the convergence. Other irregularities can be detected by monitoring the value of the log-likelihood. In normal circumstances, the log-likelihood increases at every iteration, except the first one, and the increments steadily decrease, at an approximately geometric rate. A reversal at the first iteration should be of no concern; simply, the initial solution is poorer than the OLS fit which corresponds to $\hat{\mathbf{\Omega}} = \mathbf{0}$. (At an iteration, the value is calculated for the previous, not the current solution). In fact, when the converging solution $\hat{\mathbf{\Omega}}$ vanishes the iterations merely recover the original OLS fit.

Ill-conditioning of the regression design matrix $\mathbf{X}$ causes slow convergence, and ill-conditioning of the variation design $\mathbf{Z}$ does so even more severely. Constraining some of the parameters in $\mathbf{\Omega}$ usually speeds up the convergence. However, no covariance should be constrained unless both related variances are also constrained. (Usually all three parameters would in such a case be constrained to zero.) The reason for this is that a linear transformation of a variable associated with variation alters the covariances and correlations in $\mathbf{\Omega}$.

7.4 Model selection issues

'Which model?' is the ubiquitous question in any approach that calls for a simple yet adequate description of the studied dataset. The implicit footnote of the approach is that 'if we knew which the correct model was, all our inferences would be efficient'. Unable to identify this model, we usually proceed by searching for the model that has some attributes of the correct one, or we expect that the correct model would have them. At the same time, we trim the model to have as few features as possible, to achieve parsimony, because any unimportant or redundant feature in the model erodes the efficiency of the estimates of the model parameters.

Parsimony is pursued by excluding any model parameters that do not contribute to high likelihood. That is, when they are excluded, the value of the likelihood at its maximum is reduced only slightly. The origins of this approach are in hypothesis testing using the likelihood ratio test statistic. We describe the likelihood ratio test first for a general setting, and then discuss its application to two-level models. Suppose model A involves the parameter vector $\boldsymbol{\theta}$ and let $\hat{\boldsymbol{\theta}}$ be its ML estimator. With greater rigour, we should refer to A as a *class of models*, and to $\boldsymbol{\theta}$ as a set of parameter vectors, or the *parameter space*. As an alternative to A, we consider a smaller class of models B that has fewer features than class A; B is defined by restricting a sub-vector of $\boldsymbol{\theta}$ to a specific value; no generality is lost by assuming that this vector is $\mathbf{0}$. Thus, $\boldsymbol{\theta}$ can be partitioned as $(\boldsymbol{\theta}_{\mathrm{B}}, \boldsymbol{\theta}_0)$ and B is defined as $(\boldsymbol{\theta}_{\mathrm{B}}, \boldsymbol{\theta}_0 = \mathbf{0})$, and so fully described by $\boldsymbol{\theta}_{\mathrm{B}}$. Linear constraints on $\boldsymbol{\theta}$, such as $\mathbf{c}^{\top}\boldsymbol{\theta} = \text{const}$, are accommodated by a suitable (linear) reparametrisation of $\boldsymbol{\theta}$.

Testing the (null-)hypothesis that $\boldsymbol{\theta}_0 = \mathbf{0}$ entails the following exercise. We start by presuming that $\boldsymbol{\theta}_0 = \mathbf{0}$ and, based on the data $(\mathbf{X}, \mathbf{y})$, seek evidence that contradicts this assumption. For this purpose, a statistic T is found, with a (precisely or approximately) known distribution under the assumption that $\boldsymbol{\theta}_0 = \mathbf{0}$. If the realisation of this statistic, the value of T for the dataset at hand, is in the tail of this distribution, we regard it as evidence against the null-hypothesis. Thus, the possible values of the *test statistic* T are split into values that do not contradict (*fail to reject*) the hypothesis and values that correspond to evidence against B (against $\boldsymbol{\theta}_0 = \mathbf{0}$) or contradict model B. The values of T that constitute evidence against B form the critical region. Usually, the critical region is an interval $(t_0, +\infty)$. Then t_0 is called the critical value.

The likelihood ratio test statistic for the null-hypothesis $\boldsymbol{\theta}_0 = \mathbf{0}$ against the alternative $\boldsymbol{\theta}_0 \neq \mathbf{0}$ is defined as $2(l^{(A)} - l^{(B)})$, where $l^{(A)}$ and $l^{(B)}$ are the values of the log-likelihood for the respective models (classes) A and B at their respective maxima $\hat{\boldsymbol{\theta}}_{\mathrm{A}}$ and $(\hat{\boldsymbol{\theta}}_{\mathrm{B}}, \mathbf{0})$. Under certain regularity conditions [37], the asymptotic distribution of this statistic under the null-hypothesis is χ^2 with the degrees of freedom given by the length (number of components) of $\boldsymbol{\theta}_0$. The most important of the regularity conditions is that class B is *inside* class A, that is, every model in B has a neighbourhood that is subsumed in A. (The neighbourhood may be subsumed also in B, as B $\subset$ A.) The neighbourhood of a model is defined by the Euclidean metric for the parameter vectors. The regularity condition is problematic for testing the hypothesis that a variance in $\boldsymbol{\Sigma}$ (or $\boldsymbol{\Omega}$) vanishes, because a variance matrix with a zero variance is on the boundary of the parameter space defined by class A.

The likelihood ratio test is carried out as follows. First, the classes A and B are defined. For example, class B is defined by deleting a variable from the regression part. The likelihood ratio has the asymptotic null-distribution χ^2_1. We conclude that we have evidence against B, that is, we cannot reduce A, if the value of the likelihood ratio statistic exceeds a high percentile of the χ^2_1 distribution. Conventionally, the 95th percentile is chosen; for χ^2_1 it is equal to 3.84. Thus, our conclusion is not necessarily correct, because T may exceed the critical value 3.84 even when the underlying model lies in B. Admittedly the probability of this event, conditional on being in class B, is small, approximately 0.05, specified a priori.

When $T < 3.84$, we have no evidence against class B. The logically correct interpretation of such a result is that 'we do not know' whether $\theta_0 = 0$. Yet, the conclusion drawn in practice is that $\theta_0 = 0$, and we proceed by regarding the reduction to class B as appropriate (or the expansion to class A as not warranted). Apart from the logical inconsistency, we may have committed an 'error' because the distributions of T under the various models outside B have positive probabilities of values in the range $(0, 3.84)$. In a different viewpoint, we are bound to have committed an error because $\theta_0 = 0$ is but one of innumerably many values of θ_0, so it is not rational to bet on *any one* of them, unless there is some specific prior information that supports the value as exceptional. Usually there is no such information. In the following discussion, we ignore all these inadequacies of model selection, and assume that an appropriate model has been identified.

Standard errors

A typical summary of a model fit comprises estimates $\hat{\boldsymbol{\beta}}$, $\hat{\boldsymbol{\Omega}}$ and $\hat{\sigma}^2_{\mathrm{W}}$, and estimates of the associated standard errors. For $\hat{\boldsymbol{\beta}}$, they can be interpreted in the same way as their counterparts in ordinary regression. The standard errors are the square roots of the diagonal of $\mathrm{var}(\hat{\boldsymbol{\beta}})$, and are estimated naively.

With two-level models, the standard errors involve $\boldsymbol{\Omega}$:

$$\mathrm{var}(\hat{\boldsymbol{\beta}}) = \sigma^2_{\mathrm{W}} \left(\mathbf{X}^\top \mathbf{W}^{-1} \mathbf{X}\right)^{-1} ,$$

so $\widehat{\mathrm{var}}(\hat{\boldsymbol{\beta}}) = \hat{\sigma}^2_{\mathrm{W}} \left(\mathbf{X}^\top \hat{\mathbf{W}}^{-1} \mathbf{X}\right)^{-1}$. An estimation error of $\hat{\boldsymbol{\Omega}}$ leaves its imprint as an estimation error of $\mathrm{var}(\hat{\boldsymbol{\beta}})$. Dependence of the standard errors on model parameters is a much more acute problem for the elements of $\hat{\boldsymbol{\Omega}}$. Unlike for $\hat{\boldsymbol{\beta}}$, the standard errors for the parameters involved in $\boldsymbol{\Omega}$ can be established only asymptotically, by inverting the expected information matrix given by (7.18), with the REML adjustment, if appropriate. Thus, for small samples, the standard errors (as functions of model parameters) can be established only approximately. In practice, we estimate this approximation, so estimation and approximation errors are compounded. Furthermore, the standard errors depend on $\boldsymbol{\Omega}$ — the error in estimating $\boldsymbol{\Omega}$ is committed again when estimating the standard errors. Insights are difficult to gain when $\mathbf{Z}$ contains several variables. For parallel regressions, when $\mathbf{Z} = \mathbf{1}$,

$$a\mathrm{var}(\hat{\omega}) = 2\left\{\sum_{d=1}^{D}\left(\frac{n_d}{1+n_d\omega}\right)^2\right\}^{-1} .$$

This is an increasing function of $\omega = \sigma^2_{\mathrm{B}}/\sigma^2_{\mathrm{W}}$, so if $\hat{\omega} > \omega$, then the estimate of $a\mathrm{var}(\hat{\omega})$ also exceeds its target. This greatly diminishes the value of the estimated standard error of $\hat{\omega}$. The estimates of the parameters in $\boldsymbol{\Omega}$ are correlated and the parameters are constrained by the condition of non-negative definiteness. That is another reason why the standard errors for the elements of $\boldsymbol{\Omega}$ are not very useful.

A computationally more involved method is based on the *profile likelihood*. Briefly, a range of feasible values of the parameter is established as the values for which the the log-likelihood is not much smaller than its maximum. This range contains ML estimator of the parameter, but need not comprise an interval or be symmetric around it. An example is presented in Figure 7.2. ML is attained for $\hat{\theta} = 2.0$, with $l(\hat{\theta}) = -8.12$. The confidence interval for θ is defined as the values of θ for which $l(\theta) > l(\hat{\theta}) - 1.92$, that is, $(1.265, 2.905)$. The value of 1.92 was selected as the one-half of the 95th percentile of the χ^2_1 distribution. This choice is in accord with the likelihood ratio test.

Figure 7.2. Example of using the profile likelihood. ML estimate, equal to 2.00, and the limits of the confidence interval, 1.265 and 2.905, are marked by vertical dots.

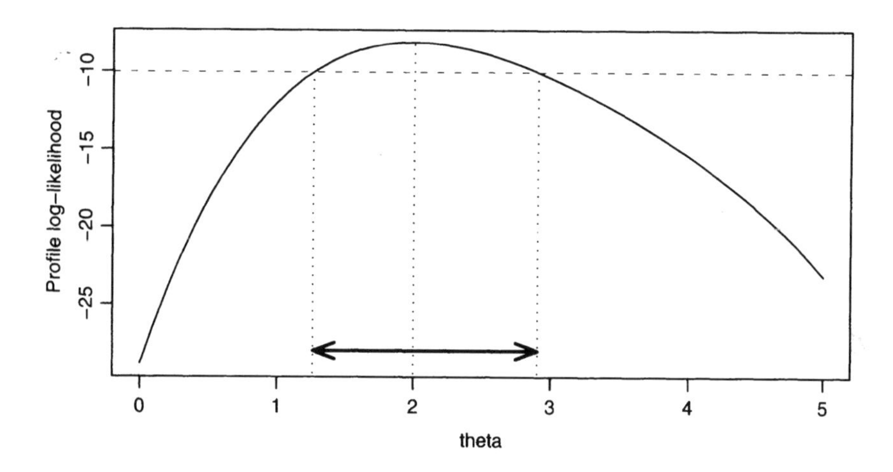

7.4.1 Residuals and model diagnostics

The purpose of diagnostic procedures is to confirm the appropriateness of the fitted model. This is done indirectly, by seeking a contradiction with the model assumptions. In such a search, the model residuals play an important role. The residuals are best motivated as replacements for the random terms γ_d and ε_{jd} in (7.9). A class of diagnostic procedures checks whether the residuals have properties we expect the random terms to have.

In ordinary regression, residuals are defined as the differences between the outcomes y and their fit $\hat{y} = \mathbf{x}\hat{\boldsymbol{\beta}}$, $e = y - \hat{y}$. In two-level models, we have to separate the two random terms, γ and ε, so that separate procedures could be applied to each set of residuals. The residuals are defined as the estimated conditional expectations of the corresponding random terms, given the data and parameter values. These expectations are estimated naively, by replacing the parameters with their ML or REML estimates.

The conditional expectation of γ_d in (7.9) is derived from the joint distribution of $\mathbf{y}_d$ and γ_d. This distribution is

$$\begin{pmatrix} \mathbf{y}_d \\ \gamma_d \end{pmatrix} \sim \mathcal{N}\left\{ \begin{pmatrix} \mathbf{X}_d\boldsymbol{\beta} \\ \mathbf{0} \end{pmatrix}, \begin{pmatrix} \mathbf{V}_d & \mathbf{Z}_d\boldsymbol{\Sigma} \\ \boldsymbol{\Sigma}\mathbf{Z}_d^\top & \boldsymbol{\Sigma} \end{pmatrix} \right\} .$$

The conditional distribution of γ_d given $\mathbf{y}_d$ is also normal,

$$(\gamma_d \,|\, \mathbf{y}_d) \sim \mathcal{N}\left(\boldsymbol{\Sigma}\mathbf{Z}_d^\top \mathbf{V}_d^{-1}\mathbf{e}_d ,\; \boldsymbol{\Sigma} - \boldsymbol{\Sigma}\mathbf{Z}_d^\top \mathbf{V}_d^{-1}\mathbf{Z}_d\boldsymbol{\Sigma}\right)$$

($\mathbf{e}_d = \mathbf{y}_d - \mathbf{X}_d\boldsymbol{\beta}$), which reduces to

$$(\gamma_d \,|\, \mathbf{y}_d) \sim \mathcal{N}\left(\mathbf{\Omega G}_d^{-1}\mathbf{Z}_d^{\top}\mathbf{e}_d \,,\, \mathbf{\Sigma G}_d^{-1}\right) \,, \tag{7.23}$$

using the identity in (7.22).

The conditional distribution of ε_d is derived similarly, from the joint distribution

$$\begin{pmatrix} \mathbf{y}_d \\ \varepsilon_d \end{pmatrix} \sim \mathcal{N}\left\{ \begin{pmatrix} \mathbf{X}_d\beta \\ \mathbf{0} \end{pmatrix}, \begin{pmatrix} \mathbf{V}_d & \sigma_{\mathrm{W}}^2\mathbf{I} \\ \sigma_{\mathrm{W}}^2\mathbf{I} & \sigma_{\mathrm{W}}^2\mathbf{I} \end{pmatrix} \right\} .$$

Using (7.21), we obtain

$$(\varepsilon_d \,|\, \mathbf{y}_d) \sim \mathcal{N}\left\{ \mathbf{W}_d^{-1}\mathbf{e}_d \,,\, \frac{1}{\sigma_{\mathrm{W}}^2}\left(\mathbf{I} - \mathbf{W}_d^{-1}\right) = \mathbf{Z}_d\mathbf{\Omega G}_d^{-1}\mathbf{Z}_d^{\top} \right\} . \tag{7.24}$$

The district- and subject-level residuals are

$$\begin{aligned} \hat{\gamma}_d &= \hat{\mathbf{\Omega}}\hat{\mathbf{G}}_d^{-1}\mathbf{Z}_d^{\top}\hat{\mathbf{e}}_d \\ \hat{\varepsilon}_d &= \hat{\mathbf{W}}_d^{-1}\hat{\mathbf{e}}_d \,, \end{aligned} \tag{7.25}$$

where $\hat{\mathbf{e}}_d = \mathbf{y}_d - \mathbf{X}_d\hat{\beta}$. The residuals satisfy the identity $\mathbf{Z}_d\hat{\gamma}_d + \hat{\varepsilon}_d = \hat{\mathbf{e}}_d$, as do their targets γ_d and ε_d ($\mathbf{Z}_d\gamma_d + \varepsilon_d = \mathbf{e}_d$).

Diagnostics can be based on the procedures for ordinary regression. Either we regard $\hat{\gamma}_d$ as if they were γ_d, or adjust them for their (estimated) variances $\hat{\mathbf{\Sigma}}\hat{\mathbf{G}}_d^{-1}$. Adjustment seems to be preferable, although it may be poorly estimated because it involves $\hat{\mathbf{\Omega}}$ and its non-linear transformations. The residuals are biased estimators of their targets; however, this bias cannot be removed without incurring substantial variance inflation. Similar problems are encountered with $\hat{\varepsilon}_d$. The normality of the random terms is checked by the normal plots of the residuals. Any patterns in the plots of residuals against the covariates indicate inadequacies in the regression part of the model.

The residuals are affected by shrinkage and are associated with unequal variances. Thus, for a parallel regression model, $|\,\hat{\gamma}_d\,|$ is unlikely to be large when n_d is small. Each γ_d is estimated optimally, but a non-linear function of them is not. Looking at patterns among the values of $\hat{\gamma}_d$ can be interpreted as forming non-linear summaries $\mathcal{F}(\hat{\gamma}_D)$ and regarding them as efficient estimators of the same summaries of the γ_d, that is, $\mathcal{F}(\gamma_D)$. In general, patterns observed among $\hat{\gamma}_d$ may reflect the method of their estimation and need not be related to the patterns among the underlying quantities.

Simulation-based diagnostics

Judging from the plots of residuals whether a particular pattern warrants a review of the model is bound to be subjective and the conclusion based on the plot not necessarily well justified. After all, patterns can occur by chance, even when the appropriate model is fitted to the data simulated from the assumed model.

This motivates a more profound way of model checking. We define a feature; this can be a plot, a table, or one or several statistics, and evaluate (or construct) the feature for the realised dataset. Then we simulate 19 datasets with the same regression and variation designs, $\mathbf{X}$ and $\mathbf{Z}$, and model parameters equal to their estimates based on the realised dataset. For the realised and each simulated dataset, we evaluate the feature. We shuffle the 20 features (one realised and 19 simulated), so that the realised feature is placed at a random location. If the realised feature stands out among them (for example, it is identified by several colleagues making independent judgements), we have evidence against the model — when the model is satisfied (as with the simulated data), such a feature is unlikely. For greater certainty, this exercise can be conducted with 49+1 or 99+1 datasets, although handling a lot of realisations of the feature may be cumbersome.

This approach is computationally rather demanding, but requires little programming additional to the method for the realised dataset. The judgement based on the features is easier to make than with the various plots of the residuals. On the one hand, the choice of the feature is crucial to the success of the method. On the other hand, the analyst has the freedom to choose one or a few features that best reflect the a priori concerns about the adequacy of the model. A set of features can be combined into a multi-feature, for instance, by setting the elementary features (say, a graph and a table) side-by-side. The advantage of a multi-feature over separate treatments of each feature is that only one assessment has to be made as to whether there is an exceptional realisation among the $M+1$ presented versions. The approach is universal; a new class of models requires for diagnostics neither any theoretical development nor intricate programming, merely computing power to repeatedly generate data according to the fitted model and evaluate the (multi-)feature.

7.5 District-level models

Fitting a random coefficient model with modern computing equipment is no longer a demanding task for the equipment or a proficient analyst. Nevertheless, reducing the data to district-level summaries, and then analysing them, remains an attractive proposition. The rationale for this is not only the greatly reduced size of the data to be analysed, but also that the analysis may be more pertinent to small-area estimation — to learn about districts, we should analyse the districts. Certainly, by aggregating (averaging) the data to district level, some information is discarded. With subject-level data, the within-district variation could be studied, but after aggregating the data it is no longer possible or has to rely on some untestable assumptions.

For the model with parallel within-district regressions, averaging yields

$$\overline{y}_d = \overline{\mathbf{x}}_d \boldsymbol{\beta} + \gamma_d + \overline{\varepsilon}_d \,, \tag{7.26}$$

where the bar indicates averaging within the district. This model should be adequate, if its originating subject-level model is, because our target is $\overline{\mathbf{x}}_d\boldsymbol{\beta} + \gamma_d$ or $\overline{\mathbf{X}}_d\boldsymbol{\beta} + \gamma_d$. We have to distinguish between the sample mean $\overline{\mathbf{x}}_d$ and the population mean $\overline{\mathbf{X}}_d$. Using the former is particularly problematic when it is based on a small sample. The district-level means $\overline{y}_d$, $d = 1, \ldots, D$, are independent but, unlike in ordinary regression, their variances are unequal. They depend on the sample size;

$$\operatorname{var}(\gamma_d + \overline{\varepsilon}_d) = \sigma_{\mathrm{B}}^2 + \frac{\sigma_{\mathrm{W}}^2}{n_d} .$$

The model in (7.26) is fitted by the Fisher scoring algorithm. The aggregation simplifies the algorithm substantially.

The log-likelihood for the model in (7.26) is

$$l = -\frac{1}{2}\left\{\log(2\pi D) + \log(\det \mathbf{V}) + \mathbf{e}^\top \mathbf{V}^{-1}\mathbf{e}\right\} , \tag{7.27}$$

where $\mathbf{V}$ is the variance matrix of $\overline{\mathbf{y}} = (\overline{y}_1, \ldots, \overline{y}_D)$. It is diagonal,

$$\mathbf{V} = \sigma_{\mathrm{B}}^2\mathbf{I} + \mathbf{n}^{-1}\sigma_{\mathrm{W}}^2 ,$$

where $\mathbf{n} = \operatorname{diag}(n_1, \ldots, n_D)$ is the diagonal matrix of the district-level sample sizes. The vector of residuals is $\mathbf{e} = \overline{\mathbf{y}} - \overline{\mathbf{X}}\boldsymbol{\beta}$, where $\overline{\mathbf{X}}$ is the $D \times p$ regression design matrix for (7.26), comprised of the district-level mean vectors $\overline{\mathbf{x}}_d$.

Since (7.27) has the same form as (7.12), the ML estimator of $\boldsymbol{\beta}$ is

$$\hat{\boldsymbol{\beta}} = \left(\overline{\mathbf{X}}^\top \hat{\mathbf{V}}^{-1}\overline{\mathbf{X}}\right)^{-1} \overline{\mathbf{X}}^\top \hat{\mathbf{V}}^{-1}\overline{\mathbf{y}} . \tag{7.28}$$

As in Section 7.3, we introduce the variance ratio $\omega = \sigma_{\mathrm{B}}^2/\sigma_{\mathrm{W}}^2$ and the scaled variance matrix $\mathbf{W} = \sigma_{\mathrm{W}}^{-2}\mathbf{V}$, so that $\mathbf{W} = \mathbf{I} + \omega\mathbf{n}^{-1}$. With this parametrisation, the ML estimator of σ_{W}^2 is

$$\hat{\sigma}_{\mathrm{W}}^2 = \frac{1}{D}\hat{\mathbf{e}}^\top \hat{\mathbf{W}}^{-1}\hat{\mathbf{e}} . \tag{7.29}$$

The Fisher scoring algorithm for ω requires the following expressions:

$$\begin{aligned}
\frac{\partial l}{\partial \omega} &= -\frac{1}{2}\left(\sum_{d=1}^{D}\frac{n_d}{1+\omega n_d} - \frac{1}{\sigma_{\mathrm{W}}^2}\mathbf{e}^\top\mathbf{W}^{-1}\mathbf{n}^{-1}\mathbf{W}^{-1}\mathbf{e}\right) \\
&= -\frac{1}{2}\left\{\sum_{d=1}^{D}\frac{n_d}{1+\omega n_d} - \frac{1}{\sigma_{\mathrm{W}}^2}\sum_{d=1}^{D}\frac{e_d^2 n_d}{(1+\omega n_d)^2}\right\} \\
-\mathrm{E}\left(\frac{\partial l^2}{\partial \omega^2}\right) &= \frac{1}{2}\left\{\sum_{d=1}^{D}\frac{n_d^2}{(1+\omega n_d)^2}\right\} .
\end{aligned} \tag{7.30}$$

The REML estimators are obtained by adjusting the log-likelihood. The adjustment is

$$l_{\mathrm{R}} = l + \frac{1}{2}\log\left\{\det\left(\overline{\mathbf{X}}^{\top}\mathbf{V}^{-1}\overline{\mathbf{X}}\right)\right\},$$

as in Section 7.3, yielding the appropriate denominator for $\hat{\sigma}_{\mathrm{W}}^2$:

$$\hat{\sigma}_{\mathrm{W}}^2 = \frac{1}{D-p}\hat{\mathbf{e}}^{\top}\hat{\mathbf{W}}^{-1}\hat{\mathbf{e}}.$$

For a given p, the change from D to $D-p$ for the district-level model is much more radical than from n to $n-p$ for the subject-level model. Therefore, the adjustment of the elements of the expected information matrix that involve ω is also more important. These are given in the Appendix. The two variances, σ_{W}^2 and σ_{B}^2, are confounded when the sample sizes n_d are identical. In general, it is much more difficult to recognise in a dataset a pattern of variation than an association by regression (correlation). Therefore, the variation in the sample sizes n_d has to be substantial, otherwise the two variances are nearly confounded. This problem can be explored more formally by inspecting the expected information matrix for σ^2 and ω. We have

$$\mathcal{I}(\sigma_{\mathrm{W}}^2, \omega) = \frac{1}{2}\begin{pmatrix} \frac{D}{\sigma_{\mathrm{W}}^4} & \frac{1}{\sigma_{\mathrm{W}}^2}U^{(1)} \\ \frac{1}{\sigma_{\mathrm{W}}^2}U^{(1)} & U^{(2)} \end{pmatrix},$$

where $U^{(h)} = (1+\omega n_1)^{-h} + \cdots + (1+\omega n_D)^{-h}$, $h = 1, 2$. This is a singular matrix when $1+\omega n_d$ are constant; that is, not only when n_d are constant, but also when $\omega = 0$. The matrix $\mathcal{I}(\sigma_{\mathrm{W}}^2, \omega)$ is a scalar multiple of the matrix of cross-products for the regression with a single covariate equal to $\sigma_{\mathrm{W}}^2/(1+\omega n_d)$.

The difficulties with simultaneous estimation of the two variances can be resolved by estimating σ_{W}^2 from the subject-level data. For example, σ_{W}^2 could be estimated before the within-district averaging from the separate within-district regressions, and the estimates pooled across the districts. For each district, the same set of regression variables have to be used. For districts with $n_d \leq p$, σ_{W}^2 cannot be estimated; such districts do not contribute to the pooled estimator of σ_{W}^2.

The residuals are evaluated as the estimated conditional expectations of γ_d and $\overline{\varepsilon}_d$:

$$\begin{aligned} \hat{\gamma}_d &= \frac{n_d\hat{\omega}}{1+n_d\hat{\omega}}(\overline{y}_d - \overline{\mathbf{x}}_d\hat{\boldsymbol{\beta}}) \\ \hat{\overline{\varepsilon}}_d &= \frac{1}{1+n_d\hat{\omega}}(\overline{y}_d - \overline{\mathbf{x}}_d\hat{\boldsymbol{\beta}}); \end{aligned} \qquad (7.31)$$

the two residuals add up to $\overline{y}_d - \overline{\mathbf{x}}_d\hat{\boldsymbol{\beta}}$.

The model in (7.26) is fitted by an iterative algorithm constructed from (7.28)–(7.30). Most comments for fitting two-level models made in Section 7.4

carry over to this model. In particular, it may be advantageous to estimate $\sqrt{\omega}$ instead of ω.

More complex patterns of variation are catered for by models

$$\overline{y}_d = \overline{\mathbf{x}}_d \boldsymbol{\beta} + \overline{\mathbf{z}}_d \boldsymbol{\gamma}_d + \overline{\varepsilon}_d ,$$

with suitably selected variables for $\mathbf{z}$. They may be selected from among $\overline{\mathbf{x}}$. The aggregate outcomes $\overline{y}_d$ are independent, with variances $\mathrm{var}(\overline{y}_d) = \sigma_{\mathrm{W}}^2 \left(1 + \overline{\mathbf{z}}_d \boldsymbol{\Omega} \overline{\mathbf{z}}_d^{\top}\right)$, where $\boldsymbol{\Omega}$ is the scaled variance matrix of the vector of district-level deviations. Thus, $\mathrm{var}(\overline{y}_d)$ is a quadratic function of $\overline{\mathbf{z}}$. Such models are identifiable, but the information about $\boldsymbol{\Omega}$ is very sparse even in sizeable data.

Model choice

In two-level models, the regression part may contain variables defined for subjects or districts. The obvious choices for the district-level variables are the within-district means of subject-level variables, although other variables, defined for districts directly (such as urbanity and other attributes of the districts) may also be included. For variables that are means (aggregates), their population versions would appear to be more appropriate. The value of a covariate should depend on the population of the district, not its sample. As we aggregate from (7.9), with $\mathbf{Z} = \mathbf{1}$, to (7.26), subject-level variables are 'converted' to sample means, whereas the values of a district-level variable are merely copied. This creates a dilemma — whether to include in (7.26) the population mean of a variable (when available) or the sample mean. We should not include both because they are similar, and would cause ill-conditioning in the regression. Both the subject-level and the population-mean versions can be included in the two-level model where, owing to the much greater sample size, there is more scope for detailed modelling using highly correlated variables. However, including many district-level variables is not appropriate; there are only D degrees of freedom for the districts.

7.6 Generalised linear models

Although the assumption of normality is key to appropriateness of many statistical methods, outcome variables that are distributed (approximately) normally are rare in sample surveys. Both respondents and interviewers are more comfortable with limited sets of response options and with various classifications, such as employment status, type of employment or housing tenure, and income brackets, even if, occasionally, 'None of the above' is the appropriate response. With such data, the ordinary regression and other models for normally distributed outcomes have a very limited scope.

Generalised linear models (GLM) are an extension of the ordinary regression that caters for distributions other than normal, and for scales on which linearity is appropriate. Dichotomous variables are an example of distinctly non-normally distributed data. A linear model is not well suited for such a variable, because no linear function can represent a good fit to outcomes that comprise zeros and ones. With GLM, a model is specified for the *expectation* underlying the outcomes, $\mathrm{E}(\mathbf{y})$. For dichotomous data, $\mathrm{E}(\mathbf{y})$ are probabilities of positive outcomes; they are in the range $[0,1]$. A linear model may fit much better to a transformation of the probabilities to $(-\infty,+\infty)$. There are several such (monotone and smooth) transformations, including the logit,

$$\mathrm{logit}(p) \;=\; \log\left(\frac{p}{1-p}\right) .$$

An example of GLM for dichotomous data $\mathbf{y}$ is

$$\mathrm{logit}\{\mathrm{E}(y)\} \;=\; \mathbf{x}\boldsymbol{\beta} .$$

A more general specification of a GLM is

$$f\{\mathrm{E}(y_j)\} \;=\; \mathbf{x}_j\boldsymbol{\beta}$$

for a set of conditionally independent outcomes y_j, $j=1,\ldots n$, with specified conditional distributions of y_j given $\mathbf{x}_j\boldsymbol{\beta}$. These distributions usually belong to the same class, such as binary with the full range of probabilities $(0,1)$. For example, the ordinary regression corresponds to the identity function f and normal conditional distribution of y_j with means $\mathbf{x}_j\boldsymbol{\beta}$ and common (unknown) variance σ^2.

Many theoretical results related to GLM are derived for the *exponential family of distributions*. The discrete or continuous densities of the distributions in this family have the form

$$f(y_j\,,\,\theta_j\,,\,\phi) \;=\; \exp\left\{\frac{y_j\theta_j - b(\theta_j)}{\phi} + c(y_j\,;\,\phi)\right\} ,$$

where b and c are some real twice-differentiable functions and ϕ is a parameter; b has positive second-order differentials. The mean and variance of an observation are $\mathrm{E}(y_j) = b'(\theta_j)$ and $\mathrm{var}(y_j) = \phi b''(\theta_j)$, respectively. The expectation b' is related to the linear predictor $\mathbf{x}_j\boldsymbol{\beta}$ through a strictly monotone *link* function η:

$$b'(\theta_j) \;=\; \eta^{-1}(\mathbf{x}_j\boldsymbol{\beta}) .$$

Many common distributions belong to the exponential family; they include the normal, binomial, Poisson, and gamma distributions. GLM can be specified by the distribution of the outcomes, the variables in the linear predictor ($\mathbf{X}$) and the link function. Sometimes it is difficult to identify a suitable distribution, but the key feature of the data that we wish to model is the dependence of the variance on the mean:

$$V\{b'(\theta)\} \;=\; \phi b''(\theta) .$$

This *variance function* V, together with the link function η and the regression design $\mathbf{X}$, is sufficient to specify a GLM, and they are often a more convenient way of defining a model.

Commonly used combinations of distribution and link function are binomial and logit, Poisson and log and, of course, normal and identity. In a logit model, the outcomes have binomial distributions with denominators m_j and their conditional distributions are given by

$$\mathrm{P}(y_j = k \,|\, p_j) = \binom{m_j}{k} p_j^k (1 - p_j)^{m_j - k} .$$

They belong to the exponential family, with $b(\theta_j) = \log(p_j) - \log(1-p_j)$. Here we set $\log(p_j) - \log(1-p_j) = \mathbf{x}_j\boldsymbol{\beta}$, so b coincides with the linear predictor and $\partial\theta_j/\partial\eta_j = \text{const}$. This is an example of a *canonical* link. In general, a linear transformation of the link function is compensated by the linear predictor, and so linearly related link functions are for all purposes equivalent.

GLM is fitted by the Fisher scoring algorithm, which is conveniently described in terms of iteratively reweighted least squares. Assuming that ϕ is known, the relevant identities are

$$l = C + \frac{1}{\phi} \sum_{j=1}^{n} \left\{ y_j\theta_j - b(\theta_j) \right\}$$

$$(\mathbf{s} =) \quad \frac{\partial l}{\partial \boldsymbol{\beta}} = \frac{1}{\phi} \sum_{j=1}^{n} \left\{ y_j - b'(\theta_j) \right\} \frac{\partial \theta_j}{\partial \eta_j} \mathbf{x}_j$$

$$(\boldsymbol{\mathcal{H}} =) \quad -\frac{\partial^2 l}{\partial \boldsymbol{\beta}\, \partial \boldsymbol{\beta}^\top} = \frac{1}{\phi} \sum_{j=1}^{n} b''(\theta_j) \left(\frac{\partial \theta_j}{\partial \eta_j} \right)^2 \mathbf{x}_j \mathbf{x}_j^\top - \frac{1}{\phi} \sum_{j=1}^{n} \left\{ y_j - b'(\theta_j) \right\} \frac{\partial^2 \theta_j}{\partial \eta_j^2} \mathbf{x}_j \mathbf{x}_j^\top , \qquad (7.32)$$

where $\eta_j = \mathbf{x}_j\boldsymbol{\beta}$ and C is a constant that plays no role in maximising l. As $\mathrm{E}(y_j) = b'(\theta_j)$, the expectation of the second term in $\boldsymbol{\mathcal{H}}$ vanishes. The expected information $\boldsymbol{\mathcal{I}}$ is given by the first term in $\boldsymbol{\mathcal{H}}$. In the Fisher scoring algorithm, the information matrix is formed as the weighted total of squares and cross-products of the covariates, with the weights related to the variances $b''(\theta_j)/\phi$. The score function can also be interpreted as the weighted totals of cross-products of the residuals $e_j = y_j - \mathrm{E}(y_j)$ and $\mathbf{x}_i$, after a suitable re-scaling of e_i.

7.6.1 Two-level GLMs

GLMs can be extended to two levels in direct analogy with the extension for models with the normality assumptions. We assume that the conditional expectations $\mathrm{E}(\mathbf{y}_d \,|\, \gamma_d)$ are related to linear predictors as

$$\mathrm{E}(y_{jd}\,|\,\boldsymbol{\gamma}_d) = \eta^{-1}\left(\mathbf{x}_{jd}\boldsymbol{\beta} + \mathbf{z}_{jd}\boldsymbol{\gamma}_d\right) .$$

Marginally, $\boldsymbol{\gamma}_d$ are a random sample from the normal distribution with mean $\mathbf{0}$ and variance matrix $\boldsymbol{\Sigma}$. The 'normal' two-level model in (7.9) is a special case of this formulation, with identity link function η.

The likelihood for a two-level GLM involves integrals,

$$l = \prod_{d=1}^{D} \int \cdots \int f\left(\mathbf{y}_d;\, \mathbf{X}_d\boldsymbol{\beta} + \mathbf{Z}_d\boldsymbol{\gamma}_d\right) \Phi(\boldsymbol{\gamma}_d; \boldsymbol{\Sigma})\, \mathrm{d}\boldsymbol{\gamma}_d ,$$

where f is the conditional joint density function for the observations of a district, given $\boldsymbol{\gamma}_d$, and $\Phi(\boldsymbol{\gamma}, \boldsymbol{\Sigma})$ is the density of the r-variate normal distribution with mean $\mathbf{0}$ and variance matrix $\boldsymbol{\Sigma}$. Evaluation of multiple integrals, D per iteration, is a formidable task even today, although a lot of headway has been made in the recent years, owing to a combination of raw computing power, suitable software and efficient algorithms. Numerical quadrature and its adaptations can comfortably tackle the problem in at most two dimensions ($r \leq 2$). Improvements on numerical quadrature with fixed sets of evaluation points incorporate information about the integrand.

Methods that are computationally much less demanding maximise an approximation to the likelihood. They are satisfactory only in some simple settings, and are particularly vulnerable when the district-level variation is substantial.

Appendix. The REML adjustment of the Hessian

This appendix gives an expression for the second-order partial differential of the REML adjustment of the log-likelihood l_{R} for two-level and district-level models.

From (7.20) in Section 7.3.1 we have

$$\frac{\partial l_\Delta}{\partial \omega} = -\frac{1}{2\sigma_{\mathrm{W}}^2} \mathrm{tr}\left\{ \left(\mathbf{X}^\top \mathbf{W}^{-1}\mathbf{X}\right)^{-1} \sum_{d=1}^{D} \mathbf{X}_d^\top \mathbf{W}_d^{-1} \mathbf{Z}_d \,\frac{\partial \boldsymbol{\Omega}}{\partial \omega}\, \mathbf{Z}_d^\top \mathbf{W}_d^{-1}\mathbf{X}_d \right\} ,$$

where $l_\Delta = \partial l/\partial\omega - \partial l_{\mathrm{R}}/\partial\omega$ is the adjustment to the log-likelihood. Denote

$$\mathbf{U} = \sum_{d=1}^{D} \mathbf{Z}_d^\top \mathbf{W}_d^{-1}\mathbf{X}_d \left(\mathbf{X}^\top\mathbf{W}^{-1}\mathbf{X}\right)^{-1} \mathbf{X}_d^\top \mathbf{W}_d^{-1}\mathbf{Z}_d ,$$

so that $\sigma_{\mathrm{W}}^2 \partial l_\Delta/\partial\omega = -\frac{1}{2}\mathrm{tr}\left(\mathbf{U}\,\partial\boldsymbol{\Omega}/\partial\omega\right)$. Then

$$\frac{\partial l_\Delta^2}{\partial\omega_1\partial\omega_2} = -\frac{1}{2\sigma_{\mathrm{W}}^2}\mathrm{tr}\left(\mathbf{U}\,\frac{\partial\boldsymbol{\Omega}}{\partial\omega_1}\,\mathbf{U}\,\frac{\partial\boldsymbol{\Omega}}{\partial\omega_2}\right)$$
$$+\frac{1}{\sigma_{\mathrm{W}}^2}\mathbf{U}\,\frac{\partial\boldsymbol{\Omega}}{\partial\omega_1}\sum_{d=1}^{D}\mathbf{Z}_d^\top\mathbf{W}_d^{-1}\mathbf{X}_d\,\mathbf{X}_d^\top\mathbf{W}_d^{-1}\mathbf{Z}_d\,\mathbf{Z}_d^\top\mathbf{W}_d^{-1}\mathbf{Z}_d\,\frac{\partial\boldsymbol{\Omega}}{\partial\omega_2} . \tag{7.33}$$

District-level models

The adjustment of the log-likelihood for the model in (7.26) has the first-order partial differentials with respect to σ_{W}^2 and ω

$$\frac{\partial l_\Delta}{\partial \sigma_{\mathrm{W}}^2} = \frac{p}{2\sigma_{\mathrm{W}}^2}$$

$$\begin{aligned}\frac{\partial l_\Delta}{\partial \omega} &= -\frac{1}{2}\mathrm{tr}\left\{\left(\overline{\mathbf{X}}^\top \mathbf{W}^{-1}\overline{\mathbf{X}}\right)^{-1}\overline{\mathbf{X}}^\top \left(\mathbf{W}\mathbf{n}\mathbf{W}\right)^{-1}\overline{\mathbf{X}}\right\} \\ &= -\frac{1}{2}\mathrm{tr}\left\{\left(\overline{\mathbf{X}}^\top \mathbf{W}^{-1}\overline{\mathbf{X}}\right)^{-1}\sum_{d=1}^{D}\frac{n_d}{(1+n_d\omega)^2}\overline{\mathbf{x}}_d\overline{\mathbf{x}}_d^\top\right\}. \qquad (7.34)\end{aligned}$$

The adjustments to the information matrix are their negative differentials:

$$-\frac{\partial^2 l_\Delta}{\partial (\sigma_{\mathrm{W}}^2)^2} = \frac{p}{2\sigma_{\mathrm{W}}^4}$$

$$\begin{aligned}-\frac{\partial^2 l_\Delta}{\partial \omega^2} = -\frac{1}{2}\mathrm{tr}&\left[\left\{\left(\overline{\mathbf{X}}^\top \mathbf{W}^{-1}\overline{\mathbf{X}}\right)^{-1}\sum_{d=1}^{D}\frac{n_d}{(1+n_d\omega)^2}\overline{\mathbf{x}}_d\overline{\mathbf{x}}_d^\top\right\}^2\right. \\ &\left. + \left(\overline{\mathbf{X}}^\top \mathbf{W}^{-1}\overline{\mathbf{X}}\right)^{-1}\sum_{d=1}^{D}\frac{n_d^2}{(1+n_d\omega)^3}\overline{\mathbf{x}}_d\overline{\mathbf{x}}_d^\top\right], \qquad (7.35)\end{aligned}$$

and

$$\overline{\mathbf{X}}^\top \mathbf{W}^{-1}\overline{\mathbf{X}} = \sum_{d=1}^{D}\frac{n_d}{1+n_d\omega}\overline{\mathbf{x}}_d\overline{\mathbf{x}}_d^\top .$$

7.7 Suggested reading

Development of methods for random-effect models was strongly simulated by research in animal breeding and genetics; see [102] and references therein. Until the emergence of abundant computing power, efficient organisation of the calculations in a model fitting procedure was an important concern; [93], [101] and [119] respond to this challenge. Bias of the maximum likelihood estimators of the variances in random coefficient models has been regarded as a deficiency from the early days; a comprehensive solution of this problem is presented by [204]; see also [94] and [95]. The influential paper on the EM algorithm, [44], suggested fitting random coefficient models by regarding the random terms as the missing data. See [45], [231] and [278] for applications of this approach. The 'contest' of the computational algorithms for random coefficient models (multilevel analysis) appears to have been won by Fisher scoring, [138] and [149], although iterative generalised least squares and its various generalisations, [85], are used by many through its implementation in the software `MLwin`. For a comprehensive Bayesian treatment of the subject, see [24]. A suite of `Splus` functions for analysis of multilevel data is described and illustrated on numerous examples in [209].

Reference [67] is generally recognised as a landmark contribution to small-area estimation, combining theoretical insights with a purposeful motivation. Reference [10] deals with a small-area problem that has since been the subject of several reanalyses and illustrations. Improved approximations to the (expected) MSEs of model-based small-area estimators are developed in [125]. Reference [210] is a collection of contributions, most of them on model-based methods, to small-area estimation by the 'who-is-who' in the subject in the 1980's. Applications of methods based on Bayesian models to U.S. Government related programmes are presented by [174] and [175]. Concerned with estimation of prevalence (percentages), they engage generalised linear models with random coefficients; see [271] for a closely related application and [82] for a more general treatment of the problem.

Reference [83] presents an authoritative review of methods for small-area estimation. It is updated by [222], although the rate of development since then has accelerated to a great extent. Reference [223] is a comprehensive treatment of the problem from a committed model-based perspective. Reference [259] reviews the current activities in small-area estimation at Statistics Canada and connects estimation with survey design issues. The Bayesian and frequentist paradigms are contrasted by [5] and [258].

7.8 Exercises

1. Describe the essential differences between (paired) ANOVA and rANOVA models with the same number of groups and the same within-group sample sizes. Simulate datasets for the two models. Assess the efficiency of the rANOVA estimator for group 1, $\hat{\mu}_1^{\mathrm{C}}$, in the paired ANOVA model, and the ANOVA estimator $\hat{\mu}_1$ in the paired rANOVA model.
2. Implement the Fisher scoring algorithm for the random-intercept model.
3. Summarise the advantages and drawbacks of the various arrangements for ensuring that intermediate- and final-iteration estimates of the between-district variance matrix in a two-level model are non-negative definite.
4. Prove the identities in (7.21), first for scalar ω (1×1 matrix $\mathbf{\Omega}$).
5. Prove in detail the various matrix versions of rules for differentiation of matrices used in Section 7.3.3, for instance, that

$$\frac{\partial \mathbf{W}^{-1}}{\partial \omega} = -\mathbf{W}^{-1} \frac{\partial \mathbf{W}}{\partial \omega} \mathbf{W}^{-1} .$$

6. Prove that the elementary- and district-level residuals, given by (7.25), add up to the model-fit deviation $\hat{e}_{jd}$.

7. Derive the score and Hessian for the two-level model with the original parametrisation ($\boldsymbol{\beta}$, σ_{W}^2, $\boldsymbol{\Sigma}$), and compare the Fisher scoring algorithm based on it with its alternative based on the relative (scaled) variance matrix $\boldsymbol{\Omega} = \sigma_{\mathrm{W}}^{-2}\boldsymbol{\Sigma}$. Make the same comparison for REML and for district-level models.
8. Simulate a dataset for small-area estimation. Suppose a country comprises $D = 400$ districts. Generate the district-level probabilities p_d of the positive outcome of a binary target variable from a beta distribution. Draw the district-level subsample sizes from a gamma distribution. (Round the values to integers.) Generate the dichotomous values of the target variable.
9. Estimate the between-district variance from the simulated data. Compare it with the variance of the probabilities p_d, $d = 1, \ldots, D$, and with the variance of the beta distribution used for generating p_d. Repeat the exercise a few times.

8

Using auxiliary information

By auxiliary information we mean any information that is not directly related to the target of estimation. The directly related information (*direct information*) for estimating a population summary of a variable in a district is the set of values of that variable on the subsample of subjects from the district. When estimating the mean μ_d of a variable Y in a population of district d, any data pertaining to subjects from outside district d, from a different population in the district, or for a different variable, constitutes auxiliary information. The values of such an *auxiliary variable* may be either from the same or a different population and either from the district or from outside the district. The auxiliary data may be in the form of (individual) subjects' records, their (national or district-level) sample summaries, or summaries that relate to other populations (or other surveys of the same population). Arguably, such information is 'second-rate'; a (sub-)sample of the values of Y from the target population, using a well designed survey, is the gold standard. Often, direct information is not available in sufficient quantity, and auxiliary information is, at a fraction of the cost of the direct information. Sometimes no special effort is required — the auxiliary data for one quantity is the direct information for another. A case in point is estimation of the population mean of several, or all, districts — the data from outside the target district is the auxiliary information.

In this chapter, we develop methods that exploit auxiliary information. 'Exploitation' should be understood as follows: with (more) auxiliary information we estimate the quantity of interest with greater or equal precision (smaller or equal MSE) than without it. Satisfying this standard will turn out to be difficult; we cannot achieve it because the auxiliary information may contain elements that are not useful, and we cannot recognise them with certainty. Nevertheless, we will identify situations in which auxiliary information contributes substantially to improved estimation. The contention will move from identifying suitable auxiliary information to how best to exploit it and how to protect our inferences from a breakdown due to inappropriate assumptions or excessive uncertainty about them.

We can draw a parallel with (ordinary) regression models, where we seek to exploit the 'explanatory' power of covariates. We prefer more explanatory variables, but each of them should contribute to the explanation of the variation in the outcomes. So, we apply a rule for selecting variables, and conclude with a sanitised list of covariates. Whichever way we do it, we have to rely on decisions (whether to include or exclude a variable) that are not correct with certainty. Although such uncertainty is usually ignored, it never should be. Such neglect may cause our inferences to be of poor quality, despite strong false indications to the contrary. Nevertheless, we start by ignoring this source of uncertainty, so as to avoid circular arguments. The problem we pose is still relevant: suppose we have identified an appropriate model for the data (the target variable) and the setting (districts within a country). How should we estimate the district-level means of the target variable?

8.1 From models to small-area estimates

In model-based estimation, we act upon the assumption that the appropriate model has been identified and the estimators derived have the claimed properties. Otherwise, we would be stuck, not knowing the properties of a model fit when the model is not appropriate. And, what is the point of using a model that is not appropriate? Actually, the argument is not quite so one-sided, because the selected model may be inappropriate, despite our best efforts, however competently applied. A defensive strategy would assume that the selected model is *not too bad.*

First we address the following task. A model has been fitted, yielding estimates of all the model parameters and some assessment of their precisions, such as the estimated standard errors. How should small-area estimates be derived from the fit, assuming that the model is appropriate? To focus the discussion, we assume that a two-level model, as in (7.9), has been fitted.

8.1.1 Synthetic estimation

In synthetic estimation we put all our faith in the model we have adopted for the population:

$$Y_{id} = \mathbf{x}_{id}^{\top}\boldsymbol{\beta} + \mathbf{z}_{id}^{\top}\boldsymbol{\gamma}_d + \varepsilon_{id} , \tag{8.1}$$

so that by averaging we obtain

$$\mu_d = \boldsymbol{\mu}_d^{(\mathrm{x})\top}\boldsymbol{\beta} + \boldsymbol{\mu}_d^{(\mathrm{z})\top}\boldsymbol{\gamma}_d + \bar{\varepsilon}_d .$$

We ignore the average of the subject-level deviations, $\bar{\varepsilon}_d$, assuming either that the population is large enough (effectively, infinite), or that it can be estimated no better than by zero. This is equivalent to drawing no distinction between the population of the district and the superpopulation implied by the model in (8.1). Next, suppose the selected model reduces the district-level variation to a level so low that we can ignore it. Or, less profoundly justified, we ignore γ_d because its expectation vanishes; $\mathrm{E}_{\mathcal{D}}(\gamma_{\mathcal{D}}) = \mathbf{0}$. With these steps, we have replaced μ_d with ${\boldsymbol{\mu}_d^{(\mathrm{x})}}^\top \boldsymbol{\beta}$ as our target of estimation. The vector of means $\boldsymbol{\mu}_d^{(\mathrm{x})}$ may be estimated elementwise directly, although whenever the population mean for a component is available it is preferred to its direct estimator. If some of the components can be estimated from other surveys, we should choose the more efficient estimator, although the estimators based on the different sources (surveys) could also be combined.

The estimator

$$\hat{\mu}_d = {\hat{\boldsymbol{\mu}}_d^{(\mathrm{x})}}^\top \hat{\boldsymbol{\beta}}\,, \tag{8.2}$$

with the various alternatives for $\hat{\boldsymbol{\mu}}_d^{(\mathrm{x})}$, is called *synthetic*. There are alternatives for $\hat{\boldsymbol{\beta}}$ also. For example, it could be based on ordinary regression. Our further development does not depend on the origins of $\hat{\boldsymbol{\mu}}_d^{(\mathrm{x})}$ and $\hat{\boldsymbol{\beta}}$. We merely assume that they are (approximately) unbiased, and denote by $\boldsymbol{\Sigma}_\mathrm{x}$ and $\boldsymbol{\Sigma}_\beta$ their respective sampling variance matrices.

The first row and column of $\boldsymbol{\Sigma}_\mathrm{x}$ comprises zeros because the corresponding variable, the intercept, entails no variation. The rows and columns that correspond to the other variables for which the (district-level) population means $\boldsymbol{\mu}_d^{(\mathrm{x})}$ are known also vanish. Variables that are constant within districts also belong to this category, although their values in districts not represented in the survey may have to be established separately from the survey.

When $\boldsymbol{\Sigma}_\mathrm{x} = \mathbf{0}$, that is, when $\hat{\boldsymbol{\mu}}_d^{(\mathrm{x})} = \boldsymbol{\mu}_d^{(\mathrm{x})}$,

$$\mathrm{var}\left({\hat{\boldsymbol{\mu}}_d^{(\mathrm{x})}}^\top \hat{\boldsymbol{\beta}} \right) = {\boldsymbol{\mu}_d^{(\mathrm{x})}}^\top \boldsymbol{\Sigma}_\beta \boldsymbol{\mu}_d^{(\mathrm{x})}\,,$$

and so, assuming that $\mathbf{Z}$ is a subset of $\mathbf{X}$,

$$\mathrm{MSE}\left({\hat{\boldsymbol{\mu}}_d^{(\mathrm{x})}}^\top \hat{\boldsymbol{\beta}} \,|\, \mu_d^{(\mathrm{x})} \right) = {\boldsymbol{\mu}_d^{(\mathrm{x})}}^\top \boldsymbol{\Sigma}_\beta \boldsymbol{\mu}_d^{(\mathrm{x})} + {\boldsymbol{\mu}_d^{(\mathrm{z})}}^\top \gamma_d \gamma_d^\top \boldsymbol{\mu}_d^{(\mathrm{z})}\,.$$

The eMSE is equal to the same expression, with $\gamma_d \gamma_d^\top$ replaced by its district-level expectation $\boldsymbol{\Sigma}_\mathrm{B}$.

When $\boldsymbol{\mu}_d^{(\mathrm{x})}$, or some of its components, are not known the MSE and eMSE are bound to be greater; less information should yield less precision. For simplicity, we assume that $\hat{\boldsymbol{\mu}}_d^{(\mathrm{x})}$ and $\hat{\boldsymbol{\beta}}$ are not correlated. This is not correct when $\hat{\boldsymbol{\mu}}_d^{(\mathrm{x})}$ and $\hat{\boldsymbol{\beta}}$ are based on overlapping sets of subjects (the district subsample and the survey sample), but the overlap is small for all but one or two of the most populous districts. If $\mathrm{cov}\left(\hat{\boldsymbol{\mu}}_d^{(\mathrm{x})}, \hat{\boldsymbol{\beta}}\right) = \mathbf{0}$,

$$\mathrm{var}\left({\hat{\boldsymbol{\mu}}_d^{(\mathrm{x})}}^\top \hat{\boldsymbol{\beta}} \right) = \mathrm{tr}\left(\boldsymbol{\Sigma}_\mathrm{x} \boldsymbol{\Sigma}_\beta\right) + \boldsymbol{\beta}^\top \boldsymbol{\Sigma}_\mathrm{x} \boldsymbol{\beta} + {\boldsymbol{\mu}_d^{(\mathrm{x})}}^\top \boldsymbol{\Sigma}_\beta \boldsymbol{\mu}_d^{(\mathrm{x})}\,; \tag{8.3}$$

the first two terms can be interpreted as the 'penalty' for not knowing $\boldsymbol{\mu}_d^{(\mathrm{x})}$. This variance inflation presents a dilemma. Should we include a covariate x in the model because it is a good predictor, without considering its impact on $\mathrm{var}\left(\hat{\boldsymbol{\mu}}_d^{(\mathrm{x})\top}\hat{\boldsymbol{\beta}}\right)$? In an orthodox two-step approach, we would establish a suitable model first, and then base the estimation on the fit of this model, disregarding any information about $\boldsymbol{\Sigma}_{\mathrm{x}}$. Note that we do not know $\boldsymbol{\Sigma}_\beta$ in advance either, so we are at the mercy of some quantities (variance matrices) we did not expect to be of much importance.

In summary, a good model (that is, a model that fits the data well) does not solve all the problems. Some worse fitting models may be more useful. Moreover, some models may be better suited for inferences about some districts and other models about other districts. These negative comments about modelling may encourage the reader to apply patently inadequate models, such as the ordinary regression, assuming $\mathbf{Z} = \mathbf{0}$ in (8.1). The approach we advocate weighs carefully what the alternative models have to offer.

Another plausible failure of the synthetic estimator is depicted in Figure 8.1. The estimator of μ_d is based on a regression with a single variable and parallel regressions ($\mathbf{Z} = \mathbf{1}$). The symbols A and B mark the sampled subjects from two districts; one with predominantly positive and one with negative deviation γ_d, so that the synthetic estimator has a substantial bias for both districts. Little comfort that the biases average out; relying on $\mathrm{E}_{\mathcal{D}}(\gamma_{\mathcal{D}}) = 0$ is not appropriate.

The variation of the means μ_d around the regression $\mathbf{x}^\top\boldsymbol{\beta}$ is a component of $\mathrm{eMSE}\left(\hat{\boldsymbol{\mu}}_d^{(\mathrm{x})\top}\hat{\boldsymbol{\beta}} \,|\, \mu_d\right)$:

$$\mathrm{eMSE}\left(\hat{\boldsymbol{\mu}}_d^{(\mathrm{x})\top}\hat{\boldsymbol{\beta}} \,|\, \mu_d\right) = \boldsymbol{\mu}_d^{(\mathrm{z})\top}\boldsymbol{\Sigma}_{\mathrm{B}}\boldsymbol{\mu}_d^{(\mathrm{z})} + \mathrm{var}\left(\hat{\boldsymbol{\mu}}_d^{(\mathrm{x})\top}\hat{\boldsymbol{\beta}}\right),$$

and the variance is given by (8.3).

Apportionment method

The apportionment method is a special case of synthetic estimation, in which the auxiliary information comprises the values of a single categorical variable on the sample. This variable may be defined for the districts (each district belonging to a category), it may be almost so (many districts belong to one category but some straddle across the categories' boundaries), or not at all. Geographical classifications, such as to regions, are examples of the former two cases, and a classification of the subjects (such as according to age or family composition) an example of the latter.

In the apportionment method, the national mean (or another population summary) is first estimated for each category, and the estimate for a district is derived by combining these estimates according to the composition of the

Figure 8.1. An illustration of a weakness of the synthetic estimator. The symbols A and B represent the samples from two districts. The solid line is the fit to the sample and the dashed line the fit to the population.

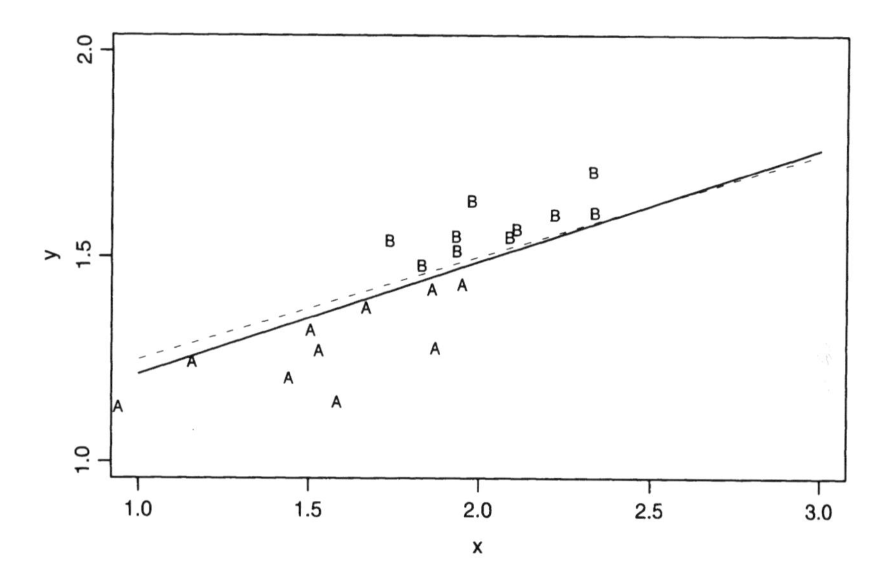

district. Suppose the categories have national means θ_k, $k = 1, \ldots, K$, and they are estimated by $\hat{\theta}_k$. The mean for a district that belongs entirely to category k is estimated by $\hat{\theta}_k$. The mean for district d that overlaps with the categories $k = 1, \ldots, K$ with respective fractions p_{dk} is estimated by

$$\hat{\mu}_d = \sum_{k=1}^{K} p_{dk} \hat{\theta}_k = \mathbf{p}_d^\top \hat{\boldsymbol{\theta}} ,$$

where $\mathbf{p}_d = (p_{d1}, \ldots, p_{dK})^\top$ are the population proportions N_{dk}/N_d of the representation of category k in district d, and $\hat{\boldsymbol{\theta}} = (\hat{\theta}_1, \ldots, \hat{\theta}_K)^\top$. The vector $\mathbf{p}_d$ is also called the *composition* of district d. In $\hat{\mu}_d$, each category's estimate is given weight according to the (population) size of its overlap with the district. The proportions p_{dk} may not be available, and have to be estimated. This is particularly problematic when the category-by-district subsamples are small and no external information about the counts N_{dk} or the composition $\mathbf{p}_d$ is available.

The apportionment method is effective when the subpopulations within the categories are relatively homogeneous, when the within-category variances are small. Apart from knowing the composition $\mathbf{p}_d$, or estimating it with high precision, another important contributor to the success of the method is that the subpopulations of the district-by-category intersections have similar means within each category. That is, $\hat{\theta}_k$ is a good estimator of μ_{dk}, the mean for the intersection of district d and category k. This condition is not directly promoted by the choice of the classification. After all, the categories may be quite heterogeneous, and yet their within-district means quite similar. A related condition, that the within-district subpopulations have similar distributions within each category, can be interpreted as *non-informative* allocation of subjects to districts. To motivate this, suppose the assignment or attribution of the category precedes the allocation, and the district of (present or future) residence itself exerts no influence on the assignment. Such a process, in which subjects from each category are assigned to the districts at random (although with varying subsample sizes), with no regard for their values of the outcome variable, might be a realistic model for how subjects have ended up in the various districts and how they have acquired their particular values. However, nobody and no identifiable force could have exercised any control over such an allocation. The apportionment method is particularly vulnerable in this regard.

A careful reader will notice that the arguments against the apportionment method run parallel with those against synthetic estimation. In summary, the synthetic estimator entails two sources or error: the replacement of μ_d by ${\boldsymbol{\mu}_d^{(\mathrm{x})}}^\top \boldsymbol{\beta}$ as the target, and estimation of ${\boldsymbol{\mu}_d^{(\mathrm{x})}}^\top \boldsymbol{\beta}$. And, as with all model-based methods, model selection is another source.

8.2 Composite estimation

Synthetic estimators use a formula derived for the whole country and apply it to each district. This may be very effective for the districts with poor representation in the survey because their direct information is of next to no use. However, for districts with substantial representation, for which the direct estimator is competitive, the synthetic estimator accords no preference to the data from the district. This iniquity can be resolved by using the direct estimator for the districts with the largest subsample sizes. To do this we would designate a threshold sample size n^*; for the districts with $n_d > n^*$ the direct estimator would be used, and for the other districts the synthetic estimator. The discontinuity (switching from one estimator to the other) is discomforting. For some districts, the method applied accords no special status to the outcomes from the district concerned; for others, data from outside the district are ignored altogether. The role of the outcomes from the district concerned can be enhanced by combining the direct estimator with the synthetic one. This can be arranged, with the coefficients satisfying a well specified criterion. The composite estimator derived in Chapter 6 can be regarded as a special case of this, with the synthetic estimator based on the trivial model $y = \mu + \varepsilon$. With it, the auxiliary information comprises the values of the target variable from outside the district. Here we will draw on more extensive auxiliary information, exploiting the association of the target variable with the covariates.

Suppose an appropriate two-level model has been identified and fitted and, having been based on a large sample, its parameters are estimated with precision so high that we need to make no distinction between estimators and underlying parameters. For further simplicity, suppose the district-level population means of the covariates, $\boldsymbol{\mu}_d^{(\mathrm{x})}$, are known. The synthetic estimator $\hat{\boldsymbol{\mu}}_d^{(\mathrm{x})\top} \hat{\boldsymbol{\beta}}$ of μ_d has bias $B_d = -\boldsymbol{\mu}_d^{(\mathrm{z})\top} \boldsymbol{\gamma}_d$, so its eMSE is

$$\mathrm{E}_{\mathcal{D}} \left(\boldsymbol{\mu}_d^{(\mathrm{z})\top} \boldsymbol{\gamma}_{\mathcal{D}} \boldsymbol{\gamma}_{\mathcal{D}}^\top \boldsymbol{\mu}_d^{(\mathrm{z})} \right) = \boldsymbol{\mu}_d^{(\mathrm{z})\top} \boldsymbol{\Sigma}_{\mathrm{B}} \boldsymbol{\mu}_d^{(\mathrm{z})} . \qquad (8.4)$$

We can estimate B_d without bias by the average residual $\overline{e}_d = \overline{y}_d - \overline{\mathbf{x}}_d \boldsymbol{\beta}$; it is unbiased and its variance is $\sigma_{\mathrm{W}}^2/n_d$. As in Chapter 6, we do not choose between the two candidates, $\hat{\boldsymbol{\mu}}_d^{(\mathrm{x})\top} \hat{\boldsymbol{\beta}}$ and $\overline{y}_d$, but combine them, aiming to estimate μ_d with minimum MSE or eMSE. The two estimators are uncorrelated, one with small variance but expected squared bias B_d^2 and the other with no bias but variance $\sigma_{\mathrm{W}}^2/n_d$. The coefficients of their combination that has minimum MSE are proportional to their respective precisions:

$$(1 - b_d^*)\overline{y}_d + b_d^* \boldsymbol{\mu}_d^{(\mathrm{x})\top} \boldsymbol{\beta} = \boldsymbol{\mu}_d^{(\mathrm{x})\top} \boldsymbol{\beta} + (1 - b_d^*) \left(\overline{y}_d - \boldsymbol{\mu}_d^{(\mathrm{x})\top} \boldsymbol{\beta} \right) , \qquad (8.5)$$

where

$$b_d^* = \frac{\sigma_{\mathrm{W}}^2/n_d}{\sigma_{\mathrm{W}}^2/n_d + \left(\boldsymbol{\gamma}_d^\top \boldsymbol{\mu}_d^{(\mathrm{z})} \right)^2} .$$

The dependence of b_d^* on $\boldsymbol{\gamma}_d$ is avoided by minimising eMSE, with the coefficient

$$b_d = \frac{\sigma_{\mathrm{W}}^2/n_d}{\sigma_{\mathrm{W}}^2/n_d + \boldsymbol{\mu}_d^{(\mathrm{z})\top} \boldsymbol{\Sigma}_{\mathrm{B}} \boldsymbol{\mu}_d^{(\mathrm{z})}} = \frac{1}{1 + n_d \boldsymbol{\mu}_d^{(\mathrm{z})\top} \boldsymbol{\Omega} \boldsymbol{\mu}_d^{(\mathrm{z})}} ,$$

where $\boldsymbol{\Omega} = \sigma_{\mathrm{W}}^{-2} \boldsymbol{\Sigma}_{\mathrm{B}}$ is the scaled variance matrix, the multivariate version of the variance ratio ω.

An alternative estimator is derived from the conditional expectation of $\boldsymbol{\gamma}_d$; see (7.23). We estimate μ_d by

$$\boldsymbol{\mu}_d^{(\mathrm{x})\top} \boldsymbol{\beta} + \boldsymbol{\mu}_d^{(\mathrm{z})\top} \boldsymbol{\Omega} \left(\mathbf{I} + \mathbf{Z}_d^\top \mathbf{Z}_d \boldsymbol{\Omega} \right)^{-1} \mathbf{Z}_d^\top \mathbf{e}_d . \qquad (8.6)$$

This estimator differs substantially from (8.5); for example, it cannot be expressed as a function of $\boldsymbol{\mu}_d^{(\mathrm{z})}$. The difference is due to the perspectives adopted in deriving the two estimators. For $\mathbf{Z} = \mathbf{1}$, the estimators (8.5) and (8.6) are

$$\frac{B_d^2}{\sigma_{\mathrm{W}}^2/n_d + B_d^2} \overline{y}_d + \frac{\sigma_{\mathrm{W}}^2/n_d}{\sigma_{\mathrm{W}}^2/n_d + B_d^2} \boldsymbol{\mu}_d^{(\mathrm{x})\top} \boldsymbol{\beta}$$

$$\frac{n_d\omega}{1 + n_d\omega} \overline{y}_d + \boldsymbol{\mu}_d^{(\mathrm{x})\top} \boldsymbol{\beta} - \frac{n_d\omega}{1 + n_d\omega} \overline{\mathbf{x}}_d^{\top} \boldsymbol{\beta} ,$$

respectively. They differ because the former minimises MSE and the latter eMSE (B_d^2 vs. $\sigma_W^2\omega$), and because the latter involves the sample mean $\overline{\mathbf{x}}_d$ instead of the population mean $\boldsymbol{\mu}_d$.

In (8.5), we acknowledge that district d has a population with a mean $\boldsymbol{\mu}_d^{(z)}$ different from its sample version $\overline{\mathbf{z}}_d$, whereas in (8.6) $\boldsymbol{\mu}_d^{(z)}$ does not appear at all, because the underlying model assumes that the values of all the covariates are fixed. The estimator in (8.6) has optimal properties with respect to replications in which $\mathbf{Z}_d$ is fixed and $\gamma_{d'}$ for $d' \neq d$ are random. The replications relevant to the small-area setting have $\mathbf{Z}_d$ random (it is outside the designer's control) and $\gamma_{d'}$ are fixed — they do not differ from one replication to the next. In (8.6), the synthetic and direct estimators are combined more flexibly than in (8.5); on the other hand, the reliance on $\overline{\mathbf{z}}_d$ is disconcerting especially when the within-district sample size n_d is small or the within-district variance of $\mathbf{z}_d$ is large. However, the properties of both estimators are contingent on appropriateness of the selected model. Such concerns about model choice and diagnostics are an unwelcome part of the 'modelling' bargain.

An undoubted advantage of composite estimation is that the 'individuality' γ_d of each district is represented. This is done by regarding γ_d as random. It is by no means a step toward a valid (or correct) model! The boundaries of the districts have been drawn up administratively, possibly with some historical precedents, so the districts may evolve their individuality over time. However, the district-level deviations γ_d are by no means random; if a replication of the survey were conducted the values of γ_d would not change for any district d. Also, other divisions of the country may have their individualities, some may be stronger than for the districts. But the complication of the model implied by this argument is not constructive and is hardly warranted.

8.2.1 Shrinkage and borrowing strength

For parallel regressions ($\mathbf{Z} = \mathbf{1}$), the district-level deviation is estimated by

$$\hat{\gamma}_d = b_d \left(\overline{y}_d - \overline{\mathbf{x}}_d^\top \hat{\boldsymbol{\beta}} \right) ,$$

where

$$b_d = \frac{n_d \hat{\omega}}{1 + n_d \hat{\omega}} .$$

Naively, we would estimate $\hat{\gamma}_d$ as the average residual $\overline{\hat{e}}_d = \overline{y}_d - \overline{\mathbf{x}}_d^\top \hat{\boldsymbol{\beta}}$. Taking the conditional expectation leads to a *shrinkage* toward zero, the (unconditional) expectation of γ_d. The raw-average residual $\overline{\hat{e}}_d$ is pulled toward zero, and the extent of shrinkage depends on the sample size n_d and the estimated district-level variance. This is easy to motivate when $\hat{\omega} = \omega = 0$. In this case, the same regression applies to each district, and so $\overline{\hat{e}}_d$ differs from zero solely because of the within-district variation and finite sample size n_d. When $\hat{\omega}$ is very large and n_d not very small, little shrinkage takes place. For intermediate values of $\hat{\omega}$ and n_d, the extent of shrinkage is a compromise that can be described as a composition of the unbiased estimator $\hat{\bar{e}}_d$ and zero. The small-area estimator of μ_d based on $\hat{\gamma}_d$ is

$$\begin{aligned}\tilde{\mu}_d &= \overline{\mathbf{x}}_d^\top \hat{\boldsymbol{\beta}} + (1 - b_d)\hat{\bar{e}}_d \\ &= (1 - b_d)\overline{y}_d + b_d \overline{\mathbf{x}}_d^\top \hat{\boldsymbol{\beta}} \,. \end{aligned} \tag{8.7}$$

This is a composite estimator, combining the direct estimator $\overline{y}_d$ and the synthetic estimator $\overline{\mathbf{x}}^\top \hat{\boldsymbol{\beta}}$. We can regard the national mean, considered in Section 6.3, as the synthetic estimator based on the regression model with no covariates. The shrinkage of $\hat{\bar{e}}_d$ toward zero converts in (8.7) to shrinkage toward the 'average' regression $\mathbf{x}^\top \hat{\boldsymbol{\beta}}$. This can be motivated as hedging bets against any idiosyncracies of district d by drawing on the information in the rest of the data, or *borrowing strength* from the other districts.

The conditional variance of $\hat{\gamma}_d$ is

$$\operatorname{var}(\hat{\gamma}_d \,|\, \mathbf{y};\, \mathbf{X}) \;=\; \frac{\sigma_{\mathrm{W}}^2 \omega}{1 + n_d \omega} \,.$$

This variance is based on averaging over the districts, and so it is comparable to eMSE in Chapter 6.

In summary, $\tilde{\mu}_d$ in (8.7) is a generalisation of the composite estimator derived in Section 6.3. The original composite estimator makes no use of auxiliary information contained in the other variables, but is applicable for any population quantity, so long as it can be estimated directly. Its straightforward application is associated with two important caveats: that the district-level variance is estimated, and that eMSE is minimised (subject to approximation) instead of MSE. On the other hand, the optimal properties of the shrinkage estimator in (8.7) rely on appropriateness of the model (including the normality of y), are based on estimates $\hat{\boldsymbol{\beta}}$ and $\hat{\omega}$, and their precision is also evaluated by the estimated eMSE. The regression model has a great potential to contribute to efficient estimation of μ_d by reducing ω, but the method is applicable only to population means and their transformations (including the population total, if the district-level population sizes are known). For a good set of auxiliary variables, ω is greatly reduced. Section 8.3 describes a method in which the strengths of the two approaches are combined — auxiliary information is exploited, but without having to rely on a model with the straitjacket of linearity and normality. Of course, these conditions can be replaced by others, as in GLM and non-linear models, but the model specification remains a difficult problem and an inconvenient caveat. The problem is further compounded by the choice of the variation part of the model, although it is often sufficient to set $\mathbf{Z} = \mathbf{1}$.

8.3 Multivariate composition

We concluded in the discussion of (8.7) that estimation of the district-level mean μ_d can be improved by combining the sample mean $\overline{y}_d$ with the synthetic estimator. The synthetic estimator is a linear combination of $\overline{\mathbf{x}}_d$, and so the estimator $\tilde{\mu}_d$ is a linear combination of $(\overline{y}_d, \overline{\mathbf{x}}_d)$. Do we need the model and the baggage of the associated assumptions? Why not tackle the problem head-on and estimate μ_d by

$$\hat{\mu}_d^{\mathrm{C}} = (1 - \mathbf{b}_d^\top \mathbf{1})\overline{y}_d + \mathbf{b}_d^\top \overline{\mathbf{x}}_d \tag{8.8}$$

for a suitably selected vector $\mathbf{b}_d$? This formulation has several advantages: first, having the same form as in (8.7), $\hat{\mu}_d^{\mathrm{C}}$ in (8.8) is more general because the coefficients $\mathbf{b}_d$ are not imposed by a possibly inappropriate model. The assumptions of normality and linearity are dispensed with. Further, we have the option to replace any component of $\overline{\mathbf{x}}_d$ with a different estimator of its subpopulation version (based on an external source), or even with the subpopulation quantity itself. In the two-level model, we could not use any variable without its values for each sampled subject. Related to this is the flexibility in incorporating the sampling design. In two-level models, this entails some difficulties; in the newly formulated task, this amounts to replacing $\overline{\mathbf{x}}_d$ with the direct estimator of the corresponding population mean. And finally, we can dispense with the (iterative) computational routines for model fitting that, in the end, yield estimators of μ_d by an indirect route.

We restate the problem in a slightly more general form, mainly to introduce a simpler notation, but also to indicate the versatility of the approach. Suppose $\hat{\boldsymbol{\mu}}_d$ is an unbiased estimator of the district-level mean $\boldsymbol{\mu}_d$ and $\hat{\boldsymbol{\mu}}$ is an unbiased estimator of the national mean $\boldsymbol{\mu}$. To estimate a linear combination $\mu_d = \mathbf{u}^\top \boldsymbol{\mu}_d$, with a known vector $\mathbf{u}$, we consider the estimators of the form

$$\hat{\mu}_d^{\mathrm{C}} = (\mathbf{u} - \mathbf{b}_d)^\top \hat{\boldsymbol{\mu}}_d + \mathbf{b}_d^\top \hat{\boldsymbol{\mu}} . \tag{8.9}$$

This is the multivariate analogue of the estimator in (6.4), even though the target μ_d is a scalar. For example, estimating the first component of $\boldsymbol{\mu}_d$ corresponds to setting $\mathbf{u} = (1, 0, \ldots, 0)^\top$. As in Section 6.3, we first find the minimum MSE estimator $\hat{\mu}_d^{\mathrm{C}}$, and then address the problem of estimating the optimal vector of coefficients $\mathbf{b}_d^*$, as it depends on unknown parameters. Since we consider several versions of $\hat{\mu}_d^{\mathrm{C}}$, defined by the vector of coefficients $\mathbf{b}_d$, we write $\hat{\mu}_d^{\mathrm{C}}(\mathbf{b}_d)$ to emphasize the dependence on $\mathbf{b}_d$. In most cases, $\mathbf{b}_d$ depends on some parameters that have to be estimated, and so we will also work with $\hat{\mu}_d^{\mathrm{C}}(\hat{\mathbf{b}}_d)$, using an estimator in place of $\mathbf{b}_d$.

The notation we use parallels its univariate version introduced in Chapter 6: $\mathbf{V}_d$ is the sampling variance matrix of $\hat{\boldsymbol{\mu}}_d$ and $\mathbf{V}$ the sampling variance matrix of $\hat{\boldsymbol{\mu}}$; $\mathbf{C}_d = \mathrm{cov}(\hat{\boldsymbol{\mu}}, \hat{\boldsymbol{\mu}}_d)$ and $\boldsymbol{\Delta}_d = \boldsymbol{\mu} - \boldsymbol{\mu}_d$. The MSE of $\hat{\mu}_d^{\mathrm{C}}$ in (8.9) is

$$\begin{aligned}
\mathrm{MSE}\left\{\hat{\mu}_d^{\mathrm{C}}(\mathbf{b}_d)\right\} &= (\mathbf{u} - \mathbf{b}_d)^\top \mathbf{V}_d(\mathbf{u} - \mathbf{b}_d) + \mathbf{b}_d^\top \mathbf{V} \mathbf{b}_d + 2\mathbf{b}_d^\top \mathbf{C}_d(\mathbf{u} - \mathbf{b}_d) \\
&\quad + \mathbf{b}_d^\top \boldsymbol{\Delta}_d^\top \boldsymbol{\Delta}_d \mathbf{b}_d \, . \\
&= \mathbf{u}^\top \mathbf{V}_d \mathbf{u} - 2\mathbf{b}_d^\top \left(\mathbf{V}_d - \mathbf{C}_d\right) \mathbf{u} \\
&\quad + \mathbf{b}_d^\top \left(\mathbf{V}_d + \mathbf{V} - \mathbf{C}_d - \mathbf{C}_d^\top + \boldsymbol{\Delta}_d^\top \boldsymbol{\Delta}_d\right) \mathbf{b}_d \\
&= \mathbf{u}^\top \mathbf{R}_0 \mathbf{u} - 2\mathbf{b}_d^\top \mathbf{R}_1 \mathbf{u} + \mathbf{b}_d^\top \mathbf{R}_2 \mathbf{b}_d \, ,
\end{aligned} \tag{8.10}$$

with the implicitly defined matrices $\mathbf{R}_0$, $\mathbf{R}_1$ and $\mathbf{R}_2$ that are the obvious multivariate analogues of R_0, R_1 and R_2 introduced in Section 6.3; see (6.5). The MSE in (8.10) is minimised for

$$\begin{aligned}\mathbf{b}_d^* &= \mathbf{R}_2^{-1}\mathbf{R}_1\mathbf{u} \\ &= \left(\mathbf{V}_d + \mathbf{V} - \mathbf{C}_d - \mathbf{C}_d^\top + \boldsymbol{\Delta}_d\boldsymbol{\Delta}_d^\top\right)^{-1}(\mathbf{V}_d - \mathbf{C}_d)\mathbf{u}\,;\end{aligned}$$

the inverse is well defined because $\mathbf{R}_2 = \mathrm{E}\left\{(\hat{\boldsymbol{\mu}}_d - \hat{\boldsymbol{\mu}})(\hat{\boldsymbol{\mu}}_d - \hat{\boldsymbol{\mu}})^\top\right\}$ is positive definite. The minimum attained is

$$\begin{aligned}&\mathbf{R}_0 - \mathbf{R}_1^\top\mathbf{R}_2^{-1}\mathbf{R}_1 \\ &= \mathbf{u}^\top\mathbf{V}_d\mathbf{u} - \mathbf{u}^\top(\mathbf{V}_d - \mathbf{C}_d^\top)\left(\mathbf{V}_d + \mathbf{V} - \mathbf{C}_d - \mathbf{C}_d^\top + \boldsymbol{\Delta}_d\boldsymbol{\Delta}_d^\top\right)^{-1}(\mathbf{V}_d - \mathbf{C}_d)\mathbf{u}\,.\end{aligned}$$

If $\mathbf{b}_d^*$ were available, $\mathbf{u}^\top\boldsymbol{\mu}_d$ would be estimated by

$$\hat{\mu}_d^{\mathrm{C}} = \mathbf{u}^\top\left(\mathbf{I} - \mathbf{R}_1^\top\mathbf{R}_2^{-1}\right)\hat{\boldsymbol{\mu}}_d + \mathbf{u}^\top\mathbf{R}_1^\top\mathbf{R}_2^{-1}\hat{\boldsymbol{\mu}}\,.$$

As this holds for an arbitrary vector $\mathbf{u}$, we can omit it and state that the vector $\boldsymbol{\mu}_d$ is estimated efficiently by

$$\hat{\boldsymbol{\mu}}_d^{\mathrm{C}} = (\mathbf{I} - \mathbf{B}_d^*)^\top\hat{\boldsymbol{\mu}}_d + \mathbf{B}_d^{*\top}\hat{\boldsymbol{\mu}}\,, \qquad (8.11)$$

where $\mathbf{B}_d^* = \left(\mathbf{V}_d + \mathbf{V} - \mathbf{C}_d - \mathbf{C}_d^\top + \boldsymbol{\Delta}_d\boldsymbol{\Delta}_d^\top\right)^{-1}(\mathbf{V}_d - \mathbf{C}_d)$. The estimator $\hat{\boldsymbol{\mu}}_d^{\mathrm{C}}$ is called *multivariate composite*; it is a generalisation of the *univariate* composite estimator introduced in Section 6.3. We refer to $\mathbf{B}_d^*$ as the shrinkage matrix.

Practical implementation of (8.11) is hindered by our inability to estimate $\boldsymbol{\Delta}_d$ with any appreciable precision for most districts. We can adopt the solution proposed in Section 6.3 — to replace the squared bias $\boldsymbol{\Delta}_d\boldsymbol{\Delta}_d^\top$ with its district-level expectation $\boldsymbol{\Sigma}_{\mathrm{B}}$. As a consequence, we switch the assessment of efficiency from MSE to eMSE, as we have done in the univariate setting.

8.3.1 How to choose x?

Although multivariate composition involves no models, the variables in $\mathbf{x}$ that constitute the auxiliary information still have to be selected. More variables should yield a more efficient estimator. This is the case with the *ideal* composite estimator (8.11) because the MSE attains a lower minimum when optimised over a wider range of convex combinations.

In practice, the (co-)variance matrices $\mathbf{V}_d$, $\mathbf{V}$ and $\mathbf{C}_d$, as well as the vector of biases $\boldsymbol{\Delta}_d$ or the district-level variance matrix $\boldsymbol{\Sigma}_{\mathrm{B}}$, have to be estimated. Many variables in $\mathbf{X}$, especially when some of them are highly correlated, introduce an instability in $\hat{\mathbf{B}}_d^*$ and, as a result, a paradox — more auxiliary information leads to less efficiency. However, for a single auxiliary variable, the intuition is confirmed. A variable that has a higher district-level correlation with y, smaller sampling variance and smaller district-level variation leads to greater efficiency. To show this, suppose $\mathbf{u} = (1, 0)$ and let

$$\mathbf{V}_d = \begin{pmatrix} V_d^{(1)} & V_d^{(12)} \\ V_d^{(21)} & V_d^{(2)} \end{pmatrix},$$

and similarly for $\mathbf{\Sigma}_\mathrm{B}$, $\mathbf{V}$ and $\mathbf{C}_d$. (Note that $\mathbf{C}_d$ is not symmetric.) We explore how $\mathrm{eMSE}\left\{\hat{\mu}_d^\mathrm{C}(\mathbf{b}_d)\right\}$ depends on $V_d^{(2)}$, $V^{(2)}$ and $\Sigma_\mathrm{B}^{(2)}$, the variances associated with the auxiliary variable. Suppose $\hat{\boldsymbol{\mu}} = \sum_d q_d \hat{\boldsymbol{\mu}}_d$ and the two components of $\boldsymbol{\mu}$ are estimated from the same survey. Then $\mathbf{C}_d = q_d \mathbf{V}_d$, and $\mathbf{R}_1 = (1 - q_d)\mathbf{V}_d$ and $\mathbf{R}_2 = (1 - 2q_d)\mathbf{V}_d + \mathbf{V} + \mathbf{\Sigma}_\mathrm{B}$. The reduction of the eMSE by the bivariate shrinkage is by

$$(1 - q_d)^2 (0 \;\; 1) \mathbf{V}_d \left\{\mathbf{V}_d (1 - 2q_d) + \mathbf{V} + \mathbf{\Sigma}_\mathrm{B}\right\}^{-1} \mathbf{V}_d (0 \;\; 1)^\top ,$$

that is, the $(1 - q_d)^2$-multiple of the (2,2) element of the matrix

$$\mathbf{V}_d \left\{\mathbf{V}_d (1 - 2q_d) + \mathbf{V} + \mathbf{\Sigma}_\mathrm{B}\right\}^{-1} \mathbf{V}_d .$$

This is

$$\frac{(1 - q_d)^2 V_d^{(1)2}}{F_d^{(1)} - \Sigma_\mathrm{B}^{(12)2} / F_d^{(2)}} ,$$

where $F_d^{(h)}$, $h = 1, 2$, is the diagonal element of the 'denominator' matrix $\mathbf{V}_d + \mathbf{V} - \mathbf{C}_d - \mathbf{C}_d^\top + \mathbf{\Sigma}_\mathrm{B}$. This expression enables a simple discussion of when an auxiliary variable is useful in bivariate composite estimation. First, large district-level covariance $\Sigma_\mathrm{B}^{(12)}$ (its sign is immaterial) is preferred. Second, small $F_d^{(2)}$ is preferred; that is, small sampling variance $V_d^{(2)}$ and small district-level variance $\Sigma_\mathrm{B}^{(2)}$. The variance $V^{(2)}$ and covariance $C_d^{(12)}$ are of much smaller magnitude than $V_d^{(2)}$, so their values have only a minor impact.

Next, suppose the auxiliary information originates from a different survey, so that the direct estimators of the two components of $\boldsymbol{\mu}_d$ are independent. The same algebra applies as above, except that $\mathbf{V}_d$, $\mathbf{C}_d$ and $\mathbf{V}$ are diagonal. Now $\hat{\boldsymbol{\mu}} = \sum_d \mathbf{Q}_d \hat{\boldsymbol{\mu}}_d$ and $\mathbf{C}_d = \mathbf{Q}_d \mathbf{V}_d$, where $\mathbf{Q}_d$ are diagonal matrices containing the sampling fractions in the two surveys.

Estimating the sampling (co-)variance matrices $\mathbf{V}_d$, $\mathbf{V}$ and $\mathbf{C}_d$ is a task from standard sampling theory, and so we do not address it here. However, we explore the impact of uncertainty about them on small-area estimation. The only other quantity required in composite estimation is the district-level variance matrix $\mathbf{\Sigma}_\mathrm{B}$.

Estimators of μ_d based on two-level models with random slopes involve within-district totals of cross-products, $\mathbf{Z}_d^\top \mathbf{X}_d$, see (7.25). The estimator in (8.9) maintains its generality over model-based estimators if the corresponding within-district mean cross-products are included in the vector μ_d. Note that the constituent variables, $\mathbf{Z}$ and $\mathbf{X}$, are also represented in the auxiliary information, so $\hat{\boldsymbol{\mu}}_d$ may contain several highly correlated estimators. It is easier to see in composite estimation that this is not conducive to efficient estimation. In the model-based approach, the problem appears not to arise because $\hat{\mu}_d^{\mathrm{C}}$ is based on an expression derived by assuming known district-level variance matrix $\boldsymbol{\Sigma}_{\mathrm{B}}$, and model choice and assessment are made by exploring the overall fit.

In model-based approach, we have to be careful about explanatory variables that are recorded (observed) subject to error. In multivariate composition these auxiliary variables can be used as any other, so long as the measurement error is duly reflected in $\mathbf{V}_{d,}$, $\mathbf{C}_d$ and $\mathbf{V}$, or their estimators. This is a much simpler problem than the correction for attenuation in regression.

8.3.2 Estimating $\boldsymbol{\Sigma}_{\mathrm{B}}$

The auxiliary variables in $\mathbf{X}$ are not necessarily normally distributed, neither within nor across districts. It is therefore advantageous to avoid any methods that rely on normality. The district-level variance matrix can be estimated by moment matching, without any distributional assumptions. We describe the estimation of a variance and a covariance in $\boldsymbol{\Sigma}_{\mathrm{B}}$.

For a variable X, we define the weighted sum of squares

$$S_{\mathrm{B}} = \sum_{d=1}^{D} w_d (\hat{\theta}_d - \hat{\theta})^2 \,,$$

evaluate its expectation as a function of the district-level variance $\sigma_{\mathrm{B}}^2 = \mathrm{var}_{\mathcal{D}}(\mu_{\mathcal{D}})$ and the sampling (co-)variances c_d, v_d and v, and then solve the equation that matches the statistic S_{B} to its expectation. The weights $w_1, \ldots, w_D$ can be any positive constants; their choice is discussed below. By w_+ we denote their total; $w_+ = w_1 + \cdots + w_D$.

We have

$$\mathrm{E}(S_{\mathrm{B}}) = \sum_{d=1}^{D} w_d \left\{ v_d + v - 2c_d + (\theta_d - \theta)^2 \right\} \,,$$

and

$$\mathrm{E}_{\mathcal{D}} \left\{ \mathrm{E}(S_{\mathrm{B}}) \right\} = w_+ \sigma_{\mathrm{B}}^2 + \sum_{d=1}^{D} w_d (v_d + v - 2c_d) \,.$$

Hence the estimator

$$\hat{\sigma}_{\mathrm{B}}^2 = \frac{1}{w_+} \left\{ S_{\mathrm{B}} - \sum_{d=1}^{D} w_d (v_d - 2c_d) \right\} - v \,. \tag{8.12}$$

An obvious choice for the weights w_d are the sample sizes n_d, so that more precise contributions to S_{B} are assigned greater weights. This choice is not without problems. When some variables are associated (correlated) with the sample size, some bias is incurred. When no such associations are present, the choice is appropriate. When all the estimators $\hat{\theta}_d$ are normally distributed S_{B} has the χ^2 distribution with $D-1$ degrees of freedom.

To estimate a covariance, we form the weighted sum of cross-products

$$S'_{\mathrm{B}} = \sum_{d=1}^{D} w_d(\hat{\theta}_d - \hat{\theta})(\hat{\theta}'_d - \hat{\theta}') ,$$

for a suitable set of weights w_d. Its expectation over sampling and across the districts is

$$\mathrm{E}_{\mathcal{D}}\left\{\mathrm{E}(S'_{\mathrm{B}})\right\} = w_+\Sigma_{12} + \sum_{d=1}^{D} w_d(V_{d,12} + V_{12} - 2C_{d,12}) ,$$

where the subscript 12 indicates the covariance in the matrix $\mathbf{V}_d$, $\mathbf{V}$ or $\mathbf{C}_d$. The relative precisions of $\hat{\theta}_d$ and $\hat{\theta}'_d$ vary across the districts when $\hat{\theta}_d$ and $\hat{\theta}'_d$ are based on different sources of data, but may differ even when based on the same survey. Then there is no obvious choice of the weights w_d.

The moment-matching formula requires not only the sampling variances of the direct estimators, but their entire variance matrix for every district d. In some circumstances, the covariances vanish; in other cases, they are related to the sampling variances. Some examples are discussed in the next section.

8.4 Applications

In multivariate composite estimation, we can mix auxiliary information from several sources of different types: other surveys, censuses or administrative information (population registers). This section discusses a few generic examples.

8.4.1 Related variables in a survey

The analysed survey usually contains the target variable, the variable for which inferences (estimates of its district-level means) are desired. Often other, closely related, variables are also recorded. This may be because they are the target variables for other analyses, are used for constructing such variables, are used for data editing (by identifying inadmissible combinations of values), or the like.

It is a time-honoured tradition to plan the analysis of a variable X by using only the values of that variable. However, drawing inferences about a district by using only the data from the district may be similarly 'natural', yet we have dismissed this approach in Section 8.2 as inefficient. The involvement of variables other than the target can be motivated by (linear) regression and the associated synthetic estimators. Without a reference to a model, consider the following setting. Variables X and Z are highly correlated, but the district-level variance of Z, $\sigma^2_{\mathrm{B,Z}}$ is smaller than its counterpart for X, σ^2_{B}. Thus, we could estimate the district-level means of Z and derive estimates of the means for X by adjusting for the national (overall) differences between X and Z. This scheme leads to a biased estimator, but the bias may be preferred if the sampling variance is substantially reduced. The univariate shrinkage estimator, which would be applied if Z were ignored, is also biased.

Variable Z, together with others, can be used as auxiliary information in multivariate shrinkage. Instead of a single one, several auxiliary variables may be considered. Let $\mathbf{X} = (X, Z, \ldots)^\top$ be the random vector of the variables considered, with the target variable as its first component. In multivariate shrinkage, estimation of the district-level means corresponds to setting the vector of coefficients in (8.9) to $\mathbf{u} = (1, 0, \ldots, 0)^\top$. The optimal shrinkage is given by the vector $\mathbf{b}_d$ equal to the first column of $\mathbf{R}_{2,d}^{-1}\mathbf{R}_{1,d}$. When the variables in $\mathbf{X}$ are highly correlated, the correlations in $\mathbf{V}_d$, $\mathbf{V}_d - \mathbf{C}_d$ and $\mathbf{V}$ are also high, and so are the correlations in the district-level variance matrix $\mathbf{\Sigma}_{\mathrm{B}}$. Then all the elements 2, 3, ... of $\mathbf{b}_d = \mathbf{R}_{2,d}^{-1}\mathbf{R}_{1,d}$ vanish only in some esoteric situations. As the optimal shrinkage vector $\mathbf{b}_d$ is not a multiple of $(1, 0, \ldots)^\top$, the auxiliary information contributes to efficiency in estimating the district-level mean of X.

More precisely, it has the potential to contribute, because some losses are incurred as the matrices $\mathbf{V}_d$, $\mathbf{V}$, $\mathbf{C}_d$ and $\mathbf{\Sigma}_{\mathrm{B}}$ have to be estimated. That suggests that we should be sparing in the formation of the vector $\mathbf{X}$, considering only variables that are highly correlated with X. When there are several such variables it is not useful to include in $\mathbf{X}$ variables that are highly correlated with one another. At an extreme, instability in the calculation of $\hat{\mathbf{b}}_d$ can be expected when two variables that are almost copies of one another are included in $\mathbf{X}$. So, whereas it is advantageous to have a near-singular matrix $\mathbf{\Sigma}_{\mathrm{B}}$, it is not as useful to have an almost singular matrix $(\mathbf{\Sigma}_{\mathrm{B}})_{-1,-1}$, that is, the matrix $\mathbf{\Sigma}_{\mathrm{B}}$ with its first row and column removed.

Note that the target and auxiliary variables need not in fact be highly correlated. It suffices that their district-level means are highly correlated. Of course, high within-district correlation is usually accompanied by high district-level correlation, but only the latter is required.

8.4.2 Estimation for several subpopulations

Inferences are often sought not only for the entire districts, but also for their subpopulations, such as all men and all women, certain age groups (possibly defined for men and women separately), ethnic groups, heads of households, children, and for various attributes that are defined in the entire country.

If men and women have the same district-level means, the inferences for either sex could be based on the analysis of all the data, with no regard for sex. As the sample sizes in such analyses are nearly doubled compared to the analysis of the sex-specific subsets, the gains would be obvious. In practice, there are some differences between men and women, but when they are small, we should prefer the bias brought on by lumping men and women together to the variance inflation due to (approximately) halving the sample size.

In other contexts, the differences between men and women may be non-trivial. If the district-level means for men and women are highly correlated, the data for men can serve as auxiliary information for women, and vice versa. A simple way of realising some of the gains is by adjusting the results of the analysis that ignores sex for the average differences between men and women. Multivariate shrinkage exploits the similarity of the district-level means for men and women more completely, as the combination of the estimated district-level means for men and women is set more flexibly. Let $\hat{\boldsymbol{\mu}}_d$ be the vector of direct estimators of the district-level means for men and women, $\mathbf{V}_d$ their sampling variance matrix, and $\hat{\boldsymbol{\mu}}$ and $\mathbf{V}$ their 'national' counterparts. The district-level variance matrix $\boldsymbol{\Sigma}_{\mathrm{B}}$ has high correlations, for example, when the district-level means between men and women differ little from a constant, or their subpopulation means are almost perfectly linearly related. In (8.9), the vector $\mathbf{u}$ is set to $(1,0)$ and $(0,1)$ for estimating the mean for either sex, and to $(1,-1)$ for estimating their difference in district d.

Districts represented by many men in the sample tend to be represented also by many women. So, where there is a lot of direct information (many men for estimating the mean for men), there is also a lot of auxiliary information. This is an unsatisfactory feature of the application: we have little auxiliary information where we need it most, and a lot where we need it least.

As a contrasting example, suppose the targets of estimation are the district-level means for an (ethnic) minority group that constitutes a small fraction of the nation's population. If the data for the minority were analysed in isolation the sample sizes would be very small. They would fail to exploit the similarity of the minority with the majority. In effect, we might estimate the quantities of interest for the minority more efficiently by an appropriate adjustment of the corresponding estimates for the majority. The substantial increase in the effective sample size may well be worth the bias that is incurred in the process.

Men and women and minority and majority are two examples of partitioning the target population into a set of (mutually exclusive and non-overlapping) subpopulations. The means, proportions, or other district-level summaries for such subpopulations can be estimated simultaneously by multivariate shrinkage. The estimates for each district are given by the shrinkage matrix $\mathbf{B}_d$ given by (8.11). The covariances in $\mathbf{V}$ and $\mathbf{V}_d$ are difficult to estimate with designs that involve sizeable dependence of inclusion of subjects in the sample. Such designs are employed very rarely and, in practice, the correlations can be assumed to vanish. Then the covariance in $\boldsymbol{\Sigma}_{\mathrm{B}}$ is estimated without bias by the sample covariance of the district-level sample means. The cross-products for the covariances can be added up with sampling weights when appropriate.

8.4.3 Estimating compositions

In this section, another meaning of the term 'composition' is considered, unrelated to the term used in small-area estimation.

A categorical variable (a classification) defines a partition of the population into subpopulations of subjects that have the same value of the variable. Men and women are such subpopulations, as are various classifications into industrial sectors, levels of educational attainment, states of health, ownership of certain goods, age groups, and the like. The obvious quantities of interest for such classifications are the within-district proportions (percentages) of subjects who belong to each class. Such vectors of proportions, denoted by $\mathbf{p}_d$, are called (district-level) *compositions*. Their outstanding property is that each of them adds up to unity (100%); $\mathbf{p}_d^\top \mathbf{1} = 1$.

The national composition $\mathbf{p}$ is estimated by its sample version, denoted by $\hat{\mathbf{p}}$. With simple random sampling, the sample composition has a multinomial distribution. Its components are negatively correlated,

$$\mathrm{var}(\hat{\mathbf{p}} \,|\, \mathbf{p}) = \frac{1}{n} \left\{ \mathrm{diag}(\mathbf{p}) - \mathbf{p}\mathbf{p}^\top \right\} .$$

The correlation is a consequence of the negative association of the categories; if a randomly drawn subject belongs to one category, then he or she does not belong to any other. The district-level direct estimator $\hat{\mathbf{p}}_d$ is defined by restricting $\hat{\mathbf{p}}$ to district d. The negative covariances in $\mathbf{V}_d$ have to be reflected in the estimation of the district-level variance matrix $\mathbf{\Sigma}_\mathrm{B}$. This matrix is singular, as the components of $\mathbf{p}_d$ are linearly dependent, since $\mathbf{p}_d^\top \mathbf{1} = 1$.

The district-level (population) percentages of the categories may be positively correlated (where one category is in excess of the national percentage, so is the other one) or negatively (one category complements the other in the district). Multivariate shrinkage estimation of the district-level composition exploits such associations among the categories. The associations are captured by $\mathbf{\Sigma}_\mathrm{B}$ or its estimate. Estimation is improved most for the sparsely represented categories, as it exploits the association of the district-level percentages and draws on relatively abundant information from the other categories. In contrast, little gains beyond univariate shrinkage are realised for the populous categories in the district, because the other categories provide little auxiliary information. Multivariate shrinkage may obviate complex sampling designs that aim to over-represent certain subpopulations in the sample. More even representation of the subpopulations is not detrimental when the composition is estimated by multivariate shrinkage, but some efficiency may be lost in other inferences that are not directly related to the subpopulations, or are related to other subpopulations. However, more even representation is useful also for estimating $\mathbf{\Sigma}_\mathrm{B}$.

8.4.4 Survey and register

By the strict standards of statistical theory, surveys deliver an imperfect product — estimates based on a sample drawn *approximately* according to the planned design using an imperfect sampling frame. The information collected is temporal, losing its value over time. This puts a premium on the speedy conduct of all the operations, putting pressure on the process of eliciting information from the sampled subjects.

An alternative, taken up with varying levels of enthusiasm in the developed countries, are population registers. The expenditure for setting them up is much higher than for a typical survey, but analysis of their data can be conducted for the fraction of the cost of a survey, especially when the register is stored electronically, in a format accessible to the analyst.

Surveys require expensive concentrated efforts of data collection, with only fractional savings when the survey is repeated (e.g., annually). A register requires even greater initial expenditure, takes a few years until the procedures for recording the relevant data (events) are ironed out, various difficulties resolved, and incentives or other control mechanisms put in place, so that (almost) all the intended information is entered in the register, and done so in a timely fashion. When this period is over, the register can be regarded as a continual census, a data source much richer than a sample survey.

Registers have the potential to make censuses redundant. The problems with national censuses, which are special cases of sampling with inclusion probabilities equal to 1.0, are well documented. However, by its nature, data format and the information collected, a register is rather inflexible and cannot be altered at a relatively short notice to satisfy newly identified needs. A regularly conducted survey is much more flexible in this regard.

Comparing the costs of a survey and a register is meaningful only over a very long term and by taking into account all their uses. A survey is usually conducted for the specific purpose of making inferences about a population. In contrast, a register may be compiled and maintained for an administrative purpose that fully justifies the expense involved. Thus, the access to the register data may involve only administrative or commercial costs. The existence and quality of this resource is not necessarily related to its usefulness for population inferences.

Consider a setting in which a variable is recorded in a sample survey and a similar variable is recorded in a register. For example, an interview can establish the subject's employment status with sufficient detail, but at a considerable cost, and do so only for a sample of subjects. A national or regional register may hold information about each member of the labour force, using a classification based on a different definition. For example, the administrative purpose of the register is for payment of unemployment and other benefits and pensions. There is a strong incentive for the subjects to provide the relevant information, and for the authorities to verify it promptly.

How should we draw inferences about the unemployment rates in the districts? With the survey, we record the variable as defined, subject to correct responses from each subject in the sample. In contrast, the register contains closely related information, leading to biased estimation even by direct methods, but the status is available for (almost) the entire population, even if with some delay, possibly adding slightly more to the bias. A solution that chooses between the two sources is not as effective as combining the estimators based on them.

Bivariate shrinkage does not require subject-level data from the register, so the register may not need to be accessed directly if the district-level population means and percentages are publicly available. No data protection (confidentiality) issues arise in such an application, unless some districts are so small that their summaries inform about each subject in the district. The quantities derived from the register are associated with no variation, although administrative errors, delays in reporting and imperfect coverage can be represented by a token sampling variance, such as $(0.1\%)^2$ for the percentage of an event that is neither very rare nor very frequent. The survey and register are independent, so estimation of the quantities $\mathbf{V}_d$, $\mathbf{V}$ and $\mathbf{C}_d$, required for multivariate shrinkage, does not present any difficulties specific to the nature of the register. The benefits of the register as auxiliary information are obvious when the survey and register-based variables have highly correlated district-level means. Estimation would then rely almost solely on the register, except for an adjustment by the difference between the survey-related and register-based proportions. If this difference is estimated with high precision (using a survey with large sample size), and the difference varies little across the districts, the estimates for each district are very precise, even for districts not represented in the sample.

The survey- and register-based estimators can be combined for estimating *any* population target, including national population quantities. To illustrate this, suppose the target is the national mean (or rate/percentage) μ of a variable recorded in the register, and the same variable is recorded by a sample survey. The register yields the mean $\mu_\dagger$; suppose it has been established (with a high degree of confidence) that the bias of the register-based estimator, $|\mu_\dagger - \mu|$, does not exceed $\Delta_\dagger$. The survey yields the estimator $\hat{\mu}$ with sampling variance $\mathrm{var}(\hat{\mu})$. The two estimators, $\mu_\dagger$ and $\hat{\mu}$, should not be regarded as alternatives, because μ can be estimated more efficiently by their composition

$$\hat{\mu}^{\mathrm{C}} = (1-b)\hat{\mu} + b\mu_\dagger \,.$$

The 'shrinkage' coefficient b is chosen so that $\hat{\mu}^{\mathrm{C}}$ is most efficient in the least favourable feasible setting, when $|\mu_\dagger - \mu| = \Delta_\dagger$. The resulting estimator turns out to have the minimax property.

When $\mu_\dagger$ differs from μ by $\pm\Delta_\dagger$ the composite estimator $\hat{\mu}^{\mathrm{C}}$ has MSE

$$\mathrm{MSE}\{\hat{\mu}^{\mathrm{C}}(b);\, \mu\} = (1-b)^2 v + b^2 \Delta_\dagger^2 \,,$$

where $v = \mathrm{var}(\hat{\mu})$, so its minimum is attained for

$$b^* = \frac{v}{v + \Delta_\dagger^2}$$

and the resulting MSE is

$$\mathrm{MSE}\{\hat{\mu}^{\mathrm{C}}(b^*);\, \mu \,|\, \Delta_\dagger\} = \frac{v\Delta_\dagger^2}{v + \Delta_\dagger^2} \,.$$

When the shrinkage coefficient b^* is applied, even though $|\,\mu_\dagger - \mu\,| < \Delta_\dagger$, $\hat{\mu}^{\mathrm{C}}(b^*)$ is no longer the optimal composition of $\hat{\mu}$ and $\mu_\dagger$. The MSE of $\hat{\mu}^{\mathrm{C}}(b^*)$ is

$$\mathrm{MSE}\{\hat{\mu}^{\mathrm{C}}(b^*); \mu\,|\} = \frac{\mathrm{var}(\hat{\mu})}{\{\mathrm{var}(\hat{\mu}) + \Delta_\dagger^2\}^2} \left\{\Delta_\dagger^4 + (\mu_\dagger - \mu)^2 \mathrm{var}(\hat{\mu})\right\} \,.$$

This is an increasing symmetric quadratic function of the absolute bias $|\,\mu_\dagger - \mu\,|$ and, for $\mu - \Delta_\dagger \le \mu_\dagger \le \mu + \Delta_\dagger$, it attains its maximum at $\mu_\dagger = \mu \pm \Delta_\dagger$. Therefore, $\hat{\mu}^{\mathrm{C}}$ is uniformly more efficient than $\hat{\mu}$. With $\mu_\dagger$ it does not compare quite so favourably; after all, when $\Delta_\dagger = 0$ it is hard to outperform $\mu_\dagger$ — its MSE vanishes. However, $\mathrm{MSE}(\mu_\dagger\,;\, \mu)$ increases more steeply than $\mathrm{MSE}(\hat{\mu}^{\mathrm{C}})$. So, $\hat{\mu}^{\mathrm{C}}$ outperforms $\mu_\dagger$ exactly when it is most valuable, when the (absolute) bias of $\mu_\dagger$ is the largest possible. The price paid for this is that when $\mu_\dagger$ is not biased we lose some efficiency. Such a trade-off guarantees that the MSE is not large, as opposed to retaining a chance that the MSE might be small, but not being able rule out large MSE.

Figure 8.2 gives an illustration with $v = \mathrm{var}(\hat{\mu}) = 6$ and $\Delta_\dagger = 2$. The MSEs of the estimators $\hat{\mu}$, $\mu_\dagger$ and $\hat{\mu}^{\mathrm{C}}(b^*)$ are drawn in the diagram by thick solid lines in the range of biases $0 \le |\,\mu_\dagger - \mu\,| \le \Delta_\dagger$ and extended by thin dashes to $\Delta = 2.5$. The composite estimator $\hat{\mu}^{\mathrm{C}}$ (marked in the graph by symbol 'C') is uniformly more efficient than the direct estimator $\hat{\mu}$ ('S'), and is more efficient than the register-based estimator $\mu_\dagger$ ('R') when the bias is close to 2.0. It remains more efficient than both $\mu_\dagger$ and $\hat{\mu}$ well beyond the largest feasible bias of 2.0. The MSEs of $\mu_\dagger$ and $\hat{\mu}^{\mathrm{C}}$ cross at the bias of $\sqrt{1.5}$.

Now suppose $\Delta_\dagger = 1.0$ is justified. The MSE of the corresponding composite estimator is drawn in Figure 8.2 by dots and dashes and marked by symbol C$'$. For biases not exceeding 1.0 (in absolute value), this estimator is uniformly more efficient than its counterpart derived by assuming that $\Delta_\dagger = 2.0$. However, the composite estimator with $\Delta_\dagger = 1.0$ is less forgiving. It is more efficient than its counterpart for $\Delta_\dagger = 2.0$ only for bias $|\,\mu_\dagger - \mu\,| < 1.495$. Thus, 'tighter' information about the bias is rewarded by greater efficiency. But it does not pay to gamble by stating a value of $\Delta_\dagger$ that is not justified, because less efficiency is gained over the single-source estimators.

8.4.5 Historical data as auxiliary information

Many large-scale surveys are conducted regularly (annually), and they document the modest changes in various national, regional and district-level quantities of interest over the years. After constructing the year's survey database,

Figure 8.2. The composite estimator $\hat{\mu}^{\text{C}}$, combining the estimators based on a survey and an imperfect register. The symbols C, R, and S mark the MSEs of the composite and register- and survey-based estimators, respectively. $v = 6$ and $\Delta_\dagger = 2$. The line drawn by dots and dashes and marked as C′ represents the composite estimator based on $\Delta_\dagger = 1$.

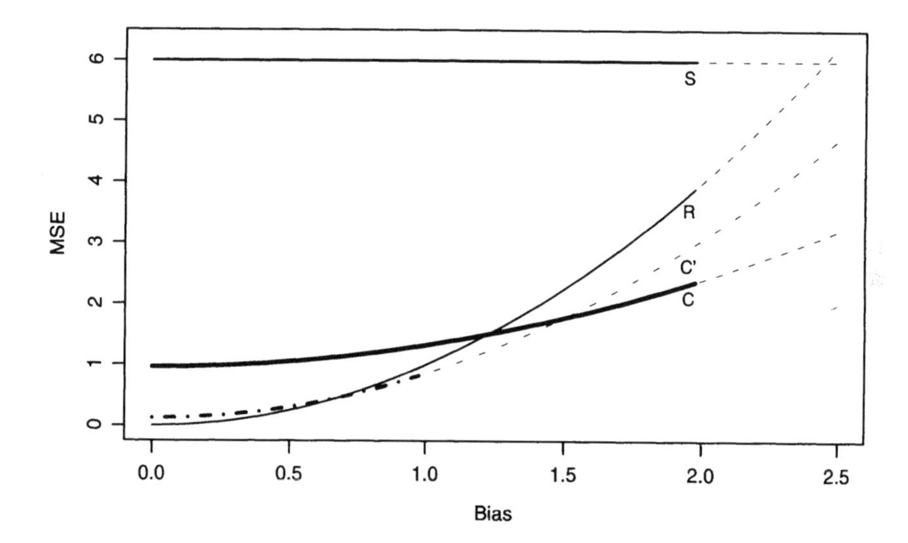

it is analysed on its own, with no input from the surveys in the past years. If the survey were not conducted in a year, the last year's estimates would be regarded as reasonable for the current year.

Analysing such a (current) survey in isolation represents a waste of resources, comparable to discarding the knowledge and experience accrued over the years. We can exploit the stability of the quantities of interest over the years by using the past years' values of the target variable as auxiliary information. Let $\mu_{d,t}$ be the population mean of the target variable in district d and year $t = 0, -1, \ldots, -T$, where the current year is $t = 0$, the previous year $t = -1$, and so on, till $t = -T$, T years ago. Denote by $\hat{\mu}_{d,t}$ the direct estimator of $\mu_{d,t}$. When a different sample is drawn each year, $\hat{\boldsymbol{\mu}}_d = (\hat{\mu}_{d,0}\,, \hat{\mu}_{d,-1}\,, \ldots, \hat{\mu}_{d,-T})$ has independent components, as does the national estimator $\hat{\boldsymbol{\mu}}$. Therefore $\mathbf{V}_d\,, \mathbf{C}_d$ and $\mathbf{V}$ are diagonal and the covariance of the district-level sample means (direct estimators) across the years is solely due to the covariance of the district-level population means.

Similarity of the district-level means usually decays with time, so using more recent surveys as auxiliary information is more important. Data from the previous year is likely to make a lot of difference, nearly doubling the effective sample size (reducing the standard errors of the direct estimators nearly $\sqrt{2}$-fold). Data from two years ago will contribute less. At some point, the gains become very small, or even inflate the MSE of the multivariate shrinkage estimators as the inverse $\hat{\mathbf{R}}_{2,d}$ becomes unstable for some districts.

In surveys with rotating panel design, a subject (or household) drawn into the sample remains in it for the next K years (or, more generally, waves). Such a design is very useful for longitudinal comparisons, obviating the need for subjects to recall events in the distant past. It is rather misleading to refer to the data collection at a particular time point as one survey, because the sample at the next time point is very similar; only about $\frac{1}{K}$th part of the sample from the previous time point has been replaced. Nevertheless, the direct estimator of a district-level quantity at the current time point can be improved, by using the data from the previous waves as auxiliary information. The data on the same subjects, about $100(1 - t/K)\%$ from t waves ago, makes little contribution, so the data from more recent past may provide less information than from earlier surveys.

8.4.6 Summary. Using all the relevant information

The applications outlined in the previous sections can be combined. For example, the current rates of unemployment in the various subpopulations can be estimated using a composition of the direct estimators from earlier years, or from a (decennial) census or a register, exploiting the temporal similarity and the similarity of the district-level rates of unemployment across the age-by-sex groups. In ideal circumstances, combining estimators from several sources, from several variables recorded in the same survey, or in related surveys, enables us to take advantage of all the information relevant for a particular target. In practice, it does not pay to use all the information because the first source (on its own) is very useful, the next one less so, and at some point the logistical difficulties make further gains more and more difficult to realise. Also, composition fails to exploit every last bit of information, and so using many auxiliary variables may be counterproductive.

Multivariate composition can be motivated by the dilemma of having several sources of information for estimating the same target. We dismiss the old-fashioned solution of selecting the best-suited source, the 'best' variable, the most efficient of the candidate estimators, and look for ways of exploiting each source, variable or estimator, by combining them. The format in which such information is presented has no impact on our capacity to use it. The data may be available as values for subjects, subjects in a different survey, direct estimates or district-level population quantities.

For the composition, we require the precisions of the direct estimators from each source. If uncertain, we should underestimate the precisions (overestimate their MSEs), so that we avoid assigning too important a role to the corresponding source. If we underrate the importance of a source we fail to exploit it fully, but do not render the resulting estimator invalid.

8.5 Planning and design for small-area estimation

Designing a survey for estimating one or a small number of quantities is a well appreciated problem, addressed comprehensively by the survey sampling theory. Nowadays, some of the theory is redundant because the population and the survey sampling mechanism can be simulated on the computer and the properties of the estimators considered evaluated empirically. In any case, the theoretically formulated problem is a gross simplification of what the survey is intended for. Inferences are usually sought by several parties (secondary analysts) about different aspects of the studied population. Of course, one cannot please everybody, and some trade-off has to be made between the conflicting demands. Analytical solutions for this more complex setting are hard to construct, partly because the relative priorities of the various inferential goals are difficult to formulate or classify. Nevertheless, the solutions for some simple problems provide insights into how to deal with realistic problems that are more complex.

Small-area estimation is an example of estimating many population quantities, in which the goals of estimation for each district are in an apparent conflict. Given limited resources, operationalised by a fixed sample size, greater subsample size in one district is bound to come at the expense of a smaller subsample size in another district. Thus, the task at hand is to strike an intelligent compromise and make the best use of the resources for the planned inferences.

Let s_d^2, $d = 1, \ldots, D$, be the MSEs of small-area estimators of population quantities θ_d. They depend on the sampling design which, for simplicity, we represent by the within-district subsample sizes $\mathbf{n} = (n_1, \ldots, n_D)$. The problem of setting the sampling design for a fixed overall sample size $n = \mathbf{n}^\top \mathbf{1}$ can be formulated as finding the minimum of a summary

$$\sum_{d=1}^{D} f\left\{s_d^2(\mathbf{n};\, d)\right\} , \tag{8.13}$$

subject to the constraint $\mathbf{n}^\top \mathbf{1} = n$. We write $s_d^2 = s_d^2(\mathbf{n})$ because s_d^2 depends on $\mathbf{n}$; on n_d obviously, but also on the other $n_{d'}$ because districts $d' \neq d$ may provide auxiliary information about district d. The function f may contain some other arguments as well, such as the district's population size N_d. By adding attributes of the district as further arguments, f may reflect the relative priorities with regard to the inferences about the districts. However, the key choice to be made is what values we attach to high and low precisions. For example, if a given precision is required for every district, precision higher than required is not any more valuable, and not reaching it would render the estimator useless. In this highly discrete setting, $f(s_d^2)$ is a step function, equal to zero up to a certain precision, and to unity otherwise. The value of f can be interpreted as a penalty for insufficient precision. The optimal design for such a function f assigns the minimum sufficient sample size to as many districts as resources allow, and represents no other districts in the survey. This is highly unsatisfactory not only for estimating other population quantities, but even for some small-area estimators. For example, synthetic and composite estimators are based on a model fitted for the whole country, and that requires a good representation of the country in the survey sample. An important factor ignored in this is that the sampling variance (as a function of the design) is not known. Usually it depends on one or several parameters that have to be estimated.

If estimation for each district has the same priority, allocating the same sample size to each district appears to be reasonable and well motivated. When the districts have very different population sizes, such a design may undermine the estimation of the national mean. (This can be addressed by using the sampling weights, but not having to resort to it is preferred.) A compromise solution is to under-represent the dispersion of the population sizes in the sample — to oversample the less populous districts and undersample the more populous ones. This can be implemented by splitting the overall sample size (or the available resources) to a component devoted to efficient estimation of the national quantity and another to efficient estimation of the small-area quantities. The relative priority of the two goals has to be reflected in how the overall sample size or the resources available are split.

A flexible class of functions f for (8.13) is given by

$$f(s_d) = N_d^q s_d^2 \,,$$

where q is a non-negative constant, referred to as the priority exponent. For $q = 0$, the population size N_d is not involved in f, and so it has no influence on the priority. For high powers q, the precision for the more populous districts becomes relatively more important. This counters the emphasis on the precision for the least populous districts.

We illustrate first how direct estimation in a simple stratified sampling design is optimised, and then proceed to more complex settings. Suppose only stratified sampling designs, with strata coinciding with the districts, and simple random sampling within each district, are considered as candidates for a survey. Then $s_d^2 = \sigma_d^2/n_d$, where σ_d^2 is the within-district variance (a population quantity). We seek the minimum of the objective function

$$\sum_{d=1}^{D} N_d^q \frac{\sigma_d^2}{n_d} \,,$$

subject to the constraint $n_1 + \ldots + n_D = n$. This problem is solved by the method of Lagrange multipliers, or by substituting $n_1 = n - n_2 - \ldots - n_D$. Either way we obtain the conditions

$$\frac{N_d^q}{n_d^2} \sigma_d^2 = \frac{N_1^q}{n_1^2} \sigma_1^2 \,,$$

$d = 2, 3, \ldots, D$, which have the unique solution

$$n_d = \frac{n\, N_d^{q/2} \sigma_d}{\sum_{d'=1}^{D} N_{d'}^{q/2} \sigma_{d'}} .$$

When no information about the relative sizes of the within-district variances σ_d^2 is available assuming that they are all equal is the obvious default. Then, for $q = 2$, n_d is proportional to N_d; $n_d = cN_d$. For $q > 2$, the more populous districts are assigned greater sample sizes, proportional to $N_d^{q/2}$. This does not lead to a reasonable allocation for any purpose, so it is meaningful to consider only $q \leq 2$. Similarly, $q < 0$ is not meaningful, as the optimal subsample sizes would be negatively correlated with the district-level population sizes.

8.5.1 Optimal design for the composite estimator

The calculations for the composite estimator are somewhat more complex, and so we assume that the within-district variances are constant; $\sigma_d^2 \equiv \sigma_{\mathrm{W}}^2$. The variance ratio $\sigma_{\mathrm{B}}^2/\sigma_{\mathrm{W}}^2$ is denoted by ω. The optimality criterion for the univariate shrinkage estimator minimises the expression

$$\sum_{d=1}^{D} N_d^q \frac{\sigma_{\mathrm{B}}^2}{1 + n_d \omega} ,$$

in which, for simplicity, we ignore the correlation of the national and direct estimator. This leads to the identity

$$\frac{N_d^{q/2}}{1 + n_d \omega} = \text{const} , \tag{8.14}$$

which has the explicit solution

$$n_d^* = \frac{(D + n\omega) N_d^{q/2}}{\omega U} - \frac{1}{\omega} . \tag{8.15}$$

where $U = \sum_{d'=1}^{D} N_{d'}^{q/2}$. In addition to rounding, an adjustment is needed when the solution contains one or several negative values of n_d^*.

For $\omega = 0$, the expression in (8.15) is not defined. In this case, however, the national estimator $\hat{\theta}$ is used for each district, and so we should focus on optimising the sampling design for $\hat{\theta}$ only.

An alternative approach to optimisation is based on the Newton method. An initial solution is defined by setting n_1, which determines the other subsample sizes by (8.14). If the resulting total $n_1 + \cdots + n_D$ exceeds n, n_1 is reduced; otherwise it is increased. The optimum is then located by linear inter- or extrapolation, as appropriate. This usually takes only a handful of iterations, even with a very poor starting solution. As the district-level subsample sizes have to be integers, the exact total sample size n is usually not reached.

Yet another approach explores elementary changes in the sampling design. Suppose a sampling design has been agreed on, but there is some leeway to adjust it so that it would be better suited for small-area estimation. An elementary change is a re-allocation of a unit sample size from one district to another. Small-area estimation prefers more even district-level subsample sizes, so a desirable re-allocation is from a district with a large (the maximum) subsample size to a district with a small (the minimum) subsample size. Analytically, or by simulations, we can establish the overall gains in precision of the small-area estimators and the losses for other estimators. We continue with elementary changes until the improvements diminish or the losses in precision of the other estimators begin to prevail. With the univariate shrinkage estimator, the most favourable elementary changes re-assign a unit from a district with the largest subsample size, $d_{\max}$, to a district with the smallest subsample size, $d_{\min}$. The changes in the eMSEs are, approximately, from $c/(1+n_{d_{\max}}\omega)$ to $c/\{1+(n_{d_{\max}}-1)\omega)\}$ and from $c/(1+n_{d_{\min}}\omega)$ to $c/\{1+(n_{d_{\min}}+1)\omega)\}$, for districts $d_{\max}$ and $d_{\min}$ with the respective sample sizes $n_{d_{\max}}$ and $n_{d_{\min}}$. Increasing the subsample size by one brings about a reduction of eMSE by approximately

$$g(n_d) = \frac{\omega}{(1+n_d\omega)\{1+(n_d+1)\omega\}} .$$

This is a decreasing function of n_d. The consequences of a unit reduction are derived similarly; the eMSE is increased by approximately $g(n_d-1)$. Hence, the increase in eMSE for district $d_{\max}$ is smaller than the reduction for district $d_{\min}$. Comparison of the multiplicative changes leads to a similar conclusion.

In summary, efficient design for small-area estimation prefers more generous allocation to less populous districts. However, the need for such evenness (preference for equalising the district-level subsample sizes) is less acute with composite than with direct estimation, because the shrinkage estimators compensate for small subsample size by drawing on auxiliary information.

Disparity of the subsample sizes

An important feature of the sampling designs optimal for small-area estimation is that less populous districts are sampled with higher sampling proportions. We refer to this feature as *disparity* of the subsample sizes. Figure 8.3 displays the optimal sample sizes for an artificial setting of a country with population of 32.15 million in its 100 districts. The curves in the left-hand panel connect the optimal sample sizes for the direct estimator for a range of priority exponents q. The population sizes are marked on the horizontal bar at the bottom of the graph. About half the districts have population sizes in the range 125–200 thousand and only 20 districts have population sizes in excess of half a million. The right-hand panel contains the curves for the composite estimator, assuming that $\omega = 0.05$. The allocation proportional to population

Figure 8.3. The optimal subsample sizes for the direct and composite estimators $\hat{\theta}_d^{\mathrm{C}}$ for a range of priority exponents q in a country with 100 districts. The dashes in the right-hand panel indicate the allocation proportional to population size.

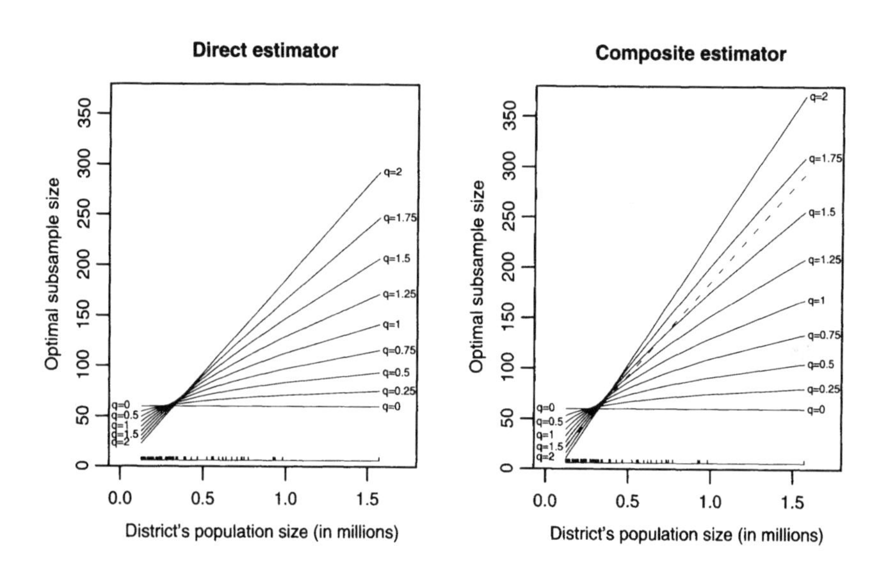

size, optimal for the direct estimator with $q = 2$, is indicated by dashes. The overall sample size is 6000.

The panels show that for exponents $0 < q < 1.75$ the sampling design optimal for composite estimation allocates subsample sizes with less disparity (closer to the proportional allocation) than the sampling design for direct estimation. For the largest values of q, the more populous districts are allocated even greater sample sizes than by the design with subsample sizes proportional to population sizes. This is a consequence of the 'handicapping' of the districts with above average sample sizes in composite estimation. These districts have relatively less auxiliary information, and the improvement in their estimation (composite vs. direct) is, on average, smaller than for the districts with below-average sample sizes.

For greater ω there is less similarity, and so the optimal design approaches its counterpart for the direct estimation. At the other extreme, as ω approaches zero, the allocation favours more and more the most populous districts because the least populous districts draw greater benefits from the similarity. However, substantial changes in the allocation make little difference in efficiency, until the sample-size allocation becomes irrelevant for $\omega = 0$.

These comments have to be qualified by the assumption that the national mean θ is estimated with high precision. However, as the sample allocation departs from proportionality, some efficiency in estimating θ is lost. This has an impact on small-area estimation that is not taken into account, even though estimation of θ may be another goal of the survey.

As the subsample-size calculations are made with some simplifying assumptions that include the value of ω, the use of eMSE instead of MSE, reference to the ideal composite estimation, and a priority exponent q that is bound to be set subjectively, it is essential to explore the dependence of the sampling design on these factors. In principle, this is straightforward; little or no additional programming is required, although the processing of extensive output by the (human) analyst may be difficult.

Estimation of the national quantity θ can be formally incorporated in the problem of optimising the sampling design. Its estimator $\hat{\theta}$ has to be associated with a priority G. Then the objective function to be optimised is

$$\sum_{d=1}^{D} f\left\{s_d^2(\mathbf{n};\, d)\right\} + G\mathrm{var}(\hat{\theta} \,|\, \mathbf{n}) \,. \tag{8.16}$$

For most settings f, s_d and $\hat{\theta}$, the solution cannot be expressed in a closed form, but the optimum can be located by simple iterative algorithms, such as the Newton method.

8.5.2 Variable subsample sizes and several divisions

So far, we have assumed that the district-level sample sizes are fixed and under the designer's control. They are random, for example, in clustered designs in which clusters either coincide with districts or contain them. In such designs, chance controls whether a district is represented in the sample at all. Of course, the probability of a less populous district not being represented is greater. Thus, clustering is poorly suited for small-area estimation; under-representation of 'small' districts is more costly than under-representation or 'large' (populous) districts. Clustering should therefore be replaced by stratification, to the extent that this is feasible. When strata coincide with districts the district-level subsample sizes are easier to control, and designs can be selected in which the strata have either fixed subsample sizes, or the subsample sizes have small variances across replications. Ideally, each district should be represented in the sample.

Sometimes the division of the domain into districts is not known, or cannot be fully considered when setting the sampling design. This may be the case when analysing historical data or when the domain has several divisions. A play-safe strategy pursues *even representation* of any district in the sample. That is, the distribution of the sample size n_d (over hypothetical replications) would be tightly concentrated around an ideal subsample size that reflects the population size of the district. Such a design is not particularly economic, involving a high average cost per subject because of the absence of tight clustering of the observations.

A further step toward realism in setting the sampling design is to express the overall cost of the survey in terms of the subsample sizes, and optimise the design with a fixed cost. Different allocations may result in different overall sample sizes. For example, priority for small-area estimation may call for many districts with small sample sizes, but the unit costs of collecting data from only a few subjects in a district may be higher than collecting data from many subjects. Thus, the pressures on resources suggest that sampling in some districts be abandoned and other districts be sampled more densely, in variance with the simplified objectives of small-area estimation that represent the resources by a fixed sample size.

Analytical approaches are limited, but their imperfect solutions are very useful for communication with the client who has difficulty in conveying all the nuances of the survey management and cost control. The analyst should find the appropriate level of complexity for the optimisation problem, so that incorporating the remaining factors subjectively would not erode the analytical contribution.

8.6 Suggested reading

Reference [65] discusses an application in which small-area estimation of the median for one subpopulation (four-member families) is assisted by information about other subpopulations (families of different sizes). A reanalysis is presented by [81].

The MSEs of the small-area estimators depend on some parameters. They depend on the targets as well, but that problem is sidestepped by referring to eMSEs. The eMSEs are usually estimated by conditioning on the estimated values of the parameters. This is appropriate only when there are many well represented small areas. Estimators of eMSEs that take into account the uncertainty about the estimated parameters are developed in [212]. A problem endemic in estimating variances is that the MSEs of the estimators depend on the target itself. The consequences of this are elaborated by [158].

Generalised linear models (GLM) with random coefficients, also known as generalised mixed linear models (GMLM), have a long history of attempts at fitting them by maximum likelihood with the computing resources available at the time. References [197] and [22] derive approximations to the log-likelihood that are easy to maximise. The partial derivatives required by the Newton-Raphson algorithm are approximated by [151]. The methods for approximation are critically reviewed by [227]; see [86] for an indirect response and [134] for an example with a cautionary tale. Most of these references focus on binary outcomes, but many of the conclusions carry over to other GMLM.

Reference [131] develops an alternative for the likelihood, called the h-likelihood, in which taking margins over the random coefficients does not involve any integration, and so model fitting with it is much easier. A generalisation is described in [132].

An application of the composite estimator described in Section 8.4.4 to clinical trials is presented in [162]. A similar theme, combining an unbiased and a biased estimator, is the subject of [89].

Diagnostics for for random coefficient models have to deal with the random terms (or residuals) at each level. Reference [129] addresses this issue by developing tests for normality of the deviations and [130] describes approaches for identifying outliers in multilevel data. With abundant computing power, the simulation approach proposed by [232] has a better control over the rate of false positive findings. See also [77], Chapter 6, and [161] for an application to random-effect models.

An approach to optimising the sampling design by splitting the overall sample size to two parts and optimising the allocation of each with respect to a different inferential goal is described by [52].

8.7 Exercises

1. Prove that the statistic S_{B} is distributed according to χ^2_{D-1} when the direct estimators $\hat{\theta}_d$ are unbiased, mutually independent and normally distributed, with sampling variances $\sigma^2_{\mathrm{W}}/n_d$, and $w_d = n_d$.
2. Show that small-area estimation using random coefficient models with random slopes, (8.1) with non-trivial $\mathbf{z}_i$, is closely related to composite estimation with auxiliary variables that are products (interactions) of variables in $\mathbf{x}$ and $\mathbf{z}$.
3. Derive the univariate composite estimator for a dichotomous target variable, assuming simple random sampling within districts and a known district-level variance σ^2_{B}.
4. Draw a random sample of size 100 from a distribution of your choice and regard it for the population means of the districts of a country. Draw another random sample (not necessarily independent from the first) from a distribution with positive values and, after rounding, regard it as the subsample sizes within the districts. For a given value of the common within-district variance σ^2_{W}, generate direct estimators of the district-level means. Apply the univariate composite estimator for each district, and count the number of 'winners' — districts in which the composite estimate is closer to the target than the direct estimate. Apply the composite estimator with a reduced coefficient, such as $0.9\hat{b}_d$, and compare its number of 'winners' with the original composite estimator based on $\hat{b}_d$. Repeat the exercise several times to estimate the distribution of the number of 'winners' for the two settings as well as for their difference. Apply a criterion for the quality of the estimators that takes into account the size of the estimation error.
5. Apply the sample size optimisation for the direct estimator with a given priority exponent q and a range of priorities G for the national estimator using the objective function in (8.16) for the fictitious country in the

previous exercise. Draw suitable graphs to show that higher priority G results in more precise estimation of the national mean.

6. Draw graphs of optimal sample allocations for the composite estimator with a range of variance ratios ω. Suppose your client prefers each subsample size to be a multiple of 20, the workload of an interviewer. Being short of a multiple of 20 is not as problematic as being slightly in excess. Consider ways of incorporating such a preference formally and informally in the setting the sampling design. With your choice, assess how much efficiency is lost because of this preference.
7. Devise a method for optimising the sampling design for univariate composite estimation with a given priority exponent q and a priority G for the national mean estimator. For a particular setting (country and its districts, real or simulated) establish the range of values of G which yield solutions that are for all practical purposes (e.g., after rounding) indistinguishable from the sampling designs that are optimal for the extreme priorities: the national estimator only ($G = +\infty$) and the district-level estimators only ($G = 0$).
8. Show that the multivariate composite estimator reduces to the vector of univariate estimators when each of the variance matrices $\mathbf{V}_d$, $\mathbf{V}$ and $\mathbf{\Sigma}_{\mathrm{B}}$ is diagonal. Describe a setting in which this would happen.
9. Find a source of some socio-economic indicators for the districts or regions of your country for a few consecutive years and study the differences among the regions across the years. Compare them with the sizes of the standard errors (margins of error), if available. Assess how effective the information from the preceding years would be for improving the estimation for the most recent year.

9

Using small-area estimators

Small-area estimators are essentially small-sample, the opposite of asymptotic. Their MSEs are usually non-trivial, and the uncertainty involved demands a careful treatment in how the estimates are used.

In an asymptotic setting, transformation and efficient estimation are commutative; that is, if $\hat{\theta}$ is efficient for θ, then so is $f(\hat{\theta})$ for $f(\theta)$ for any (continuous or differentiable) function f. Under some mild regularity conditions, maximum likelihood (ML) estimators are asymptotically efficient. In practice, the qualifier 'asymptotic' is dropped and forgotten. This is how ML has become the generally accepted standard for efficient estimation. We often claim that some of the asymptotic properties of ML apply universally, in particular unbiasedness and the commutative property of transformation and estimation. Estimators based on small or moderate sample sizes, including small-area estimators, do not have this property.

This chapter reinforces this negative conclusion on examples from small-area estimation and derives an estimator of the ranks of districts. As an aside to small-area estimation, a section discusses small-sample estimation of collections of variances and precisions, highlighting the non-asymptotic nature of the estimators. Insisting on no bias would result in unacceptable losses of efficiency, reducing our choices to direct estimators.

9.1 Non-linear transformations of the estimates

The analyst's goal is efficient estimation of a population quantity. With its evaluation, the analyst's work would appear to be concluded. A typical client, confident in the analyst's product, will treat the estimate as if it were the population quantity, being unaware of the pitfall outlined in the introduction — that an efficient estimator remains efficient only while it is subjected to linear transformations.

The multivariate version of this statement is particularly relevant to small-area estimates. Comparing two districts, by the difference $\hat{\mu}_d - \hat{\mu}_{d'}$ is appropriate. If $\hat{\mu}_d$ and $\hat{\mu}_{d'}$ are efficient for their respective targets μ_d and $\mu_{d'}$, then the difference $\hat{\mu}_d - \hat{\mu}_{d'}$ is efficient for $\mu_d - \mu_{d'}$. Similarly, the comparison of a district with the national mean is appropriate, because the target is a linear function of the estimator of μ_d. Examples of inappropriate use of the estimates are identifying the area with the smallest (or, generally, an extreme) mean, assessing the variation by the sample variance of the estimates $\hat{\mu}_d$, and ranking of the district-level means. More generally, any outstanding feature of the estimates $\hat{\mu}_d$ need not indicate the same or even a similar outstanding feature of the underlying quantities μ_d because the observation of such a feature can usually be expressed as a non-linear (and often not even continuous) function of $\hat{\mu}_{\mathcal{D}}$.

The district-level variance of the direct estimates, $\mathrm{var}_{\mathcal{D}}(\hat{\mu}_{\mathcal{D}})$, exceeds the variance of the district-level population means, $\sigma^2_{\mathrm{B}} = \mathrm{var}_{\mathcal{D}}(\mu_{\mathcal{D}})$, by a random variable with a distribution related to the sampling variances of the estimators $\hat{\mu}_d$. In fact, the variance σ^2_{B} is estimated in composite estimation; see Section 6.4. The district-level distribution of $\mu_{\mathcal{D}}$ should not be confused with the distribution of $\hat{\mu}^{\mathrm{C}}_{\mathcal{D}}$. Related to this is a weakness of all maps of estimates, in which the colour or shading of each district's area is a function of the district's estimate. For the direct estimator, the map will have more sudden switches of colour or shading from one district to its neighbour, while with a shrinkage estimator more smoothness can be expected. Shrinking less, so that the district-level estimates would have the right amount of variation (equal to $\hat{\sigma}^2_{\mathrm{B}}$), is not a good solution either.

A practical solution is offerred, indirectly, in Part I. If the targets μ_d were known the task at hand, whatever its details (e.g., drawing a map, counting the number of districts that have means above a certain value, and the like), would be relatively simple. Consider μ_d as the missing information, either in an EM or a multiple-imputation setting. In the EM algorithm, we estimate the expectation of the summary used in the M-step, and the M-step is trivial — quoting the summary from the E-step. When the summary is difficult to estimate in the E-step, or difficult to formulate algebraically (e.g., an inspection of the map, with a vaguely formulated inferential agenda), multiple imputation may be easier to implement. It entails drawing a *plausible vector* $\tilde{\boldsymbol{\mu}}$ of district-level population quantities from their joint distribution. A small number of replications of the plausible vector are drawn and the map, or the summary of interest, is constructed for each vector. The results will differ, reflecting the uncertainty about the estimates used. Averaging the vectors of plausible values, to construct a single map or feature, is not appropriate.

An unpleasant complication is that the estimators $\hat{\mu}^{\mathrm{C}}_d$ are correlated, through the national mean estimator $\hat{\mu}$ and the estimated district-level variance $\hat{\sigma}^2_{\mathrm{B}}$, or their multivariate counterparts. A short-cut ignores the correlations among the estimators. This may lead to a gross error when a lot of shrinkage takes place for many districts, even though the sampling variance of the estimators would be reflected. This may be resolved by drawing plausible values of the parameters used in composite estimation, resulting in plausible shrinkage coefficients (or matrices) and evaluating 'plausible' estimates based on them.

9.1.1 How important is bias?

Unbiasedness is generally regarded as a valuable property of an estimator. So far, we have seen that insisting on it in small-area estimation would not be very constructive. Nevertheless, we should explore how important it is to estimate without bias some of the parameters contributing to small-area statistics. To simplify the discourse, we assume that the outcomes are normally distributed.

Suppose a variance σ^2 is estimated with q degrees of freedom, that is,

$$q\frac{\hat{\sigma}^2}{\sigma^2} \sim \chi^2_q \,.$$

(χ^2_q is the χ^2 distribution with q degrees of freedom.) Although $\hat{\sigma}^2$ is unbiased, its non-linear transformation is not. We sometimes work with variance ratios, estimated by the ratios of two independent variance estimators. If $\hat{\sigma}^2$ is in the denominator, it might be preferable to substitute an unbiased estimator of $1/\sigma^2$ instead of the reciprocal of $\hat{\sigma}^2$. We have

$$\mathrm{E}\left(\frac{\sigma^2}{\hat{\sigma}^2}\right) = \frac{q}{q-2}\,,$$

so long as $q > 2$. This suggests an obvious correction for bias,

$$\tilde{\sigma}^2 = \frac{q}{q-2}\hat{\sigma}^2 \,.$$

The bias correction is unimportant when we have hundreds of degrees of freedom. At the other extreme, $\tilde{\sigma}^2$ is not defined for $q = 2$. The bias is as detrimental to estimation as variance inflation, caused by large $\mathrm{var}(\hat{\sigma}^{-2})$;

$$\mathrm{var}\left(\frac{\sigma^2}{\hat{\sigma}^2}\right) = \frac{2q^2}{(q-2)^2(q-4)}\,,$$

so that $\mathrm{var}(\sigma^2/\tilde{\sigma}^2) = 2/(q-4)$. This implies that dividing by an estimator $\hat{\sigma}^2$ that is based on fewer than five degrees of freedom is extremely unwise if small MSE of the ratio is the ultimate goal. Dividing by $\Delta + \hat{\sigma}^2$ for a suitably chosen Δ reduces the variance of the ratio, without introducing a substantial bias. In conclusion, unbiasedness is fragile; it is lost by non-linear transformations. Its pursuit may detract from the aim of efficient estimation.

9.2 Ranking and ordering

It is in our nature to order a set of related quantities and establish the identity (label) of the largest and smallest values, or to sort them in the ascending or descending order. When each quantity is estimated the order of the quantities differs from the order of the estimated quantities. This section discusses estimation of the ranks of district-level population means and similar quantities. Its starting point are the estimators based on the rank of the direct and shrinkage estimators, and the solution developed, although motivated by the idea of shrinkage, dismisses both proposals.

The rank of a quantity θ_d among $\theta_1, \ldots, \theta_D$ is defined as the number of the quantities that do not exceed θ_d:

$$R(\theta_d\,;\,\theta_D) = \sum_{d=1}^{D} I(\theta_d \geq \theta_{d'})\,. \tag{9.1}$$

(I is the identity function, equal to unity if the logical statement in its argument is correct, and to zero otherwise.) The definition assumes that there are no ties ($\theta_d \neq \theta_{d'}$ whenever $d \neq d'$); otherwise some arrangement has to be made, such as defining $I(\theta_d \geq \theta_{d'}) = \frac{1}{2}$ when $\theta_d = \theta_{d'}$ and $d \neq d'$. But we set $I(\theta_d \geq \theta_d) = 1$, irrespective of the arrangement that is made.

Naive estimation of ranks entails ranking the estimates:

$$\hat{R}(\theta_d\,;\,\theta_D) = \sum_{d=1}^{D} I(\hat{\theta}_d \geq \hat{\theta}_{d'})$$

$$\hat{R}^{\mathrm{C}}(\theta_d\,;\,\theta_D) = \sum_{d=1}^{D} I(\hat{\theta}_d^{\mathrm{C}} \geq \hat{\theta}_{d'}^{\mathrm{C}})\,.$$

Their trivial advantage is that the set of estimated ranks is a permutation of the integers $1, 2, \ldots, D$ — they *look* like genuine ranks. In general, the two sets of estimators do not agree, and they tend to differ more when the extent (and direction) of shrinkage for $\hat{\theta}_d^{\mathrm{C}}$ vary a great deal across the districts. The sampling distribution of these estimators for a fixed district d is difficult to derive or approximate analytically, especially for $\hat{R}^{\mathrm{C}}(\theta_d\,;\,\theta_D)$, because the contributing events $(\hat{\theta}_d^{\mathrm{C}} \geq \hat{\theta}')$ are dependent even after conditioning on $\hat{\theta}_d^{\mathrm{C}}$.

An alternative to these methods is based on estimating each elementary contribution $I(\theta_d \geq \theta_{d'})$. This can be formulated as an application of the EM algorithm in which $\hat{\theta}_d$ or $\hat{\theta}_d^{\mathrm{C}}$ form the incomplete information and θ_d are the missing data. Thus, the rank of θ_d is estimated as

$$\widetilde{R}^{\mathrm{C}}(\theta_d\,;\,\theta_D) = \sum_{d'=1}^{D} \mathrm{P}\left\{\theta_d \geq \theta_{d'} \,|\, \hat{\theta}_D^{\mathrm{C}}\right\} \tag{9.2}$$

or as

$$\widetilde{R}(\theta_d\,;\,\theta_D) = \sum_{d'=1}^{D} \mathrm{P}\left\{\theta_d \geq \theta_{d'} \,|\, \hat{\theta}_D\right\}\,,$$

where the probabilities are conditional not only on the sets of estimates, but also on the joint distribution of the D estimators. The probabilities are evaluated at the estimates (setting $\theta_d = \hat{\theta}_d$ or $\theta_d = \hat{\theta}_d^{\mathrm{C}}$) and normality of the estimators is assumed. For $\widetilde{R}^{\mathrm{C}}$, the conditional expectation of the difference $\theta_d - \theta_{d'}$ is estimated naively, by the difference $\hat{\theta}_d - \hat{\theta}_{d'}$. For $\widetilde{R}$, the estimators $\hat{\theta}_d$ are independent (for most sampling designs), so $\mathrm{var}(\hat{\theta}_d - \hat{\theta}_{d'}) = v_d + v_{d'}$. For $\widetilde{R}^{\mathrm{C}}$, we require the conditional distribution of the difference $\Delta_{dd'} = \theta_d - \theta_{d'}$. The difference is estimated by

$$\hat{\Delta}_{dd'} = (\mathbf{b}_d - \mathbf{b}_{d'})^\top \hat{\mathbf{p}} + (\mathbf{w} - \mathbf{b}_d)^\top \hat{\mathbf{p}}_d - (\mathbf{w} - \mathbf{b}_{d'})^\top \hat{\mathbf{p}}_{d'} .$$

Assuming normality of all the estimators involved, the conditional distribution of $\hat{\Delta}_{dd'}$ is normal, with expectation

$$(\mathbf{b}_d - \mathbf{b}_{d'})^\top \mathbf{p} + (\mathbf{w} - \mathbf{b}_d)^\top \mathbf{p}_d - (\mathbf{w} - \mathbf{b}_{d'})^\top \mathbf{p}_{d'}$$

and variance

$$(\mathbf{b}_d - \mathbf{b}_{d'})^\top \mathbf{V}(\mathbf{b}_d - \mathbf{b}_{d'}) + \{\mathbf{w} - \mathbf{b}_d + 2q_d(\mathbf{b}_d - \mathbf{b}_{d'})\}^\top \mathbf{V}_d(\mathbf{w} - \mathbf{b}_d)$$
$$+ \{\mathbf{w} - \mathbf{b}_{d'} - 2q_{d'}(\mathbf{b}_d - \mathbf{b}_{d'})\}^\top \mathbf{V}_{d'}(\mathbf{w} - \mathbf{b}_{d'}) .$$

The conditional probability $\mathrm{P}\left\{\theta_d \geq \theta_{d'} \mid \hat{\theta}_{\mathcal{D}}^{\mathrm{C}}\right\}$ is estimated from the approximation

$$\hat{\Delta}_{dd'} \hat{\sim} \mathcal{N}\left\{\hat{\Delta}_{dd'}, \widehat{\mathrm{var}}\left(\hat{\Delta}_{dd'} \mid \hat{\mathbf{p}}_{\mathcal{D}}^{\mathrm{C}}\right)\right\} .$$

The sampling variance of the estimator of a rank is

$$\mathrm{var}\left(\widetilde{R}_d^{\mathrm{C}}\right) = \sum_{d'} \mathrm{var}\left\{I(\theta_d \geq \theta_{d'}) \mid \hat{\theta}_{\mathcal{D}}^{\mathrm{C}}\right\}$$
$$+ \sum_{d' \neq d} \sum_{d'' \neq d \,\&\, d'' \neq d'} \mathrm{cov}\{I(\theta_d \geq \theta_{d'}),\, I(\theta_d \geq \theta_{d''}) \mid \hat{\theta}_{\mathcal{D}}^{\mathrm{C}}\} .$$

As each of the $(D-1)(D-2)/2$ distinct covariances has to be evaluated, this is a formidable expression. Each variance is equal to $p_{dd'}(1 - p_{dd'})$, where $p_{dd'} = \mathrm{P}(\theta_d \geq \theta_{d'})$, and each covariance to $p_{d,d'd''} - p_{dd'}p_{dd''}$, where

$$p_{d,d'd''} = \mathrm{P}(\theta_d > \theta_{d'} \text{ and } \theta_d > \theta_{d''}) .$$

In practice, the sampling variances do not have to be evaluated. A good overall impression of the uncertainty about the ranks can be gained by inspecting their spread. To motivate this, consider scenarios that result in a district being assigned an extreme rank, 1 or D. The estimated rank for district d is equal to 1.0 only when $\mathrm{P}(\hat{\Delta}_{dd'} < 0) = 0$ for all $d \neq d'$, that is, when we are certain that $\theta_d < \theta_{d'}$ for every district d'. When the uncertainty about the signs of $\Delta_{dd'}$ (fixed d, and $d' \neq d$) is considerable many of the probabilities $p_{dd'}$ are distant from both zero and unity, and the estimated rank is therefore distant from both 1 and D. In fact, when there is little or no information about θ_d, each probability $p_{dd'}$ is close to or equal to 0.5, so the estimated rank for district d is close to $(D+1)/2$, the median of the ranks. This estimate should not be interpreted as 'district d is (near the) average'. Such a statement would be well qualified only if the MSE of the estimator were small or many of the contributing comparisons $(\theta_d \geq \theta_{d'})$ had high or low conditional probabilities. As $\hat{\theta}_d^{\mathrm{C}}$ (or $\hat{\theta}_d$) contributes with its uncertainty to the ranks of all the other districts, their estimated ranks have many elementary contributions in (9.2) that are distant from both zero and unity. For a district with a relatively small $\hat{\theta}_d^{\mathrm{C}}$, say, with $\hat{R}_d^{\mathrm{C}} = 5$ among $D = 500$ districts, the probabilities $p_{dd'}$ exceed 0.5 for the four districts with smaller values of $\hat{\theta}_{d'}^{\mathrm{C}}$, and are smaller than 0.5 for the remaining 495 districts. The former four probabilities add up to less than 4.0, and the latter 495 to much less than 495.0, especially if many probabilities $p_{dd'}$ for such districts are much greater than zero, and some are even close to 0.5. Thus, the estimated ranks $\widetilde{R}_d^{\mathrm{C}}$ tend to be greater than $\hat{R}_d^{\mathrm{C}}$ when $\hat{R}_d^{\mathrm{C}}$ is small and smaller than $\hat{R}_d^{\mathrm{C}}$ when $\hat{R}_d^{\mathrm{C}}$ is large. In other words, the ranks are shrunk toward the median $(D+1)/2$. In general, probabilities $p_{dd'}$ less concentrated around zero and unity result in greater shrinkage. The level of concentration can be measured by the sample variance of the estimated ranks, compared to the variance of the set of integers 1, 2, ..., D, equal to $(D^2-1)/12$.

9.2.1 Inference about selected districts

A particular set of estimates $\hat{\theta}_d^{\mathrm{C}}$ is rarely the end-product of an analysis. The estimates, together with their estimated MSE's, are inspected for any unusual features, in search of contradictions that would point to an error in the calculations, but principally for substantive inferences, such as to identify unusual districts.

Suppose district d is identified as having an exceptionally large estimate. This is a signal for many a researcher to formulate hypotheses about this district, regarding it as an opportunity for 'noteworthy' findings and claims. Care has to be exercised because the sampling distribution of any estimator associated with a claim depends on the process that led to the formulation of the hypothesis and to the decision to evaluate the estimator. The properties of estimators, such as their sampling distribution, are contingent on their unconditional evaluation. Thus, a hypothesis formulated about district d^*, as a result of inspecting the estimates $\hat{\theta}_d^{\mathrm{C}}$, $d = 1, \ldots, D$, should be treated differently from an a priori formulated plan to test the 'same' hypothesis about district d^*. Without this plan, the hypothesis is not about district d^*, but about a district identified by a particular *process of data inspection*. In other words, d^* is a (discrete) random variable that should not be confused with its realisation, because the analysis of a replication of the survey may identify a different, or indeed no, district as exceptional.

As an example, suppose the smallest value $\hat{\theta}_d^{\mathrm{C}}$, attained for $d = d^*$, is much smaller than the next smallest estimate. A test of the hypothesis comparing the mean for district d^* with its national counterpart θ is not appropriate if we base it on the unconditional distribution of $\hat{\theta}_d^{\mathrm{C}}$. We say that district d^* has been *personalised* by confusing it with the district with the smallest value θ_d. It is more appropriate to compare the distributions of the minimum of the D estimators $\hat{\theta}_d^{\mathrm{C}}$ with the national mean, but this comparison is still not valid, because it is conditional on having found the minimum of the estimates $\hat{\theta}_d^{\mathrm{C}}$ as exceptional. Would it be exceptional in a hypothetical replication? If not, would we still wish to compare it with the national mean?

If we have a long list of configurations of the estimates that we would regard as exceptional if they occurred, the estimates may conform to a few of these configurations. In such a case, a configuration has been personalised. The minimum value of $\hat{\theta}_d^{\mathrm{C}}$ being much smaller than the next smallest value is an example of personalising a configuration. We would have made a different comparison (tested a different hypothesis) had the maximum value of $\hat{\theta}_d$ stood out, the estimates were in a narrow range, or the values of $\hat{\theta}_d$ for most districts in a region were close to the maximum.

Although it is usually informal, a typical process of inspection can be described by features considered and thresholds that classify them as noteworthy. A feature is defined as any function of the estimates (not estimators!). On the one hand, thoroughness of the inspection, considering many features, ensures that we identify more features that are remarkable, and increases the likelihood that we find a feature that would have been observed also among the targets $\theta_{\mathcal{D}}$. On the other hand, with thoroughness we raise the likelihood of flagging features that are not present among the population quantities θ_d. One way of reducing the likelihood of this is by raising the threshold for what we regard as 'remarkable' among the estimates. Even though many inferences based on ad hoc exploration of the estimates $\hat{\theta}_{\mathcal{D}}^{\mathrm{C}}$ are (meant to be) regarded as informal, they have a strong element of betting on results of past races about the outcome of which we have some (not necessarily complete) information. We should match, and preferably exceed, the probabilistic and logical rigour of the betting industry.

The analysis may suggest that the list of targets (inferences) compiled a priori is incomplete. Should targets identified after data inspection and analysis be treated as if they were specified a priori? They should if the omission can be regarded as a genuine error, but not otherwise. A target may be specified after the analysis; in general, the distribution of its estimator has to be adjusted for the process of inspection. However, when the decision to specify a target is not influenced by the values of the estimates, the process of inspection has no impact on the distribution of the estimator. Such a process is called *non-informative*. Non-informativeness of a process cannot be established empirically. It is left to the transparency and integrity of the analysts and clients to confirm it when appropriate. Being clear about the purpose of the analysis and the perspective adopted at the outset, and the background information available at that point, helps to document that the improvisation with the inferential agenda is non-informative.

9.3 Estimating many variances and precisions

Subpopulation means and proportions are the most common targets for a collection of districts or other aggregate units, but occasionally other quantities are estimated, such as variances and their reciprocals (precisions). This section describes shrinkage estimation of a collection of variances, exploiting their similarity.

Suppose districts $d = 1, \ldots, D$ are associated with respective variances σ_d^2. Two approaches to their estimation may be contemplated: direct estimation, by the sample variance of the n_d observations in district d, and by the sample variance pooled across the districts. The direct estimator, the sample variance $\hat{\sigma}_d^2$, is unbiased but has a large sampling variance. When the values of the target variable are normally distributed and the within-district sampling design is simple random, $\hat{\sigma}_d^2$ has a scaled χ^2 distribution with $n_d - 1$ degrees of freedom:

$$(n_d - 1)\frac{\hat{\sigma}_d^2}{\sigma_d^2} \sim \chi^2_{n_d-1} ;$$

$\mathrm{E}(\hat{\sigma}_d^2) = \sigma_d^2$ and $\mathrm{var}(\hat{\sigma}_d^2) = 2\sigma_d^2/(n_d - 1)$.

When the district-level variances coincide, $\sigma_d^2 \equiv \sigma^2$, each variance σ_d^2 is estimated with much greater precision by pooling the sample variances across the districts,

$$\hat{\sigma}^2 = \frac{1}{n - D'} \sum_{d';\, n'_d > 0} (n'_d - 1)\hat{\sigma}^2_{d'} ,$$

where the summation is over the districts represented in the sample and D' is the number of such districts. The pooled estimator $\hat{\sigma}^2$, associated with $n - D'$ degrees of freedom, has sampling variance $2\sigma^4/(n - D')$. When the variances σ_d^2 vary, $\hat{\sigma}^2$ estimates each of them with bias, but this drawback may still be outweighed by the substantially reduced sampling variance.

We estimate each variance σ_d^2 by the composition

$$\tilde{\sigma}_d^2 = (1 - b_d)\hat{\sigma}_d^2 + b_d\hat{\sigma}^2 , \qquad (9.3)$$

in which the coefficient b_d is to be set for each district d. For notational simplicity, we assume that each district is represented in the sample by at least two subjects, so that the direct estimator $\hat{\sigma}_d^2$ has a finite variance. We denote by σ^2 the (pooled) variance that is estimated by $\hat{\sigma}^2$ without bias:

$$\sigma^2 = \frac{1}{n - D} \sum_{d=1}^{D} (n_d - 1)\sigma_d^2 .$$

The MSE of $\tilde{\sigma}_d^2$ is

$$\begin{aligned} \mathrm{MSE}(\tilde{\sigma}_d^2;\, \sigma_d^2) &= \frac{2(1-b_d)^2\sigma_d^4}{n_d-1} + \frac{2b_d^2\sigma^4}{n-D} + 4b_d(1-b_d)\frac{\sigma_d^4}{n-D} + b_d^2(\sigma_d^2-\sigma^2)^2 \\ &= \sigma^4(R_{2,d}b_d^2 - 2R_{1,d}b_d + R_{0,d}) \,, \end{aligned} \tag{9.4}$$

where

$$\begin{aligned} R_{2,d} &= 2r_d^2\left(\frac{1}{n_d-1} - \frac{2}{n-D}\right) + \frac{2}{n-D} + (r_d-1)^2 \\ R_{1,d} &= 2r_d^2\left(\frac{1}{n_d-1} - \frac{1}{n-D}\right) \\ R_{0,d} &= \frac{2r_d^2}{n_d-1} \end{aligned} \tag{9.5}$$

and $r_d = \sigma_d^2/\sigma^2$ is the ratio of the within-district and pooled variances. In what follows, no generality is lost by assuming that $\sigma^2 = 1$, so that r_d coincides with σ_d^2. We also assume that $n_d - 1 < (n-D)/2$ for every district. This condition can be violated by at most two districts in very esoteric settings in which the subsample size of a district is close to one-half of the overall sample size. For such a district, composition would not be useful in any case because its variance would be estimated directly by $\hat{\sigma}_d^2$ with precision rivalling the precision of the pooled variance estimator $\hat{\sigma}^2$.

As $\mathrm{MSE}(\tilde{\sigma}_d^2\,;\,\sigma_d^2)$ is a quadratic function with a negative linear coefficient $-2R_{1,d}$, we can always improve on the direct estimator $\hat{\sigma}_d^2$ by choosing a small enough coefficient $b_d > 0$. The optimal coefficient b_d is equal to $R_{1,d}/R_{2,d}$, and the corresponding minimum MSE is $R_{0,d} - R_{1,d}^2/R_{2,d}$. The coefficient b_d is always positive, and exceeds 1.0 only when $1 < r_d < 1 + 4/(n-D-2)$. This is a narrow interval when $n \gg D$.

The composite estimator $\tilde{\sigma}_d^2$ can be interpreted as a shrinkage estimator; it is constructed by pulling the direct estimator toward the pooled estimator. Apart from the sample size, the extent of shrinkage depends on the target variance σ_d^2 itself; the gains in precision of the ideal estimator $\tilde{\sigma}_d^2(b_d^*)$ cannot be fully realised because the optimal coefficient b_d^* has to be estimated. This we do in Section 9.3.1. First we explore the properties of the ideal shrinkage estimator $\tilde{\sigma}_d^2$.

The optimal shrinkage coefficient is $b_d^* = \frac{1}{2}$ when $R_{2,d} = 2R_{1,d}$. In this case, $\hat{\sigma}_d^2$ and $\hat{\sigma}^2$ are equally efficient for σ_d^2 and *any* shrinkage coefficient $b_d \in (0,1)$ yields an improvement over both $\hat{\sigma}_d^2$ and $\hat{\sigma}^2$. This occurs when

$$\left(1 - \frac{2}{n_d-1}\right) r_d^2 - 2r_d + 1 + \frac{2}{n-D} = 0.$$

The solutions of this quadratic equation are

$$r_d^* = \frac{1 \pm \sqrt{2/(n_d-1) - 2/(n-D) + 4/\{(n-D)(n_d-1)\}}}{1 - 2/(n_d-1)} . \tag{9.6}$$

When the number of degrees of freedom $n - D$ is large the solution is adequately approximated by

$$r_d^* \doteq \frac{1}{1 \pm \sqrt{2/(n_d-1)}} ,$$

not depending on n or D. The approximation is very close even when $n - D = 100$ and $n_d < 20$.

When some prior information is available about the variances σ_d^2 they may be estimated by the following strategy. If we believe that σ_d^2 is close to σ^2 we use the pooled estimator $\hat{\sigma}^2$; otherwise we use $\hat{\sigma}_d^2$. The *critical ratios* r_d^* give us the bounds; within them, $\hat{\sigma}^2$ should be selected and outside them $\hat{\sigma}_d^2$. This approach has a lot in common with the tailored choice in Section 6.2.2, and that includes all its drawbacks.

In a typical setting, with many districts D and the subsample from each of them forming a small fraction of the entire sample, $1/(n-D)$ can be ignored in (9.5). Then $R_{2,d} \doteq R_{0,d} + (r_d - 1)^2$ and $R_{1,d} = R_{0,d} \doteq 2r_d^2/(n_d - 1)$. This approximation is very good even for $n_d = 10$ and $n - D = 100$. The overall degrees of freedom, $n - D$, have only a slight influence on $\mathrm{MSE}(\tilde{\sigma}_d^2; \sigma_d^2)$ or b_d^*. These and related properties are illustrated in Figure 9.1, where the shrinkage coefficient (panels A and B) and the minimum MSE (panels C and D) are plotted as functions of the ratio r_d for several sample sizes n_d. The solid lines represent $n - D = 100$ and the adjacent dashed lines $n - D = +\infty$; the sample sizes $n_d = 4, 6, 8$ and 10 are indicated at the margins of the panels. Instead of the minimum MSE, which is strongly related to r_d^2, the minimum relative MSE, MSE/r_d^2, is plotted. Panels A and C are on the linear scale of r_d and panels B and D on the log scale.

When $r_d = 1$, $\tilde{\sigma}_d^2$ almost coincides with the pooled estimator $\hat{\sigma}^2$, and so its sampling variance is very small. Greater subsample size n_d is associated with less shrinkage and smaller MSE, but the differences are small for r_d close to unity. With the relative MSE metric, shrinkage is more useful for very high than for very low r_d.

9.3.1 Estimated or guessed variance ratio

In practice, the ratio r_d is estimated or a guess of its value is made, so that the composite estimator $\hat{r}_d^{\mathrm{C}}$ could be evaluated. The MSE of the estimator $\hat{r}_d^{\mathrm{C}}$ based on such a value u_d is denoted by $\mathrm{mse}(u_d\,; r_d)$. We use lowercase 'mse' to distinguish it from the MSE in (9.4) and elsewhere, which is a function of the estimator. We have

$$\mathrm{mse}(u_d\,; r_d) = R_{2,d}\,\frac{U_{1,d}^2}{U_{2,d}^2} - 2R_{1,d}\,\frac{U_{1,d}}{U_{2,d}} + R_{0,d} ,$$

Figure 9.1. The ideal shrinkage coefficient b_d^* and the minimum relative MSE for a range of variance ratios r_d and numbers of observations $n_d = 4, 6, 8$ and 10 (indicated at the margins of the panels), with $n - D = 100$ (solid lines) and $n - D = +\infty$ degrees of freedom (dashes).

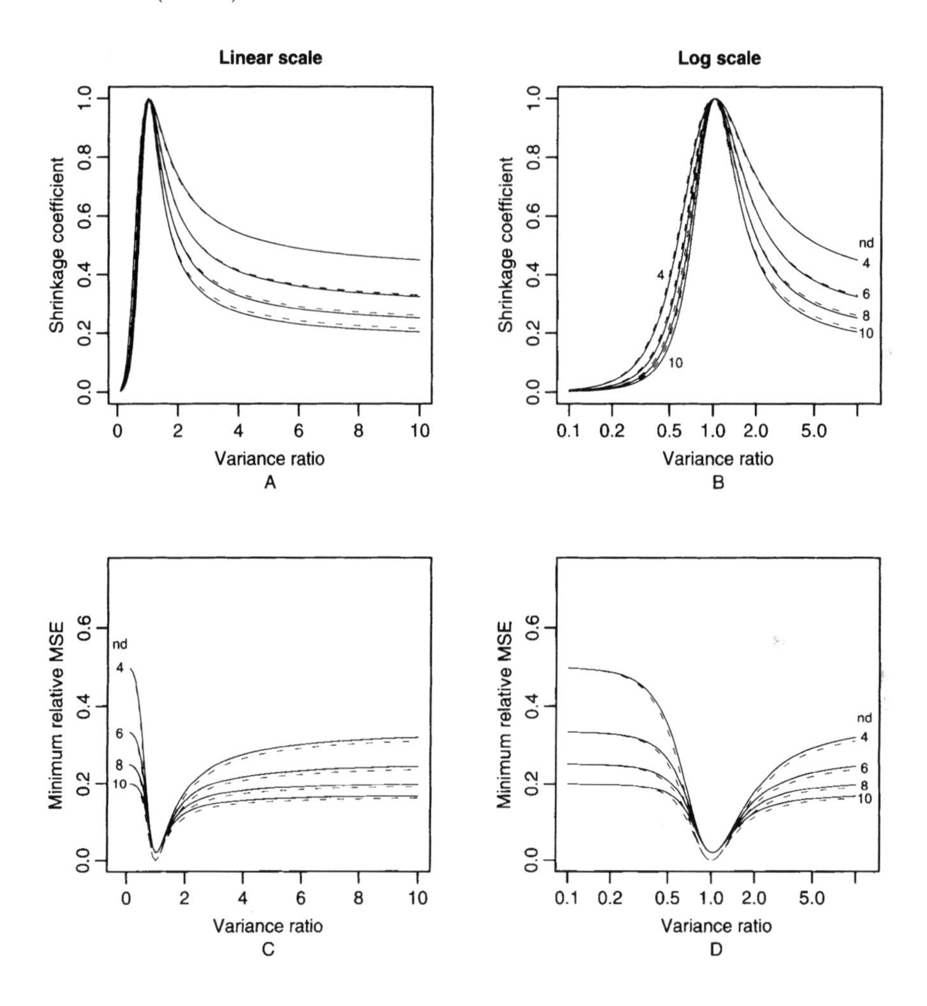

where $U_{h,d}$ are defined as $R_{h,d}$, $h = 0, 1, 2$, with u_d substituted for r_d. When $n - D$ is large, the function mse is well approximated by

$$\operatorname{mse}(u_d\,;\,r_d) \doteq R_{0,d}\left\{\frac{U_{0,d}}{U_{0,d} + (u_d - 1)^2} - 1\right\}^2 + \frac{U_{0,d}^2(r_d - 1)^2}{\{U_{0,d} + (u_d - 1)^2\}^2}$$

$$= \frac{R_d^* + U_d^{*2}}{(1 + U_d^*)^2}(r_d - 1)^2\,, \qquad (9.7)$$

where $R_d^* = R_{0,d}/(r_d - 1)^2$ and $U_d^* = U_{0,d}/(u_d - 1)^2$.

To assess the impact of the error in the setting of u_d as an initial estimator of r_d, we explore the behaviour of mse(u_d; r_d) as a function of u_d. We are interested in circumstances when a large distance $|u_d - r_d|$ is associated with a small loss of efficiency mse(u_d; r_d) − mse(r_d; r_d) or mse(u_d; r_d)/mse(r_d; r_d). When no prior information about either value of r_d is available it may be practical to choose the same value of u_d for each district d, or a value that depends only on n_d.

The extremes of mse(u_d; r_d) can occur only where its derivative vanishes or where it is not defined. It is easier to differentiate log(mse);

$$\frac{\partial \log(\mathrm{mse})}{\partial u_d} = \frac{2(U_d^* - R_d^*)}{\left(R_d^* + U_d^{*2}\right)(1 + U_d^*)} \frac{\partial U_d^*}{\partial u_d}$$

and

$$\frac{\partial U_d^*}{\partial u_d} = \frac{-4u_d}{(n_d - 1)(u_d - 1)^3} .$$

Hence, the candidate points are the solutions of $R_d^* = U_d^*$ (where $\partial \mathrm{mse}/\partial u_d = 0$), $u_d = 0$ (where $\partial U_d^*/\partial u_d = 0$) and $u_d = 1$ (where U_d^* has a singularity). The equation $R_d^* = U_d^*$ has solutions at $u_d = r_d$ and $u_d = r_d/(2r_d - 1)$. As our search is restricted to positive values of u_d, the latter solution is relevant only when $r_d > \frac{1}{2}$. At $u_d = 0$, mse has a local maximum. It corresponds to using no shrinkage.

The behaviour of mse(u_d; r_d), summarised in Table 9.1, is derived by elementary analysis. The function is decreasing at $u_d = 0$ for all values of r_d, so very small values of u_d should never be selected, because larger values of u_d yield greater gains. As $u_d \to +\infty$,

$$\mathrm{mse}(u_d\,;\, r_d) \to \frac{2r_d^2}{n_d + 1} - \frac{4(2r_d - 1)}{(n_d + 1)^2} ,$$

so mse is smaller than $R_{0,r} = 2r_d^2/(n_d - 1)$ whenever $r_d > \frac{1}{2}$. Therefore, shrinkage with a large enough assumed ratio u_d is superior to the direct estimator $\hat{r}_d$, unless the true ratio r_d is very small. But shrinkage with a smaller u_d is superior for a wider range of ratios r_d because mse is increasing for large values of u_d.

For large values of r_d, n_d and u_d, mse is smaller than $(r_d - 1)^2 =$ mse(1; r_d), the squared bias of $r = 1$ as an estimator of r_d. For example, for $r_d = 1.5$, n_d has to be at least 16, but for $r_d = 2$, $n_d > 5$ suffices, and for $r_d = 2.72$, mse is smaller than $(r_d - 1)^2$ for any sample size n_d. In these settings, we estimate r_d with greater precision than the pooled estimator by using large u_d.

Example

The MSEs of $\tilde{\sigma}_d^2$ for a set of 20 variances, based on sample sizes n_d ranging from five to ten (average 7.6), are plotted as functions of the assumed ratio u_d

Table 9.1. The behaviour of the function $\text{mse}(u_d\,;\,r_d)$, with fixed r_d, for large overall sample size n.

Condition (r_d)	$\text{mse}(r_d\,;\,u_d)$	Interval (u_d)	Values From	Values To
$r_d < \frac{1}{2}$	decreasing	$0 < u_d < r_d$	$R_{0,d}$	$\frac{R_{0,d}}{1+R_d^*}$
	increasing	$r_d < u_d < 1$	$\frac{R_{0,d}}{1+R_d^*}$	$(r_d-1)^2$
	decreasing	$1 < u_d < +\infty$	$(r_d-1)^2$	$\frac{2r_d^2}{n_d+1} - \frac{4(r_d-1)}{(n_d+1)^2}$
$\frac{1}{2} < r_d < 1$	decreasing	$0 < u_d < r_d$	$R_{0,d}$	$\frac{R_{0,d}}{1+R_d^*}$
	increasing	$r_d < u_d < 1$	$\frac{R_{0,d}}{1+R_d^*}$	$(r_d-1)^2$
	decreasing	$1 < u_d < \frac{r_d}{2r_d-1}$	$(r_d-1)^2$	$H(r_d)$
	increasing	$\frac{r_d}{2r_d-1} < u_d < +\infty$	$H(r_d)$	$\frac{2r_d^2}{n_d+1} - \frac{4(r_d-1)}{(n_d+1)^2}$
$r_d > 1$	decreasing	$0 < u_d < \frac{r_d}{2r_d-1}$	$R_{0,d}$	$H(r_d)$
	increasing	$\frac{r_d}{2r_d-1} < u_d < 1$	$H(r_d)$	$(r_d-1)^2$
	decreasing	$1 < u_d < r_d$	$(r_d-1)^2$	$\frac{R_{0,d}}{1+R_d^*}$
	increasing	$r_d < u_d < +\infty$	$\frac{R_{0,d}}{1+R_d^*}$	$\frac{2r_d^2}{n_d+1} - \frac{4(r_d-1)}{(n_d+1)^2}$

Note: $H(r_d) = 2r_d^2 \frac{(n_d-1)(3r_d-1)^4+2(r_d-1)^2 r_d^2}{\{(n_d-1)(3r_d-1)^2+2r_d^2\}^2}$.

in Figure 9.2. The two panels illustrate the same setting, generated artificially, but in panel A the overall sample size $n = 152$ and in panel B $n = 1020$ is assumed. The variance ratios r_d are indicated in the plots by diamonds at the height $y = 0.0$. The greatest differences between the panels arise in the neighbourhood of $r_d = 1$ and $u_d = 1$, where full shrinkage, $b_d^* = 1$, is optimal. But even these differences are minute.

The two panels show that for unknown r_d we run much smaller risk by choosing some value $u_d > 1$ than choosing $u_d < 1$. The MSEs have a local minimum to the left of $r = 1.0$, but the dip is in a rather narrow range and we could not locate it based on $\hat{r}_d$ that involves only a handful (4–9) of degrees of freedom. Therefore, to estimate r_d efficiently when we have no information about it other than $\hat{r}_d$ and $\hat{\sigma}^2$, we should choose a large u_d. Otherwise we run the risk of inefficient estimation for many districts.

When $r_d = 1$ we cannot improve on the pooled variance estimator $\hat{\sigma}^2$ for σ_d^2. Although by choosing $u_d > 1$ we do not rule out a large MSE, a reasonable conservative strategy sets u_d to an a priori upper bound on the variance ratios r_d. Then we incur losses in estimating the small variances σ_d^2, those for which $r_d < 1$, but gain precision in estimating the large variances. Of course, this 'socialist' policy of reducing the inequalities in the precisions of

Figure 9.2. MSEs of the variance estimators, as functions of the assumed variance ratio. No external information (left-hand panel) and v estimated with $n - D = 1000$ degrees of freedom (right-hand panel). The variance ratios are marked by diamonds $\diamond$. The thick curve is the average MSE over the 20 estimators $\widetilde{\sigma}_d^2$. Simulated data.

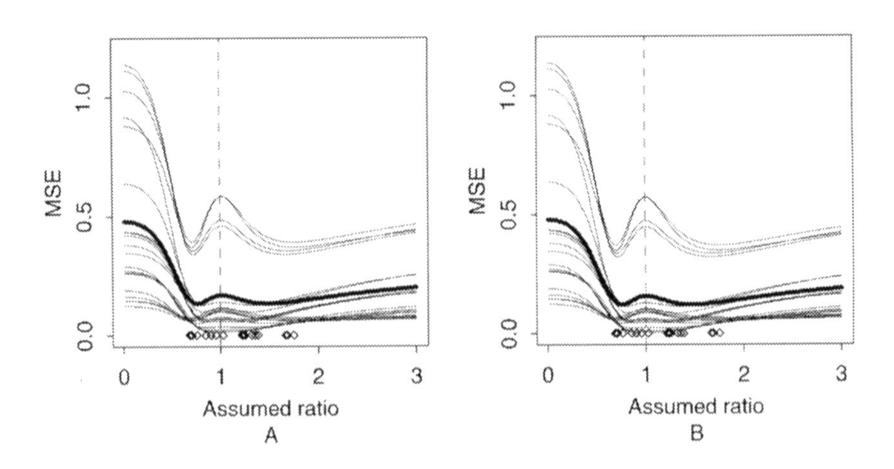

the estimators should be moderated by the sample sizes n_d. Direct estimation of each σ_d^2 corresponds to $u_d \equiv 0$. This estimator is clearly not competitive for most variances, although not for all of them.

9.3.2 Estimating precisions

The shrinkage estimator developed in Section 9.3.1 is applicable when the (within-group) sample sizes are small. We therefore cannot presume that efficient estimation of a variance, say of σ_d^2 by $\widetilde{\sigma}_d^2$, implies that $1/\widetilde{\sigma}_d^2$ is an efficient estimator of the precision $1/\sigma_d^2$. Shrinkage estimation of precisions can be derived by the same steps as in Section 9.3.1, although the relevant moments are different and yield a different way of combining the direct and pooled estimators.

Let Q be a random variable distributed according to χ_p^2, with $p > 4$. Then $1/Q$ has expectation $1/(p-2)$ and variance $2/\{(p-2)^2(p-4)\}$. Therefore, the precision $1/\sigma_d^2$ is estimated without bias by

$$\hat{\varrho}_d = \frac{n_d - 1}{(n_d - 3)\hat{\sigma}_d^2},$$

with variance

$$\operatorname{var}(\hat{\varrho}_d) = \frac{2}{(n_d - 5)\sigma_d^4}.$$

Similarly, the pooled precision is estimated without bias by

$$\hat{\varrho} = \frac{n-D}{(n-D-2)\hat{\sigma}^2}\,,$$

with variance $\mathrm{var}(\hat{\varrho}) = 2\sigma^{-4}/(n-D-4)$. Since the estimated precision has an infinite variance for $n_d \le 5$, we should estimate the precision for the groups with five or fewer units always by the pooled precision $\hat{\varrho}$. The covariance of the direct and pooled estimators of the precision cannot be derived analytically, so we resort to an approximation by the Taylor expansion. We have

$$\begin{aligned}
\mathrm{cov}(\hat{\varrho}_d\,,\,\hat{\varrho}) &\doteq \frac{n_d-3}{n_d-1}\,\frac{n-D-2}{n-D}\,\frac{2}{\sigma_d^4\sigma^4}\,\mathrm{cov}(\hat{\sigma}_d^2;\,\hat{\sigma}^2) \\
&= \frac{(n_d-3)(n-D-2)}{(n_d-1)(n-D)^2}\,\frac{4}{\sigma^4}\,.
\end{aligned}$$

In analogy with the pooled variance σ^2, we define the variance $\sigma_\circ^2$ by pooling the precisions σ_d^{-2}:

$$\frac{1}{\sigma_\circ^2} = \frac{1}{n-3D}\sum_{d=1}^{D}\frac{n_d-3}{\sigma_d^2}\,.$$

The shrinkage estimator

$$\hat{\varrho}_d^{\mathrm{C}} = (1-b_d)\hat{\varrho}_d + b_d\hat{\varrho}$$

has the approximate MSE

$$\mathrm{MSE}(\hat{\varrho}_d^{\mathrm{C}}) \doteq \sigma_\circ^4\varrho^2\left(R_{2,d}^\circ b_d^2 - 2R_{1,d}^\circ b_d + R_{0,d}^\circ\right),$$

with

$$\begin{aligned}
R_{2,d}^\circ &= \frac{2}{n_d-5}\,\frac{1}{r_d^2} + \frac{2}{n-D-4} - \frac{4(n_d-4)(n-D-2)}{(n_d-1)(n-D)^2} + \left(\frac{1}{r_d}-1\right)^2 \\
R_{1,d}^\circ &= \frac{2}{n_d-5}\,\frac{1}{r_d^2} - 2\frac{(n_d-3)(n-D-2)}{(n_d-1)(n-D)^2} \\
R_{0,d}^\circ &= \frac{2}{n_d-5}\,\frac{1}{r_d^2}\,.
\end{aligned}$$

We refer to $1/r_d$ as the *relative precision*. The minimum MSE is attained for $b_d^\circ = R_{1,d}^\circ/R_{2,d}^\circ$. Note that b_d° differs from b_d^*, especially when n_d is small. This illustrates that the optimal shrinkage coefficient depends not only on the sample sizes and variance ratios, but also on the target of estimation.

As in Section 9.3.1, we consider an estimated or guessed relative precision $1/u_d$ and assess its sensitivity vis-à-vis $1/r_d$. Since the derivations are very similar, we summarise them briefly. Assuming large D, the mse using an 'incorrect' relative precision $1/u_d$ is

$$\mathrm{mse}(u_d^{-1};\,r_d^{-1}) \doteq \frac{R_d^\circ + U_d^{*2}}{(1+U_d^\circ)^2}\,(r_d^{-1}-1)^2\,,$$

where $R_d^\circ = 2R_d^2/(R_d - 1)^2/(n_d - 5)$ and $U_d^\circ = u_d^{-2}/(u_d^{-1} - 1)^2/(n_d - 5)$. This expression differs from $\mathrm{mse}(u_d\,;\, r_d)$ in (9.7) only by the additional four degrees of freedom subtracted from the sample sizes n_d in R_d° and U_d°. Therefore, a guess of the upper bound of the relative precisions $1/r_d$ is a conservative choice for $1/u_d$. This corresponds to the lower bound on the variance ratios r_d. Thus, a substantially different choice of shrinkage is made for the precisions than for the variance ratios, unless the variances are distributed symmetrically on the log scale. The loss of the four degrees of freedom also introduces a further substantial difference in shrinkage, especially for groups that have small subsample sizes. In this sense, estimation of precisions requires more data than estimation of variances.

9.4 Suggested reading

League tables of administrative units and institutions (schools, hospitals, economic performances of countries or regions, and the like) are often treated by the straightforward comparison of summaries for the units concerned. Methods that adjust for differences in the context, such as the background of the school's students, are illustrated by [87]. Some of the intuition required for their application to be appropriate is replaced by formal criteria in [43]. Reference [126] is the original source of the method described in Section 9.2. The problematic nature of using small-area estimates is highlighted by [256]. They propose estimators that are specific for each of the three purposes they consider.

Related to ranking is the problem of identifying units with outstandingly good or poor performance; [260] presents a case study concerned with confirming the unsatisfactory performance of a surgical unit. Reference [31] is a suitable entry point to the literature on extremes. The context of extremes in small-area estimation corresponds to 'observations' (estimates) that are subject to estimation error.

The most natural graphical presentation of small-area estimates might be by maps in which the (estimated) values are represented by shades or colours. Reference [79] argues cogently that (replicate) maps composed of estimates are systematically different from the map that would have been composed of the target values.

9.5 Exercises

1. Suppose a variance σ^2 is estimated by $\hat{\sigma}^2$ and $q\hat{\sigma}^2/\sigma^2$ is distributed according to χ_q^2. Find the scalar multiple of $\hat{\sigma}^2$ that estimates σ^2 with the smallest MSE. Describe the solution as a shrinkage estimator.
2. Solve the analogous problem for estimating the precision $1/\sigma^2$.

3. Explore by simulations the bias of $1/(1 + n\hat{\omega})$ in estimating $1/(1 + n\omega)$ when $50\hat{\omega}/\omega \sim \chi^2_{50}$. Compare the biases and MSEs of $1/(1 + cn\hat{\omega})$ for a range of values of c around 1.0.
4. On a simulated example of small areas in the Exercises of Chapter 8, compare the ranks of the population means with their direct and composite estimates. Define a distance between two sets of ranks (for instance, by their mean squared difference), and establish by simulations which set of ranks (derived from the direct or composite estimates) is closer to the ranks of the population means. If your definition of the distance can be applied to any set of D numbers, apply it to the estimated ranks $\widetilde{R}^{\mathrm{C}}$.
5. Alter the simulated population mean for a district so that it would become an outlier. Estimate by simulations how frequently would the district be regarded as an outlier based on its estimate. How frequently is another district 'detected' as an outlier? How does the detection rate depend on the sample size?
6. Discuss how composite estimation of the sampling variances could be used (to estimate v_d) in composite estimation of population-means of small areas. Explain why efficient estimation of v_d may not lead to efficient estimation of the ideal shrinkage coefficient b_d.
7. Verify all the identities in Section 9.3.2. Describe the difficulties that would be encountered when estimating the function $(a_1 + \sigma^2)/(a_2 + \sigma^2)$ for some constants a_1 and $a_2 > 0$.

10

Case studies

This chapter describes four applications of small-area estimation. The sections are self-contained and can be read in any order, although Section 10.1 is much more extensive than the other three.

10.1 The UK Labour Force Survey

The rate of unemployment is a key indicator of the state of the labour force and the economy in general in every industrialised country. High unemployment is a sign, or a correlate, of crisis, indicating that a lot of the nation's capacity to generate wealth is unused, as was the case during the Great Depression in the United States. More recently, in the 1970's and 80's, the unemployment rate was anxiously watched by politicians, labour unions, employers and the public at large, interpreting any change as an improvement or worsening of their country's economic climate. Having established itself as a well understood and easy to interpret figure, professionals and laymen alike are comfortable making comparisons of their country's unemployment rate over time, or with countries of similar level of economic development.

The unemployment rate is far from constant in the regions of most countries, despite extensive migration of labour, transfer of employment opportunities across the regions, and intervention of governments. Some migration is initiated by new employment and retirement, although commuting to work across regional or even national boundaries is quite common, especially in the continental countries of the European Union. In the UK, the South-East and Home Counties have been regions of low unemployment and North-East and West Midlands regions of high unemployment, since the onset of the decline of the traditional manufacturing industries at least. A natural step from the interest in the rates of unemployment in the regions is to study the labour force with even greater geographical detail, such as in the jurisdictions of local authorities (districts) that provide services relevant to the unemployed.

There are two principal sources of information about unemployment in the UK. The Claimant Count (CC) is an administrative register of all the members of the labour force who are claiming unemployment benefit. The registers are maintained by local authorities, and the relevant figures are published regularly. They comprise the percentage of the members of the labour force who reside in each district and receive unemployment benefit. The percentages are also given separately for men and women. They are available from `www.statistics.gov.uk/neighbourhood/Downloads`.

The UK Labour Force Survey (LFS), conducted by the Office for National Statistics (ONS), is a quarterly sample survey of residential addresses in the UK. One of the variables recorded by LFS is the employment status, as defined by the International Labour Organisation (ILO). According to this definition, an individual is classified as unemployed if he or she has no employment, is willing to work and has taken active steps to find employment. An individual is *economically inactive* if he or she is not employed and does not seek employment. For example, most full-time students, housewives and the retired are economically inactive, as are the jobless who have given up search for employment. Children (up to the age of 16) are classified in a separate category. Although many working-age adults (men aged 16–64 and women 16–59 in the UK) who are classified as unemployed according to the ILO definition are also included in CC, the definitions are not identical.

LFS has a rotating panel design. An address included in the survey is kept in the sample for the next four quarters. The sample is 'refreshed' every quarter by newly selected addresses to replace the 'retiring' addresses that were included in the survey for the first time a year ago. For example, an address included for the first time in spring (March–May) 2002 is retained in the sample till spring 2003. We say that such an address, typically a household, and its occupants are in wave I in spring 2002, in wave II in the next round of the survey (three months later, in summer 2002), and so on, till retirement from the survey panel after wave V in spring 2003. The rotation is conducted in such a way that the districts are well represented in any round of the survey.

Just like any other large-scale survey that relies on the cooperation of its subjects, LFS does not collect the complete data as planned by the sampling design and interview protocol. Nonresponse in LFS was discussed in Section 5.1. The number of subjects in the survey database is around 140 000, from about 60 000 addresses. About 80 000 of the subjects are of working age. The LFS database can be obtained from ONS; see `www.statistics.gov.uk/labour_market/lfs` for details.

The estimate of the national rate of unemployment based on the LFS is one of the key products of the survey analysis. Being based on a large sample, it is estimated with high precision. If simple random sample were employed with sample size 80 000, the rate of 4% would be estimated with standard error $\sqrt{0.04 \times 0.96/8} = 0.07\%$. The standard error of the comparison of the rates in two consecutive quarters is much smaller than $0.07\sqrt{2} = 0.10\%$ because the two estimated rates are highly correlated, owing to the substantial overlap (about 80%) of the subjects in the two rounds. In fact, if the rates in the two quarters are identical, the standard error of the difference of its estimators is about 0.03%. In publications, including the media, the estimated rate of unemployment is quoted in percentages, rounded to one decimal place. Thus, an estimated difference of 0.1% in the published figures indicates that its population counterpart is highly unlikely to be negative.

Although the sample size of LFS is sufficient for estimating the national rate of unemployment, as well as the rates in the 17 regions of the UK, it is not sufficient for direct estimation of the rates in all but a few of the country's 434 districts. The average population of a district is about 140 000 and the average subsample size of working-age adults in such a district is about 200. The standard error of the direct estimator of the unemployment rate for such a sample, given that the (population-level) rate is 4%, is 1.4%. As the rate of 1% is exceptionally low and 7% exceptionally high, such precision is of next to no value because the estimates for many districts could not reliably distinguish between very low and very high rates of unemployment.

The districts' populations are in a wide range. Several cities and metropolitan areas form districts with populations exceeding half a million, and Orkneys, Shetlands, and some other outlying rural districts, as well as the City of London, have populations of less than 30 000 each. In London, each of the 32 boroughs forms a district. The sampling design, using the post-code sectors as primary sampling units, does not sample rural districts with probabilities substantially different from urban or metropolitan areas.

In the analysis, we ignore the sampling design (assume that it is simple random), and report the results for spring 2001, with item nonresponse dealt with by multiple imputation (see Section 5.1). LFS is conducted throughout the UK and the definitions of districts in LFS and CC coincide, except for Northern Ireland, which is represented as a single district in CC but as 26 districts in LFS. For consistency with analyses that use CC as auxiliary information, all the results discussed refer to the UK excluding Northern Ireland.

The estimated national rate of unemployment in spring 2001 was 3.59%, with estimated standard error 0.08%. The estimated district-level variance of the unemployment rates is 1.64, so that the district-level standard deviation of the rates is about 1.3%. The district-level rates are not symmetric around the national rate because there are relatively few districts with high rates and more (less populous) suburban and rural districts with low rates.

The standard error of the direct estimator of the unemployment rate for a district with sample size 200 is 0.7%, given that the population rate is 1%, and 1.7%, given that it is 7%. Such a precision is not satisfactory for any purpose other than the crudest assessment of unemployment. The precision of the direct estimator is comparable to the national estimator used for estimating the rate for the district (standard error 1.3%). In univariate shrinkage these two estimators are combined, resulting in an improvement over both estimators. The main difficulty in applying univariate shrinkage is that the sampling variance of the direct estimator $\hat{p}_d$ depends on the (unknown) target

p_d. As the rates are small, the variance is approximately proportional to the rate: $v_d = \mathrm{var}(\hat{p}_d) \doteq p_d/n_d$. Estimating this variance naively by $\hat{v}_d = \hat{p}_d/n_d$ is not satisfactory because the estimation error in $\hat{p}_d$ is committed again in $\hat{v}_d$. One solution is to estimate v_d by $\hat{p}(1-\hat{p})/n_d$, using the estimated national rate $\hat{p}$. In another, v_d is estimated naively, after truncating the sample rate at 2% (or a similar threshold). Thus, $\hat{v}_d = \hat{p}'_d(1-\hat{p}'_d)/n_d$, where $\hat{p}'_d = \hat{p}_d$ if $\hat{p}_d > 0.02$ and $\hat{p}'_d = 0.02$ otherwise. Another option is to apply the univariate shrinkage with one of these proposals, and then estimate v_d by $\hat{p}_d^{\mathrm{C}}(1-\hat{p}_d^{\mathrm{C}})/n_d$ using the 'provisional' shrinkage estimator $\hat{p}_d^{\mathrm{C}}$.

It is difficult to identify the estimator of v_d that leads to optimal estimation of p_d. It is not necessarily the most efficient estimator and, in any case, there is no uniformly most efficient estimator of v_d. The various ways of fine-tuning the shrinkage improve the estimation of v_d (and p_d) for some districts at the expense of others. Therefore, we should state first our priorities for distributing the precision among the districts. For example, if preference is given to districts with high unemployment, $\hat{v}_d$ should be based on their (anticipated) rates, say, $p^\dagger = 6\%$, unless there is strong evidence that the rate is different. This suggests applying shrinkage even in estimating v_d. Such a scheme would combine the estimates based on $\hat{p}_d$ or $\hat{p}_d^{\mathrm{C}}$ and on $p^\dagger$. These options are as yet very poorly explored, partly because the preferences for 'allocating' the precision to the districts are difficult to formulate.

However, the direct estimator is a weak competitor with either of the schemes, unless the rate p_d is very small. This can be illustrated by a sensitivity analysis. Consider a district represented in the sample by 50 working-age adults, none of whom is unemployed. The sample rate of unemployment is 0%, and naive estimation of v_d would lead to $\hat{v}_d = 0$, because the error in estimating p_d leads to the implausible conclusion that the estimator has no sampling variation.

The probability of no unemployed encountered in a simple random sample of size $n = 50$, $\mathrm{P}\left(\sum_i X_{id} = 0 \,|\, n_d = 50;\, p_d\right) = (1-p_d)^{n_d}$, is a decreasing function of p_d. It reaches 0.01 for $p_d = 8.8\%$. We explore the MSE of the univariate shrinkage estimator with v_d based on a range of values of p_d. In the calculations, we ignore v and c_d as they are much smaller than the estimated district-level variance $\hat{\sigma}_{\mathrm{B}}^2 = 1.64(\%)^2$.

Figure 10.1 summarises the dependence of MSE on the rate p_d by the plots of the root-MSEs for the shrinkage (solid) and direct estimators (dashes). The shrinkage applied in each panel is based on the probability $p^\dagger$ given in the subtitle (1%, 4%, 7% and 10%) and indicated by vertical dots. In all four panels, the direct estimator is more efficient than the shrinkage estimator when p_d is small. For $p^\dagger = 1\%$, the difference between $\mathrm{MSE}(\hat{p}_d)$ and $\mathrm{MSE}(\hat{p}_d^{\mathrm{C}})$ varies least dramatically with p_d, but the gains for the majority of districts which have p_d in the vicinity of the national rate $\hat{p} = 3.6\%$ are smaller than in the other panels. For higher rates of $p^\dagger$ we 'bank' more on the gains around $p_d = \hat{p}$ and 'gamble' more at the extremes where the direct estimator is more efficient. To put this in an appropriate perspective, recall that the vast

Figure 10.1. Shrinkage estimation with $v_d = \text{var}(\hat{p}_d)$ based on guessed values of p_d, indicated by vertical dots. In each panel, the MSE of the shrinkage estimator is drawn by solid line and the MSEs of the direct estimator by dashes.

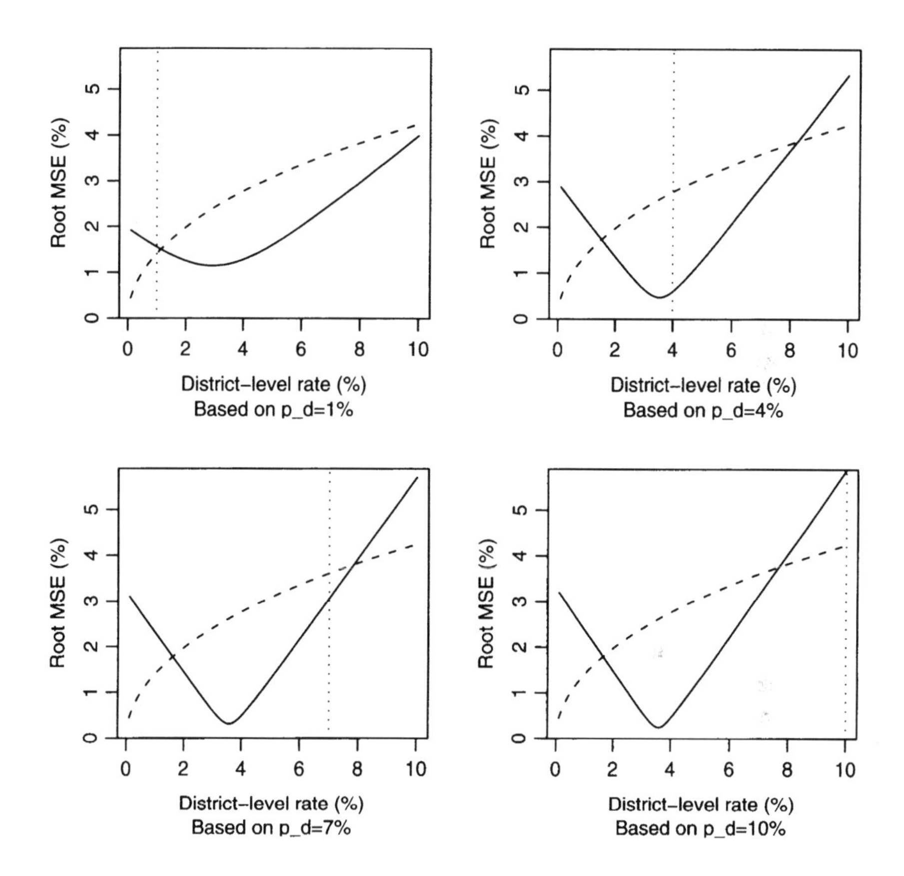

majority of the districts have rates in the range $3.6\% \pm 2 \times 1.3\%$. We need not be unduly concerned about the inefficiency of the shrinkage estimator for $p_d < 1\%$ and $p_d > 7.5\%$. The loss of efficiency when p_d is small is less serious than when p_d is large because, given n_d, $\text{MSE}(\hat{p}_d; p_d)$ increases with p_d.

Basing v_d on $p^\dagger = 4\%$, near the national rate, would be adequate. Some efficiency is gained when $p^\dagger$ is adjusted by the direct estimator $\hat{p}_d$, especially when n_d is large. If $\hat{p}_d = 0\%$, the choice of $p^\dagger = 7\%$ would be poorly justified; we may be inclined to choose $p^\dagger < \hat{p}$, recognising that the district's rate is likely to be lower than the national rate. The confidence in this depends on the sample size n_d.

10.1.1 Multivariate shrinkage

Two auxiliary variables yield gains in efficiency (on average) over univariate shrinkage: the rates of economic inactivity and the CC rates. The employed, economically inactive and unemployed are three categories of the ILO employment status, so the discussion about estimating compositions in Section 8.4.3 is applicable in this context. The rates of economic inactivity are of interest also in their own right. The district-level rates of unemployment and economic inactivity should be estimated simultaneously because they are highly positively correlated. However, the direct estimators of the two rates have identical sample sizes, so the gains in efficiency by simultaneous estimation are distributed with iniquity; districts with greater sample sizes have more auxiliary information than districts with smaller sample sizes.

In contrast, the CC rates are without any sampling variation, other than due to administrative errors and rounding. They are prima facie good auxiliary information for the unemployment rates, but may be useful also for estimating the rates of economic inactivity. The estimates of the national rates for the three variables (unemployment, economic inactivity and claiming unemployment benefit) are, in percentages, $\hat{\mathbf{p}} = (3.59, 21.22, 3.42)^\top$, with respective standard errors $(0.10, 0.34, 0.00)^\top$. For trivariate shrinkage, we require the sampling variance matrix of the national rates. Its estimate, obtained by moment matching, is

$$\hat{\mathbf{V}} = \frac{1}{100^4} \begin{pmatrix} 103 & 195 & 0 \\ 195 & 1174 & 0 \\ 0 & 0 & 0 \end{pmatrix} .$$

The scalar multiple of 100^{-4} is chosen so that the matrix entries are in hundredths of percentages squared. The national rate of CC is regarded as established with precision, but we associate the district-level CC rates with a 'token' standard error of 0.10%, to represent the rounding and administrative errors and related ambiguities. The correlation between the estimates of the unemployment and economic inactivity rates is adjusted for the negative correlation in sampling.

The district-level variance matrix is estimated by moment matching as

$$\hat{\mathbf{\Sigma}}_\mathrm{B} = \frac{1}{100^2} \begin{pmatrix} 1.64 & 5.74 & 2.19 \\ 5.74 & 26.90 & 7.01 \\ 2.19 & 7.01 & 3.76 \end{pmatrix} .$$

As anticipated, the correlation of the two unemployment rates is high, equal to $2.19/\sqrt{1.64 \times 3.76} = 0.88$. The other two correlations in $\hat{\mathbf{\Sigma}}_\mathrm{B}$ are also high; 0.86 and 0.70 for the economic inactivity rates with ILO unemployment and CC rates, respectively. Although the district-level rates of economic inactivity are widely spread, their sampling variances depend on the underlying rates much less because the rates are distant from 0% and 100%.

Instead of listing all the estimates, we illustrate trivariate shrinkage estimation on a few selected districts. District 20UH (Teesdale, county Durham) has subsample size 36, one of the smallest. The direct estimates of the unemployment, economic inactivity and CC rates are $\hat{\mathbf{p}}_{20\mathrm{UH}} = (0.0\%, 19.4\%, 3.0\%)^\top$. These estimates are associated with the respective standard errors $(2.2\%, 6.7\%, 0.10\%)^\top$. The shrinkage matrix (see Section 8.3) is

$$\hat{\mathbf{B}}_{20\mathrm{UH}} = \begin{pmatrix} 0.93 & -0.03 & -0.49 \\ -0.29 & 0.76 & -1.25 \\ 0.00 & 0.00 & 0.00 \end{pmatrix},$$

yielding the estimates $(3.09\%, 19.23\%, 3.0\%)^\top$, with estimated standard errors $(0.56\%, 3.20\%, 0.10\%)^\top$. The matrix $\hat{\mathbf{B}}_{20\mathrm{UH}}$ indicates that the rate of unemployment is estimated by the combination

$$(0.07, -0.03, -0.49)\hat{\mathbf{p}}_{20\mathrm{UH}} + (0.93, -0.03, -0.49)\hat{\mathbf{p}}\,,$$

where $\hat{\mathbf{p}}$ is the estimate of the vector of national rates. So, in estimating the unemployment rate for district 20UH, the local and national rates of economic inactivity are almost ignored (coefficients -0.03 for both), as is the direct estimate of the district's unemployment rate (coefficient 0.07). The estimate is, approximately, equal to the national unemployment rate adjusted by one-half of the national and local CC rates.

For estimating the economic inactivity rate for district 20UH, the unemployment rates are much more important. The multivariate shrinkage estimate is

$$(-0.29, 0.24, -1.25)\hat{\mathbf{p}}_{20\mathrm{UH}} + (-0.29, 0.76, -1.25)\hat{\mathbf{p}}\,.$$

In contrast to the unemployment rate, the district's direct estimator is far from ignored (coefficient 0.24). This can be interpreted as follows. The CC rates are better auxiliary information for the unemployment rates, so the direct estimator is almost redundant. For economic inactivity rate, the CC rates are less useful, so the highly unreliable (large-variance) direct estimator is relatively more useful. The fact that the coefficient associated with the CC rates is negative and so large is not remarkable. The CC rates are in a relatively narrow range compared to the economic inactivity rates, so their impact is weaker than the size of the coefficient might suggest. It may seem paradoxical that the CC rate has a greater coefficient for estimating economic inactivity than for unemployment rate (-1.25 vs. -0.49). This is a consequence of the wide range of the rates of economic inactivity and relative paucity of information about it from the other districts' rates.

And finally, shrinkage leaves the CC rates unchanged. That is a consequence of their high precision.

Next we explore estimation for district 40UE, Taunton Deane in Somerset. It is a medium-size district, with subsample size 150. The direct estimates of its unemployment and economic inactivity rates are $(2.67\%, 15.07\%)^\top$, with estimated standard errors $(1.41\%, 2.93\%)^\top$, and their trivariate shrinkage counterparts, using the CC rate for the district equal to 1.7%, are $(2.40\%, 16.28\%)^\top$ with estimated standard errors $(0.48\%, 2.24\%)^\top$. The estimated gains by shrinkage are much more modest than for district 20UH, especially for the rate of economic inactivity. There is more 'direct' information, so the auxiliary information is relatively weaker, and is made less prominent by the shrinkage. The shrinkage matrix is

$$\hat{\mathbf{B}}_{40\mathrm{UE}} = \begin{pmatrix} 0.88 & -0.07 & -0.38 \\ -0.37 & 0.40 & -0.53 \\ 0.00 & 0.00 & 0.00 \end{pmatrix} .$$

Compared to $\hat{\mathbf{B}}_{20\mathrm{UH}}$, the role of the CC rates is reduced, especially for estimating the rate of economic inactivity. The direct estimates are assigned greater weight by shrinkage for both unemployment and economic inactivity rates (0.12 and 0.60, respectively). While the unemployment rate remains an important auxiliary variable for the rate of economic inactivity, economic inactivity is not a useful auxiliary variable for the unemployment rate. In fact, the weight assigned to the unemployment rate for estimating the economic inactivity is greater (in absolute value) for district 40UE than for 20UH (-0.37 vs. -0.29). This is a consequence of the greater subsample size of district 40UE.

As the last example, we consider district 00CN, Birmingham, which has the largest subsample size, 1151. The direct estimates of its rates of unemployment and economic inactivity are $(5.54\%, 29.34\%)^\top$, with estimated standard errors $(0.67\%, 1.35\%)^\top$. Their trivariate shrinkage counterparts are $(5.49\%, 29.34\%)^\top$, with estimated standard errors $(0.37\%, 1.20\%)^\top$. The CC rate for the district is 5.9%. The shrinkage matrix is

$$\hat{\mathbf{B}}_{00\mathrm{CN}} = \begin{pmatrix} 0.69 & -0.08 & -0.25 \\ -0.51 & 0.16 & -0.01 \\ 0.01 & 0.00 & 0.01 \end{pmatrix} .$$

The role of the CC rate in estimating the unemployment rate is reduced further, and is almost eliminated for the rate of economic inactivity. The similarity of the district-level rates is not exploited reciprocally. Although the rate of unemployment contributes to estimating the rate of economic inactivity (weight -0.51), the rate of economic inactivity is all but ignored in estimating the unemployment rate (weight -0.08).

The extent of shrinkage applied for the districts is plotted against the sample size in Figure 10.2. In the left-hand panels, the shrinkage coefficients for estimating the district-level unemployment rates, and in the right-hand panels the corresponding coefficients for estimating the rates of economic inactivity are plotted against the sample size. The points for the three districts discussed earlier are marked by the symbol $\times$. The horizontal axes are on the log scale because the points are then more evenly spread. To improve the resolution,

Figure 10.2. The extent of shrinkage and the district's subsample size. The left-hand panels plot the extent of shrinkage of the three district-level rates in estimating the rate of unemployment (UN), and the right-hand panels their counterparts for estimating the rates of economic inactivity (IA). The signs are changed as indicated by the labels of the vertical axes. The points for the three districts discussed in the text are marked by the symbol $\times$.

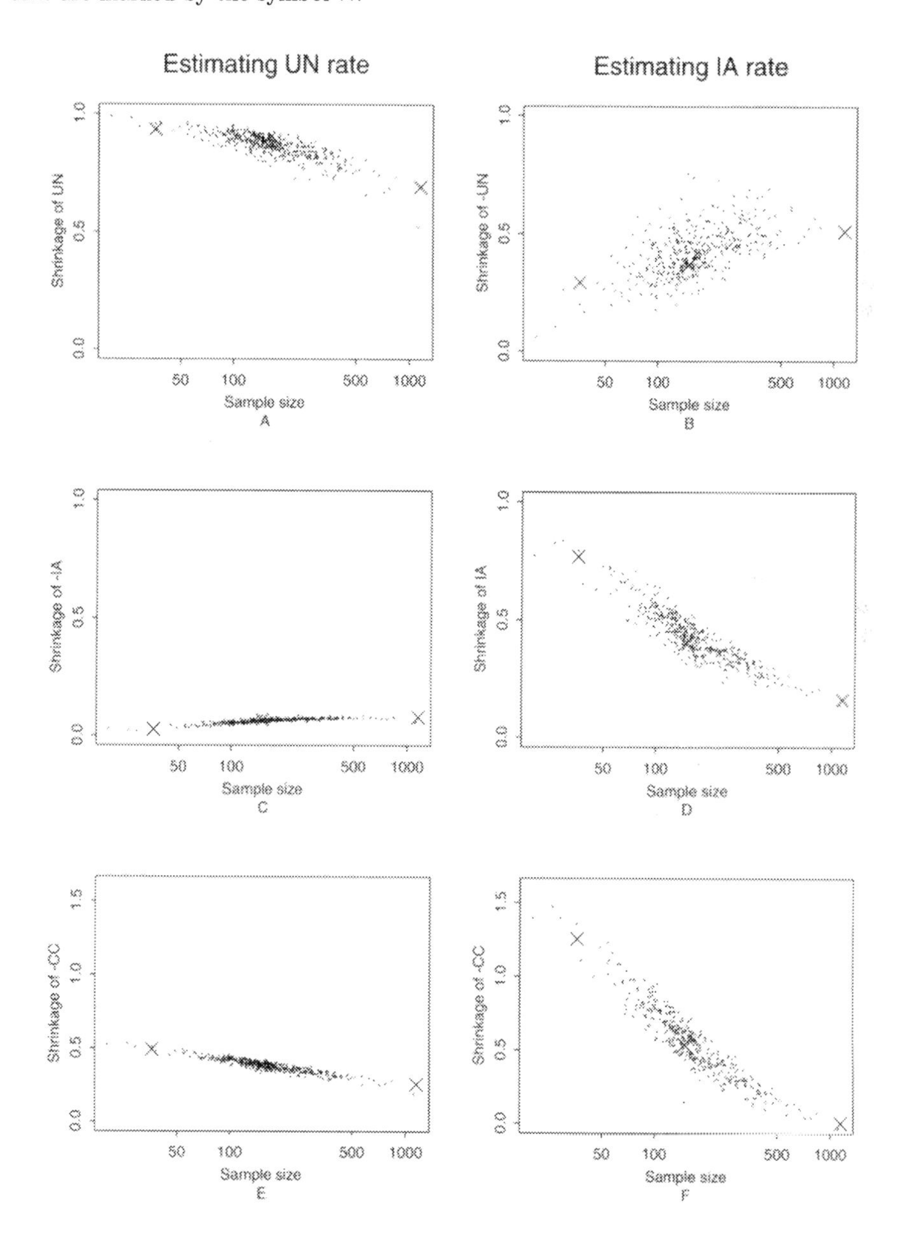

district 00AA (City of London, subsample size 4) is excluded from the plots. The signs of the coefficients are changed, as indicated by the axis labels, so that the ranges of the vertical axes of panels A–D are (0, 1).

The graphs highlight the strong association of shrinkage with the subsample size, except for the shrinkage of UN rates in estimating the IA rates. The 'self'-shrinkage (of UN to estimate UN rates and of IA to estimate IA rates) is stronger for the UN rates than for the IA rates, a consequence of the vastly greater district-level variance of the IA rates. Panels B and C document that UN rates are much more useful for estimating the IA rates than vice versa. Panels E and F show that the CC rates make a substantial contribution to estimating the IA rates for districts with small subsample sizes, but are much less useful for the districts with the largest subsample sizes. In contrast, the contribution made by the CC rates to estimating the UN rates is much smaller for the least populous districts but decreases only slightly with the district's subsample size.

The variation of the shrinkage coefficients within a given sample size is due to the differences in the (estimated) district-level rates used in calculating the shrinkage matrices $\hat{\mathbf{B}}_d$. Part of this variation is due to the differences in the population rates and part due to sampling variation. The latter is an undesirable component. Its impact can be assessed by a sensitivity analysis described by the following example.

District 22UJ, Harlow in Essex, has subsample size 97. We selected it deliberately, from the 24 districts with subsample sizes 96–104, as the district with the shrinkage coefficient for the UN rate in estimating the IA rate, −0.18, that is the smallest in absolute value for all the 24 districts. An unusual feature of the data for this district is the high sample UN rate (7.42%, with estimated standard error 2.36%), and low sample IA rate (13.40%, with estimated standard error 3.48%). Trivariate shrinkage estimation brings these rates much closer to the national trend, by reducing the estimated UN rate to 2.89% (standard error 0.52%) and increasing the estimated IA rate to 17.05% (standard error 2.51%). Shrinkage appears to be very useful for UN rate in particular, reducing its estimated standard error about 4.5 times. However, the radical change in the estimate, more than 2.5 times, may be disconcerting, especially to an analyst who appreciates the qualifier 'estimated' (used with shrinkage, standard error, and the like), or somebody skeptical about the method who is not willing to explore its details.

A pessimist would assess the error committed by estimating the shrinkage coefficients by using the coefficients for a district with a similar sample size, selecting such a district so as to obtain estimates that differ from those quoted above as much as possible. We carry out this exercise more comprehensively, by calculating the estimates based on the shrinkage coefficients for all the districts with sample sizes in the range 96–104. These values, referred to as the *plausible* estimates, of the UN rate for district 22UJ are in the range 2.95%–3.38%. Thus, there is no dispute about the direction of shrinkage — radical reduction from the direct estimate, but the shrinkage used for the estimate

$\hat{\mathbf{p}}_{22\mathrm{UJ}}^{\mathrm{C}}$ is the strongest. The explanation for this is in the rather extreme values of the direct estimates $\hat{\mathbf{p}}_{22\mathrm{UJ}}$ — the second highest for unemployment and the third lowest for economic inactivity among the 24 districts — unusual, given the high district-level correlation of the two rates.

The plausible estimates of the IA rate for district 22UJ are in the range 17.49%–19.35%. This time, the shrinkage used for $\hat{\mathbf{p}}_{22\mathrm{UJ}}^{\mathrm{C}}$ is the most conservative, because with the shrinkage based on the other districts we assume that the direct estimator is less precise. In conclusion, the sensitivity analysis shows that shrinkage is robust with respect to estimation of the sampling variance matrix $\hat{\mathbf{V}}_d$. If we assumed that the range of the plausible estimates is an indication of the sampling variance that is not accounted for, it would contribute to MSE by only about $0.015(\%)^2$ for the UN rate, and $0.31(\%)^2$ to the IA rate. Even with such an inflation, based on a rather pessimistic scenario, the shrinkage estimators remain much more efficient than their constituent direct estimators. However, the bias of $\hat{\mathbf{p}}_{22\mathrm{UJ}}^{\mathrm{C}}$ is more difficult to assess. The bias is substantial if district 22UJ is essentially different from the rest of the country. On the one hand, this is a weakness of the method; on the other, no more than a few districts may be exceptional, so the (multivariate) shrinkage is efficient for most districts. Without shrinkage, we would leave the information in the other districts of the country untapped.

Sensitivity of the estimates of the standard error could be explored similarly. However, the estimated standard error, being based on $\mathrm{e}\widehat{\mathrm{MSE}}$, is biased, so such an exercise is not as useful. The standard errors can be assessed more comprehensively by bootstrap. One implementation of the bootstrap replicates the sampling and estimation processes a large number of times, generating bootstrap replicate datasets with the same (national) sample size as in the original survey, and assesses the variation of the estimates across the replicates. For any given district, the replicates may have different district-level subsample sizes. As the assessment of the sampling variation conditions on the district-level subsample sizes, we have to restrict the sampling in the bootstrap to fixed district-level sample sizes. Carrying out the repeated sampling on the data from 80 000 subjects is perhaps an analytical overkill.

A simpler implementation of the bootstrap draws random samples only from the districts, and assumes the district-level subsamples to be fixed. Consequently, the sampling variation associated with $\hat{\mathbf{V}}_d$ is ignored, and we assess only the component of sampling variation due to estimating the district-level variance matrix $\mathbf{\Sigma}_{\mathrm{B}}$. However, the impact of the uncertainty about $\mathbf{V}_d$ was assessed earlier by a sensitivity analysis. The bootstrap indicates that the district-level variance matrix $\mathbf{\Sigma}_{\mathrm{B}}$ is estimated with very small sampling variation, adding to the standard error for a typical district 0.02 and 0.10 for the respective UN and IA rates.

10.1.2 Distribution of district-level rates

A simple way of estimating the distribution of a set of quantities, such as the district-level rates of unemployment, is by a histogram of the values, if they were available. Smoothing, for instance, by kernel density estimation, may improve the presentation and, with an appropriate level of smoothing, provides a better estimate of the density in a superpopulation represented by the D districts.

The quantities $p_{\mathcal{D}}$, that is, p_d, $d = 1, \ldots, D$, whose distribution we want to estimate, are not observed. Estimating the distribution of $p_{\mathcal{D}}$ naively from $\hat{p}_{\mathcal{D}}$ is not efficient because the target distribution is a non-linear function of $p_{\mathcal{D}}$. The values of the functions that contribute to the target as additive terms should be estimated; see Section 9.1. As we are interested in numerous features of the distribution, such as symmetry, modes, tails, and various quantiles, these functions are difficult to specify.

The direct estimates are more dispersed than the targets, so the histogram of $\hat{p}_{\mathcal{D}}$ offers a distorted view of the histogram of $p_{\mathcal{D}}$. The shrinkage estimates $\hat{p}_{\mathcal{D}}^{\mathrm{C}}$, even though (largely) more efficient, are not appropriate either; their histogram offers a view of $p_{\mathcal{D}}$ that is distorted in a different way — $\hat{p}_{\mathcal{D}}^{\mathrm{C}}$ are dispersed less than $p_{\mathcal{D}}$. The distortion with both sets of estimates can be attributed to the sampling variation of the direct estimators and the auxiliary information. We could reduce the shrinkage for the district-level estimates so that the district-level variance of the resulting estimates would match the estimated district-level variance $\hat{\sigma}_{\mathrm{B}}^2$. In univariate shrinkage, and assuming that $v = c_d = 0$, this amounts to using the shrinkage coefficient $b_d = 1/\sqrt{1 + n_d\omega}$.

We describe a more principled approach, similar to estimating the ranks of the districts in Section 9.2. For any value x, we wish to establish the proportion of the districts d for which $p_d < x$. This proportion,

$$F(x) = \frac{1}{D} \sum_{d=1}^{D} I(p_d < x) ,$$

is the empirical distribution function. The empirical density is defined as $\{F(x + \Delta) - F(x)\}/\Delta$ or, more precisely, as

$$f(x) = \frac{F(x + \frac{1}{2}\Delta) - F(x - \frac{1}{2}\Delta)}{\Delta} ,$$

where Δ is a suitable small number, set so that $f(x)$ is an efficient estimator of the underlying density. (If Δ is too small, $f(x)$ oscillates between zero and large positive values.) Each elementary contribution to $F(x)$, $I(p_d < x)$, is estimated by its probability based on the estimated distribution of $\hat{p}_d^{\mathrm{C}}$, in analogy with the the elementary contributions to the ranks in (9.1) and (9.2):

$$I(p_d < x \,|\, \hat{\mathbf{p}}_d, \hat{\mathbf{p}}, \ldots) \mathrel{\hat{\sim}} \mathcal{N}\left\{\hat{p}_d^{\mathrm{C}}, \widehat{\mathrm{eMSE}}\left(\hat{p}_d^{\mathrm{C}}\right)\right\} ,$$

Figure 10.3. Estimates of the district-level distribution function (panel A) and density (panel B) of the district-level rates of unemployment. The direct and shrinkage estimates of the density, calculated with $\Delta = 0.2$, are smoothed.

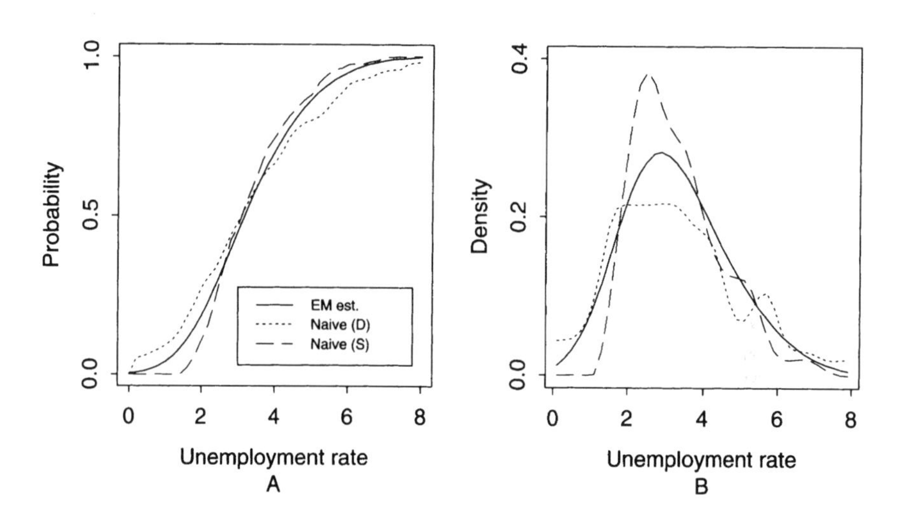

approximately. This identity can be motivated by the EM algorithm in which the district-level population rates are the complete information, and their estimation constitutes the E-step. To evaluate the sampling variance of $F(x)$, the covariances of the shrinkage estimators $\hat{p}_d^{\mathrm{C}}$ have to be taken into account. The evaluation is not necessary, as a good impression of the sampling variation of $\hat{F}$ is gained by comparing it with its trivial counterparts based on the direct and shrinkage estimates. As an alternative, the direct estimators can be used to estimate $F(x)$. The sampling variation is easier to evaluate, but it is much greater, as the contributing estimators $\hat{p}_d$ are much less efficient than the shrinkage estimators $\hat{p}_d^{\mathrm{C}}$.

The three estimates of the distribution function are plotted in Figure 10.3, together with the estimated densities derived from them. The estimator motivated by the EM algorithm (solid line) looks like a compromise of the two naive estimators, based on the direct estimates (D, dots) and shrinkage estimates (S, dashes). The fact that the EM estimate is a smooth distribution function and the naive estimates are not is not important in the context.

The differences among the estimates are illustrated more clearly on the estimated densities in panel B. The naive estimate based on the shrinkage estimators $\hat{p}_{\mathcal{D}}^{\mathrm{C}}$ is associated with much smaller district-level variance than the EM estimate, which in turn is associated with much smaller variance than the naive estimate based on the direct estimators $\hat{p}_{\mathcal{D}}$. The naive direct estimate suggests that a handful of districts have no unemployed at all, not a realistic proposition, and that some districts have unemployment in excess of 8%. The naive shrinkage estimate claims that no district has unemployment rate lower than 1.5% and that only one district has unemployment rate greater than 7%. The inefficiency of the naive estimators is best highlighted by simulating, or at least considering, how they would change if the overall sample size were increased or reduced. With a reduction, the direct estimates would be more dispersed and the shrinkage estimates less dispersed. In contrast, the EM estimator suffers only from the consequences of poorer estimation of the district-level variance matrix, which has an impact on the extent of shrinkage. The naively estimated densities in Figure 10.3, already smoothed to remove their excessive oscillation, could be smoothed even further.

The variances of the estimated densities are 3.74 for the naive shrinkage, 1.41 for naive direct, and 2.01 for the EM estimate. Neither of them agrees with the estimated district-level variance $\hat{\sigma}_{\mathrm{B}}^2$, equal to 1.64. The EM method is more efficient than the two naive alternatives for pointwise estimation, but that does not imply efficiency in estimating the shape, smoothness or any other feature that is a non-linear function of values of the density. Most likely, the EM estimator yields a density that is too smooth, and the naive methods densities that are not smooth enough. We should define a particular feature, such as skewness, and estimate it efficiently from the direct estimates. The EM algorithm and, for more complex targets, multiple imputation, are appropriate methods for this. But no single estimated distribution function or density could serve as an estimate for a multitude of features of the underlying distribution.

In principle, the density function can be estimated by the methods of functional data analysis [220]. The target density is represented by its coefficients (coordinates) q_h in an infinite basis of functions g_h, $h = 1, \ldots$, and the density $f(p_{\mathcal{D}}) = q_1 g_1 + q_2 g_2 + \cdots$ is estimated by the finite (truncated) expansion $\hat{f}(p_{\mathcal{D}}) = \hat{q}_1 g_1 + \cdots + \hat{q}_H g_H$, for a suitable integer H.

Small-area estimates are often represented by maps; the areas are shaded according to the value of the (shrinkage) estimate. The caveats attached to such maps are that they are based on estimates, with estimated precisions. This information is far from complete because it does not convey the correlations of the district-level estimators, and a typical user of such a map could not take the information about this correlation structure of the district-level estimators into account. The map displays artefacts associated with the method of estimation. Optimal estimation for each district does not imply any good properties of the collection of the estimates, even if the properties are inferred only informally, as observations (impressions) of the 'estimated' map. A universal solution is provided by simulation, closely related to multiple imputation. To motivate it, we pose the following missing-data problem. The complete-data analysis comprises drawing a map based on the district-level population means. Denote this task by $\mathcal{F}(p_{\mathcal{D}})$, indicating the argument p_d, $d = 1, \ldots, D$. Given suitable software, this is a relatively simple task. The incomplete data is the set of estimates $\hat{p}_d^{\mathrm{C}}$ for districts $d = 1, \ldots, D$. Executing $\mathcal{F}(\hat{p}_{\mathcal{D}}^{\mathrm{C}})$ is a poor replacement for $\mathcal{F}(p_{\mathcal{D}})$ because $\mathcal{F}$ can be interpreted as a non-linear operation. Instead, we execute $\mathcal{F}(p_{\mathcal{D}}^{\dagger})$, where $p_d^{\dagger}$ are *plausible values* of p_d, $d = 1, \ldots, D$. The plausible values are drawn at random from the estimated joint distribution of $\hat{p}_{\mathcal{D}}^{\mathrm{C}}$. This is done by drawing a set of plausible values of the direct estimators $\hat{\mathbf{p}}_d$, estimating the district-level variance matrix $\mathbf{\Sigma}_{\mathrm{B}}$ and evaluating the shrinkage estimators based on it. Drawing from the distributions of $\hat{p}_d^{\mathrm{C}}$ directly is not appropriate because we fail to represent the correlation of the shrinkage estimators across the districts. Strictly speaking, all vectors and matrices required for evaluating $\hat{p}_d^{\mathrm{C}}$ should be drawn from their respective distributions, but this complication is probably not warranted.

Several sets of plausible values are simulated independently, by replicating this process, and a map is drawn for each set. These *plausible maps* represent scenarios well supported by the data, and they require no caveats related to estimation of the district-level rates. It is essential to produce several maps, to represent the uncertainty about any feature of interest. We can be confident that a feature is present in the 'population' version of the map, $\mathcal{F}(p_{\mathcal{D}})$, if it is present in (almost) all the plausible maps $\mathcal{F}(p_{\mathcal{D}}^{\dagger})$.

As a summary, the direct and shrinkage estimates of the district-level rates are plotted in Figure 10.4. To illustrate how the extent of shrinkage depends on the sample size, districts with the smallest and largest subsample sizes are marked in the plots by the respective symbols $\circ$ ($n_d < 70$) and $\times$ ($n_d > 400$). The left-hand panels plot each pair of directly estimated rates and the right-hand panels their shrinkage counterparts. Unemployment and economic inactivity rates are shrunk quite radically (compare panels A and B), and the unemployment rates are aligned according to the CC rates (panels C and D) much more closely than the economic inactivity rates are (panels E and F). As discussed earlier, the estimators represented in these graphs have good properties for the rates of individual districts, and should on no account be used directly for any inferences about the bivariate distributions of the district-level population rates.

10.1.3 Estimation for age-by-sex subpopulations

Unemployment and economic inactivity are distributed very unevenly between men and women, and among the ages. Young men and women (aged 16–24) have high rates of both unemployment and economic inactivity because many of them are enrolled in education, and disproportionately many of those who are not are unemployed. The rates of economic inactivity tend to be higher among women, and the rates of unemployment higher among men in the same age category. The rates of economic inactivity drop from over 30% for 16-year-old men to around 5% for 30-year olds, then increase very slightly until the age of 50 when they rise steeply as a result of early retirements. The trend for women is similar, but the rates are much higher in the age range of 25–50 years. The age-specific national rates of unemployment and economic inactivity of working-age men and women in spring 2001 are drawn in Figure 10.5. The curves are smoothed to reduce the impact of the sampling variation.

Figure 10.4. The direct and shrinkage estimates of the district-level unemployment (UN) and economic inactivity (IA) rates. The symbols ∘ and × are used for about 5% of the districts with the smallest and largest sample sizes, respectively.

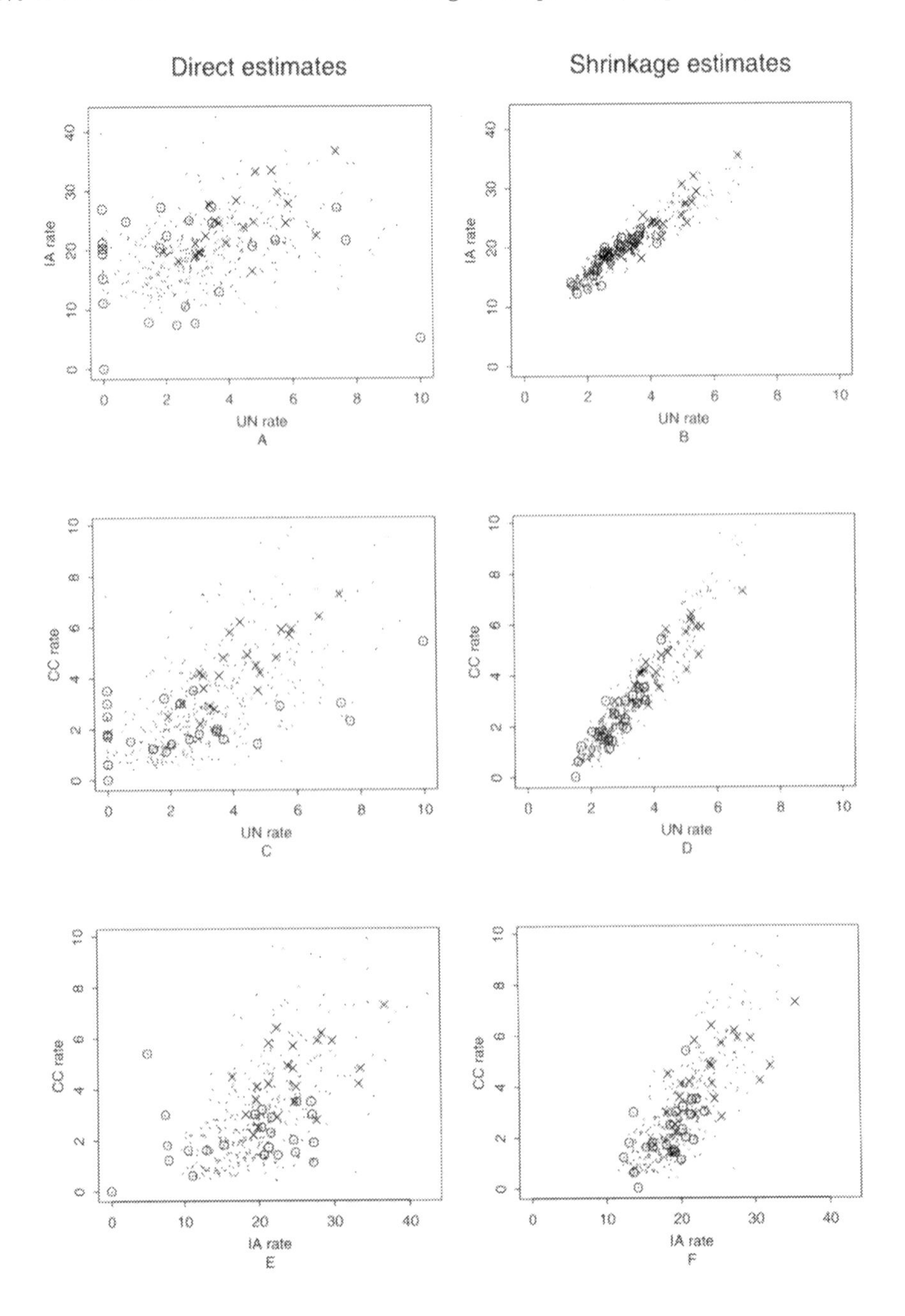

Figure 10.5. Estimates of the age-specific national rates of unemployment (UN) and economic inactivity (IA) for men and women, Spring 2001.

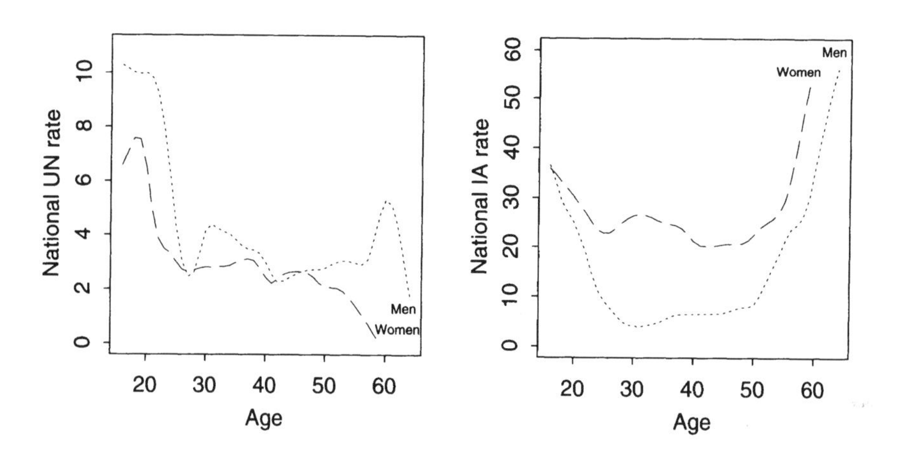

Local authorities require the rates of unemployment and economic inactivity for the youngest and oldest members of the labour force, because their employment status is associated with demand for certain services: training and support for job-seeking for the young, and the change in lifestyle and health-care needs for the retired. The sample sizes for the district-by-age groups are for most districts so small that direct estimation or estimation by univariate shrinkage (using only the subsample of subjects in the age group from all districts) is unsatisfactory. If the trends described by Figure 10.5 applied in all districts, estimation for any particular age group would be improved dramatically by exploiting such similarity. Even if the trends are not reproduced in every district, the rates for one age group are bound to be similar to the rates for the 'neighbouring' groups. This provides a strong rationale for applying multivariate shrinkage.

In principle, we can choose any age groups for the role of auxiliary information. More detail, with narrower age ranges, might provide more auxiliary information; however, as the district-level subsample sizes for these groups are small, the difficulties with estimating the sampling variances $\mathbf{V}_d$ become more and more acute and prevent us from effective exploitation of the similarity of the rates across the age groups. The district-level CC rates are available for men and women only, and for no age groups. Nevertheless, they provide powerful auxiliary information if the rates within an age group are highly correlated with the district-level rates (for the same sex).

A pragmatic choice, avoiding handling large variance matrices, is to consider as auxiliary information only the unemployment and economic inactivity rates for the complement of the target age group within the sex, together with the CC rates for the same sex, leading to five-variate shrinkage estimation.

Including the CC rate for the other sex is not useful because the two sets of rates are very highly correlated; in effect, we would duplicate the auxiliary information provided by one of them.

For young men (aged 16–24), the estimated district-level correlation matrix is

$$\frac{1}{100}\begin{pmatrix} 100 & 95 & 83 & 63 & 90 \\ 95 & 100 & 66 & 11 & 88 \\ 83 & 66 & 100 & 55 & 73 \\ 63 & 11 & 55 & 100 & 37 \\ 90 & 88 & 73 & 37 & 100 \end{pmatrix} \qquad \begin{bmatrix} \mathrm{UN-o} \\ \mathrm{UN-y} \\ \mathrm{IA-o} \\ \mathrm{IA-y} \\ \mathrm{CC-m} \end{bmatrix}$$

(the variables are indicated in the right-hand side by their obvious acronyms; 'y' stands for young and 'o' for other). The estimated district-level variances are

UN-o	UN-y	IA-o	IA-y	CC-m
1.23	11.20	28.95	69.33	8.18

(in percentages squared). The correlation matrix indicates that the UN rate for the complement (group UN-o) is good auxiliary information for the UN rate of the young men (correlation 0.95), but the IA rate for the complement is much poorer for the IA rate of young men (correlation 0.55). Ironically, the UN rate for the complement provides better auxiliary information — it has higher correlation with IA-y rate *and* its sampling variance is lower because, for a given sample size, the binomial variance decreases as the rate departs from 50%. The CC rate for men is also much better suited for estimating the UN rate of young men than for their district-level IA rates.

The direct information about the district-level UN and IA rates of young men is very sparse; the subsample size exceeds 100 only for two districts, and young men are represented in the subsamples for most districts by only a handful of subjects, or by none at all. Thus, we rely on the district-level variance matrix very heavily, and concern about the model implied by the shrinkage is well founded. However, the alternative, the direct estimator, is not practical. We can protect our inferences from over-reliance on the implied model by reducing the shrinkage. This can be done in two ways that complement one another. By reducing the covariances (e.g., by a multiplicative factor), we reduce the reliance on the similarity across the variables. By inflating the variances, we reduce the shrinkage across the districts, as if the districts were more heterogeneous. This should be done in moderation, as at the extreme, when $\mathbf{\Sigma}_{\mathrm{B}}$ is set to a diagonal matrix with large variances, little shrinkage takes place, making poor use of the similarity across both districts and variables.

10.1.4 Pooling information across time

LFS takes place every quarter, but the division into quarters is mainly for administrative and data-management purposes; approximately the same number of interviews are scheduled for every week, and a geographical balance of the interviewers' workloads is maintained throughout. Many analysts of the LFS data appreciate that the subsample sizes for direct estimation are insufficient, and respond to it by averaging over time. Thus, the unemployment figures for the UK as a whole are published every month, estimated directly from the data collected in the previous month (about a third of a survey). Rates for small subpopulations are estimated quarterly or annually, pooling the data over the relevant period. This kind of pooling can be interpreted as shrinkage, giving equal weight to each element of the auxiliary information. The formulation of (multivariate) shrinkage is much more general and flexible, allowing the analyst to reflect the relevance of the information to the target quantity.

We consider multivariate shrinkage estimation of the current district-level rates of unemployment and economic inactivity, using the (direct) estimators of these rates in the previous quarters. Surveys $t = 1, 2, 3, 4$ quarters previously share approximately $100(5 - t)\%$ of the subjects with the current survey ($t = 0$), so they are far from independent. We can avoid having to account for this sample dependence by taking only subjects in waves V in each of the previous quarters. Thus, the auxiliary information is not as extensive as might have appeared; the sample sizes associated with the auxiliary variables are only about one-fifth of the sample size of the direct estimator. However, as district-level rates are unlikely to have changed dramatically in any of the districts, and any changes have a substantial 'national' component (namely, the overall reduction of the unemployment rates in 2001–2004), it is worthwhile to include information from several quarters or even years. The task of operating with large variance matrices, one matrix inversion per district, is nowadays not regarded as excessive. It can nevertheless be avoided, without substantial loss of efficiency. Simply, we declare as auxiliary variable the direct estimates of the annual average district-level rates of unemployment and economic inactivity. This reduces the dimensionality of the problem four-fold. The average annual rates are estimated as the sample rates for subjects who were in wave V in any quarter of the year. Data would be used only for subjects from the quarter when they were in wave V. The loss of information is brought on by treating the whole year uniformly, not giving greater weight to the information from later in the year, closer to the target time point. But with the lower-dimensional shrinkage estimation, sensitivity analysis is easier to carry out and insights into how shrinkage operates are gained much more readily.

Auxiliary information need not come from the past. Estimation of the historical rates of unemployment and economic inactivity can be improved by using 'future' rates as auxiliary information. For example, estimates of the district-level unemployment rates a year ago can be updated by the information in the LFS surveys conducted since. Symmetry suggests that data from a year later are as useful as data from a year earlier.

Of course, the changes by updating are an inconvenience in an administrative setting in which estimates are treated as if they were population quantities, and consistency of appearance is rated higher than efficiency. Arguably, updating (or back-dating) may hamper the credibility of the estimates. This is a difficult problem in the interaction between the analyst and the client, because an improvement in estimation (reduction of eMSE) may be counter-productive. It is difficult to convey that estimates are subject to chance, and they depend on the information available. The more information we have, the smaller the impact of the chance. In this perspective, consistency (using the same estimate throughout) is in conflict with efficiency. Selective use of the update, using it only when the estimate has changed in a desirable direction, or its estimated MSE is reduced substantially, also amounts to bad practice because the estimator used is a mixture of the original and updated estimator. The properties of such a mixture are not estimated well by the properties of the selected estimator.

10.2 Samples of Anonymised Records

The Samples of Anonymised Records (SAR) are a database created by simple random sampling of the records in the UK Census. The Sample for individuals from the 1991 Census contains records of 2% of the UK residents at the time of the Census, around 1.16 million records. (A similar database is generated from the 2001 Census.) The database contains only a limited set of variables, so that no individuals could be identified by the pattern of their values. The sole geographical information in the database is the identifier of the resident's local area. The local areas are either local authority districts or unions of contiguous districts, amalgamated so that the population of each area exceeds 120 000. For example, the London boroughs are local areas, except for the City of London, which forms a local area together with the adjacent City of Westminster. There are 278 local areas.

This section describes estimation of the economic activity rates among young people and minorities in the local areas. (The census-based rates among all working-age adults are available from administrative sources, but they are not used here as auxiliary information.) A resident is economically active if he or she is either employed, or not employed but actively seeking employment. Full-time students, housewives and the retired are examples of persons not economically active.

The subsample size for the least populous local area is about 120 000/50 = 2400, so the standard error of its estimated rate of economic activity, given that the rate is 60%, is $100\sqrt{0.60 \times 0.40/2400} = 1.0\%$. This might be adequate for some purposes, but improvement on it is highly desirable.

Univariate shrinkage is not very useful because the standard deviation of the area-level rates, estimated by moment matching as $\hat{\sigma}_{\mathrm{B}} = 4.5\%$, is much greater than 1%. The sampling variance of the direct estimator is preferred to the bias of the national estimator of the rate. For estimating the area-level rates for subpopulations, multivariate shrinkage is much more effective, especially if suitable auxiliary information is selected. We focus first on the economic activity rates for white men aged 16–19 years. These rates tend to be lower than for middle-aged men because many 16–19 year-olds are in full-time education. The SAR database contains records of 26 963 young white men. The numbers of subjects in the least populous areas are 30 or slightly more, whereas a few cities that form a single area each have sample sizes greater than 200. Birmingham, with population in excess of 1 million, has the largest subsample size, 359. The direct estimators of the area-level rates of economic activity are in the range 35%–80%. Of course, much of this variation is due to sampling. In fact, the area-level variance of the direct estimates is $\mathrm{var}_{\mathcal{D}}(\hat{p}_{\mathcal{D}}) = 53.7(\%)^2$, whereas the estimate of the area-level variance of the underlying (subpopulation) rates is only $\hat{\sigma}_{\mathrm{B}}^2 = 21.6(\%)^2$. The estimated standard errors, calculated from the estimated eMSE, are reduced by univariate shrinkage between 1.13 and 2.15 times; the estimated gains decrease with sample size, although the estimated rate itself also exerts some influence.

It is reasonable to expect that the rates of economic activity of young men are very similar to those for women of the same age. This provides a rationale for applying bivariate shrinkage, with the young women's rates used as auxiliary information. Young men's rates can be used reciprocally to improve the estimation for young women. Indeed, the estimated area-level variance matrix for young men and women,

$$\hat{\boldsymbol{\Sigma}}_{\mathrm{B}} = \begin{pmatrix} 21.6 & 21.0 \\ 21.0 & 24.6 \end{pmatrix},$$

has a very high correlation, equal to 0.91. Although this seems very promising for bivariate shrinkage, the results are rather disappointing. The gains over univariate shrinkage are modest even for the areas with the smallest subsample sizes. For example, the subsamples for the London Borough of Hackney comprise 39 men and 57 women. The direct estimates of their economic activity rates are $(59.0\%, 42.1\%)^\top$, with estimated standard errors $(7.9\%, 6.5\%)^\top$. The univariate shrinkage estimates are $(62.1\%, 51.1\%)^\top$, with estimated standard errors $(4.0\%, 4.0\%)^\top$, and bivariate shrinkage estimates are $(58.8\%, 51.1\%)^\top$, with estimated standard errors $(3.5\%, 3.7\%)^\top$.

The gains in precision are greater for men, and their estimated standard error for bivariate shrinkage is smaller than for women, even though their subsample size is smaller. This is due to the smaller area-level variance for men and due to drawing on more auxiliary information (from women) in bivariate shrinkage. The gains in precision of bivariate over univariate shrinkage are rather disappointing because the subsample sizes for young men and women are very similar. Thus, where the direct or univariate shrinkage estimator is less precise, it is usually aided in bivariate shrinkage by less auxiliary information.

As in Section 10.1.3, using the rates of economic activity of the complement of the sample (men aged 25 and over) as auxiliary information is much more effective because these rates are based on much greater subsample sizes. To avoid near duplication of this argument, details are omitted. Instead, we illustrate multivariate shrinkage estimation of the area-level rates of economic activity of ethnic minorities (as a single group). The auxiliary information is the corresponding rate for white residents. In the UK, the minorities are very unevenly distributed across local areas. London and some large metropolitan areas in England have high concentrations of minorities, in contrast to most of the other local areas. However, not all the local areas that are part of a metropolitan area have large populations.

Figure 10.6 summarises the sample sizes for all adult subjects in SAR and all adults from ethnic minorities. Each point in panel A represents an area, and the axes correspond to the numbers of all adults and adults from minorities. Since the sample sizes are substantial, exceeding 2000 for most areas, each subsample size is close to 2% of the population size of the area. The thin solid line is drawn at the national percentage of minorities, 4.5%. The subsample sizes of the minorities are very small for many areas, especially for areas with smaller populations, and so the graph is cluttered immediately to the right of the point $(2000, 0)$. The points are spread much more evenly when presented on the log scale in panel B. In the plot, a token 0.1 is added to the numbers of minorities, to avoid the expression $\log(0)$. The diagram indicates that the proportions of minorities are smaller than the national proportion in much more than half the areas. The outlying point in the upper right-hand corner of both panels corresponds to Birmingham. Next in the descending order of sample size are the cities of Leeds, Sheffield and Glasgow; their percentages of minorities are similar to or lower than the national percentage. Several London boroughs and local areas in the Manchester Metropolitan Area have higher percentages of minorities but, as a result of the administrative division, their populations are not exceptionally large.

The direct estimates of the national rates of economic activity of minority men and women are 75.5% (estimated standard error 0.65%) and 52.2% (estimated standard error 1.15%), respectively. Although small subsample size causes difficulties with estimating the sampling variance of the direct estimator of the rate for many local areas, the problem is less acute than in Section 10.1.1, because the estimated rates are distant from zero or 100%. For such rates p_d, the dependence of $\mathrm{var}(\hat{p}_d)$ on p_d is much weaker.

Using the economic activity rates of minority men and women as the auxiliary information for one another is not effective because areas tend to have similar numbers of minority men and women. So, even if the rates for minority men and women were similar, shrinkage estimation would not be effective. In any case, the rates are not very similar. The estimated area-level variance matrix for minority men and women is

$$\hat{\boldsymbol{\Sigma}}_{\mathrm{B}} = \begin{pmatrix} 19.7 & 25.1 \\ 25.1 & 72.0 \end{pmatrix} ; \qquad (10.1)$$

the estimated correlation of the two sets of rates is 0.67. A likely explanation for the high variance for women is that the ethnic groups maintain very different attitudes to women's employment, and these attitudes, and the particular

Figure 10.6. The sample sizes of all adults and all adults from minorities in the local areas; SAR 1991. The solid line represents the national proportion.

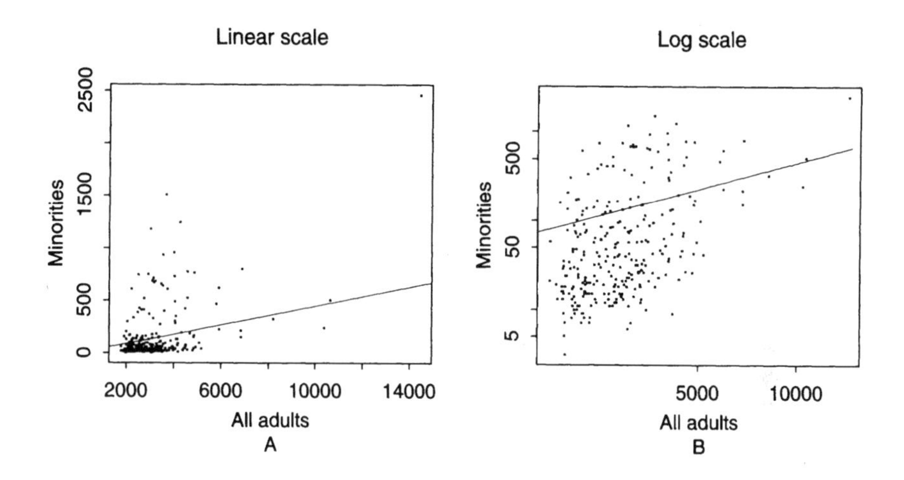

minority groups, are unevenly distributed within the minorities in the local areas. Arguably, classifying all minorities as a single group is not appropriate for administrative matters related to the labour force, but a finer classification brings about numerous other problems.

Using the rates for white men as auxiliary information is much more effective not only because of their greater subsample sizes but also because their area-level rates are much less dispersed than for minority women *and* they are more strongly correlated with the rates for minority men. The estimated area-level variance matrix for minority and white men is

$$\hat{\Sigma}_{\mathrm{B}} = \begin{pmatrix} 19.7 & 15.2 \\ 15.2 & 14.5 \end{pmatrix};$$

the estimated correlation of the two sets of rates is 0.90.

The London Borough of Haringey has a much greater proportion of ethnic minorities than the country at large. In SAR, it is represented by 386 adult men from minorities and 1428 white men; the minority men form 21.3% of the borough's subsample. The direct estimate of the rate of economic activity is 75.9%, the univariate shrinkage estimate is 75.8%, and the bivariate shrinkage estimate is 76.8%. The estimated standard errors of these estimators are 2.2%, 2.0% and 1.6%. Shrinkage is not very effective in this case because the borough's sample size in SAR is quite large. Note that the improvement by the bivariate shrinkage is greater than by the univariate shrinkage. Information from within the local area (the rate for white men, estimated from a large subsample) is more valuable than from the rates of the minorities in other local areas. This is so because many other local areas have much smaller subsample sizes for minorities, and the rates of economic activity of minorities and white men are very similar; the standard deviation of their differences is only $\sqrt{19.7 + 14.5 - 2 \times 15.2} = 1.95\%$, whereas the standard deviation of the rates for minorities is $\sqrt{19.7} = 4.4\%$. Moreover, the local-area rate for white men in Haringey is estimated with high precision (standard error 1.2%).

Next we discuss estimation of the rate for minority men in Falkirk, Scotland. The area is represented in SAR by 1671 adult men, but only four of them are from minorities, and three of these are economically active. Thus, the naive estimate of the standard error of the direct estimator exceeds 20%; four subjects yield next to no information about *any* proportion. The univariate shrinkage estimate is 75.5%, and its estimated standard error is 4.4%, a radical improvement over the direct estimator. Bivariate shrinkage increases the precision further; the estimate, 74.5%, is associated with estimated standard error 2.3%. Of course, such an estimate is based almost solely on auxiliary information. If Falkirk is an exceptional local area in some aspect related to economic activity, shrinkage would be both inappropriate and the assessment of its precision grossly incorrect. However, the direct estimator is not viable for any purpose, despite being valid, as there is no dispute about the sampling design applied to create SAR.

Estimation of the area-level rates for minority women is much less successful. The estimated area-level variance matrix for minority and white (adult) women is

$$\hat{\mathbf{\Sigma}}_{\mathrm{B}} = \begin{pmatrix} 72.0 & 16.8 \\ 16.8 & 15.3 \end{pmatrix} .$$

The correlation in this matrix, 0.51, is smaller than among the rates for minority men and women, see (10.1), but the subsample sizes of white women are so much greater than for minority men that white women provide better auxiliary information. The gains in precision for minority women are indeed much more modest than for minority men, although bivariate shrinkage still yields a substantial improvement for many areas.

Haringey is represented in SAR by 1876 adult women, 365 of them from ethnic minorities (19.5%). The direct estimate of the rate of economic activity of minority women in Haringey is 60.3% (estimated standard error 2.6%); the univariate shrinkage estimate is 59.6% (2.5%), and the bivariate shrinkage estimate 60.1% (2.4%). Here, shrinkage contributes little to the precision of the estimated rate.

For Falkirk, shrinkage is much more effective. The area is represented in SAR by six adult women from minorities and 1826 adult white women. Of course, the direct estimator is not competitive (estimate 50.0%, standard error 22.3%). The univariate shrinkage estimate is 51.9%, with estimated standard error 8.0%, and bivariate shrinkage estimate 51.8% (7.0%). The improvement by the univariate shrinkage is more modest for women than for men because the local-area rates for women are much more dispersed. The improvement by the bivariate shrinkage is only slight because the differences of the local-area rates for minority and white women are not strongly correlated. The

Figure 10.7. The direct, univariate and bivariate shrinkage estimates of the local-area rates of economic activity of the ethnic minorities; SAR 1991.

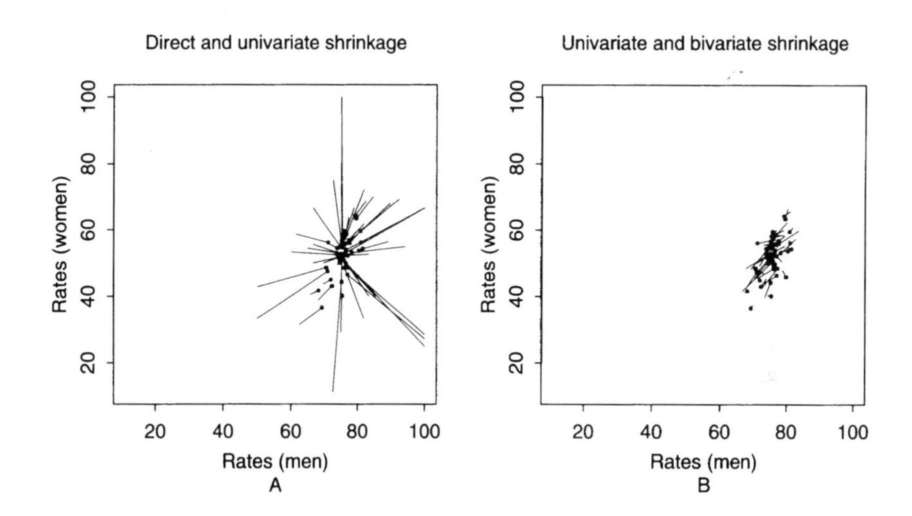

standard deviation of the differences of the local-area rates of minority and white women is 7.3%, much greater than for men (1.95%).

We conclude by graphically summarising the shrinkage estimates of the rates of economic activity for minorities in Figure 10.7, and the estimated standard errors in Figure 10.8. In panel A of Figure 10.7, local areas are represented by segments, each connecting the point with the coordinates defined by the direct estimates for minority men and women with the corresponding coordinates for the univariate shrinkage estimates (marked by black dots). The segments are plotted for a 20% systematic sample of the areas. Panel B has the same layout, connecting the univariate and bivariate shrinkage estimates for minority men and women. The panels illustrate that the changes from the direct to the univariate shrinkage estimates are much greater than from the univariate to the bivariate shrinkage estimates.

In Figure 10.8, each area is represented by a vertical segment that 'drops' from the estimated standard error of the direct estimator to the estimated standard error of the bivariate shrinkage estimator. The estimated standard error of each univariate shrinkage estimator is marked by a dash –. For men (panel A), the estimated standard errors of the univariate shrinkage estimator are in a narrow range, except for the areas for which even the direct estimator is very precise. For bivariate shrinkage, the standard errors are in an even narrower range. The gains in precision by univariate shrinkage for minority women (panel B) are much more modest, and the contribution of the white women's rates to their estimation (the improvement of the bivariate shrinkage over univariate shrinkage) is only slight.

Figure 10.8. The estimates of the standard errors for the direct, univariate and bivariate shrinkage estimators of the local-area rates of economic activity of the ethnic minorities; SAR 1991.

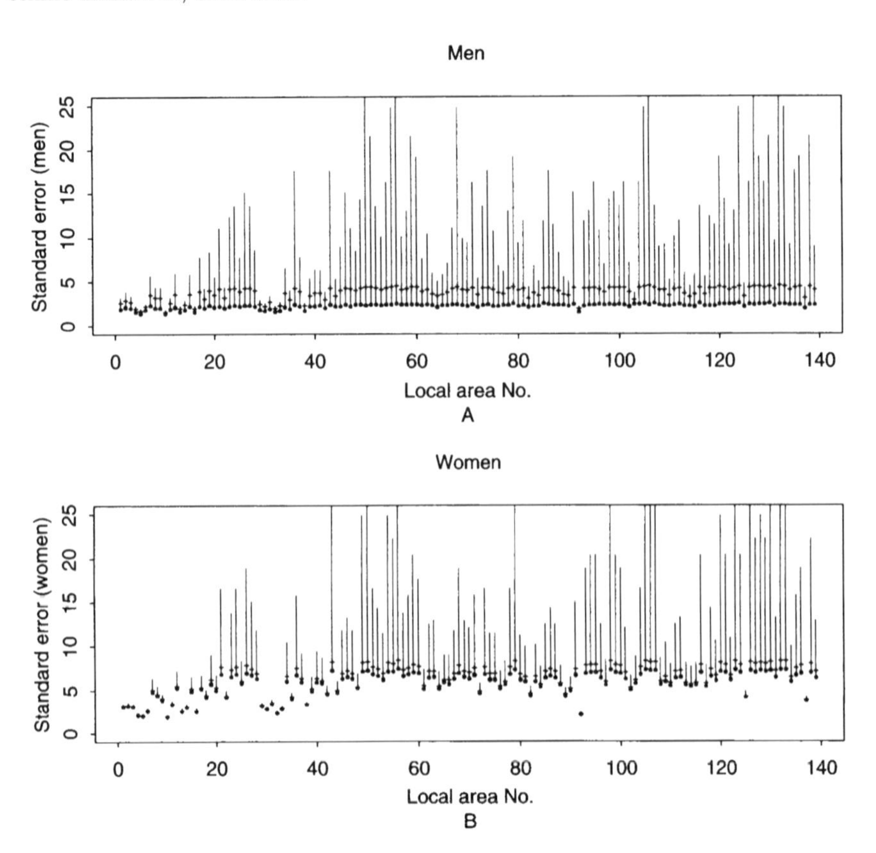

10.3 Norwegian municipalities

In the government statistics community, the Scandinavian countries are renowned for comprehensive population registers. The registers are a product of a substantial investment made decades ago, followed by years of fine-tuning of the data collection procedures, and later transferring the information to computers and arranging that their updating is as seamless as possible. The transparent benefit of these registers is that the population can be studied much more dynamically than by carefully planned extensive surveys that observe the population through a random sample at one or a few fixed time points.

This section describes the analysis of a sampling exercise carried out as part of the 1990 decenial population census in Norway. A survey embedded in the census was conducted, in which information about the employment

Table 10.1. The sampling fractions in the Norwegian municipalities.

Population range	6000–7999	8000–9999	10 000–49 999	50 000+
Municipalities	41	26	91	8
Sampling fraction	1/5	1/7	1/10	1/12

status was collected from a stratified random sample of the adult residents (aged 16 or over on the day of the Census, 3rd November 1990). We are concerned about the rates of employment within age-by-sex categories and about the composition of the employed within the Norwegian municipalities (*kommune*). Here, composition refers to the percentages of employed in the following nine industrial sectors:

AF — Agriculture, hunting, forestry and fishing;
MQ — Mining, quarrying and oil production;
MN — Manufacturing;
EW — Electricity, gas and water supply;
CB — Construction;
WR — Wholesale and retail trade, restaurants and hotels;
TC — Transport, storage and communications;
FB — Finance, insurance, real estate and business services;
SP — Social and personal services.

Each employed person, or an instance of paid employment, is associated with one of these sectors. In the survey, a binary variable was recorded indicating whether the subject was in paid employment for at least 100 days between the dates of 3rd November 1989 and 3rd November 1990.

Of the population of Norway, approximately 4.25 million, about half were members of the labour force in 1990. The population is distributed extremely unevenly over Norway's territory. Administratively, Norway is divided into 448 municipalities. Only eight (urban) municipalities had (in 1989) more than 50 000 residents; 96 municipalities had population between 10 000 and 49 999, and 275 municipalities (61%) had fewer than 6000 residents.

Except for seven municipalities, the survey sampling design comprised independent random draws in each municipality with population of at least 6000, with the sampling fractions (probabilities) given in Table 10.1. In the municipalities with population below 6000 as well as the seven 'exceptional' municipalities with greater population, full enumeration was conducted. The survey involved 595 000 subjects, 415 000 of them from municipalities in which full enumeration was conducted.

The results of the survey were reported in the form of tables of direct estimates of municipality-level rates of employment, accompanied by their estimated standard errors. The following reporting conventions were adopted, based on the relative standard error (RSE), defined as the ratio of the estimated standard error and the estimate. When the RSE is smaller than 0.2, both the estimate and standard error are reported; when the RSE is in the range 0.2–0.3, only the estimate is reported, in parentheses; and when the RSE is greater than 0.3, no figures are reported. As all the estimated proportions are distant from zero and unity, these rules for reporting direct estimates can be converted to (threshold) sample sizes that depend only on the sampling fraction. Implied in these rules is the requirement for a minimum precision of each reported estimate. We apply multivariate shrinkage and evaluate its efficiency by how many more figures would be reported than with direct estimation.

We discuss first (simultaneous) estimation of the rates of employment for the categories defined by sex and the following age groups: teenagers (16–19 years of age, T), young (20–24 years, Y), middle-aged (25–59 years, M), veterans (60–66 years, V), and retirement-aged (67 years and above, R). We refer to these groups by acronyms that code the age group (the capital letter given in parentheses) and sex (m or f, for men and women, respectively). For example, Yw denotes the group of women aged 20–24.

Our targets are the 2×5 tables of rates for the 166 municipalities in which sampling (not enumeration) was conducted. As the survey domain, we can adopt either the whole country, or only these non-enumerated municipalities. The advantage of the former is the substantially greater sample size, whereas with the latter we protect our inference against the bias due to municipalities that are different from (less populous than) the target municipalities. We choose the former solution; otherwise a lot of useful information would be discarded. The impact of the data from the enumerated municipalities can be reduced by associating their rates with a positive sampling variance, for instance, the variance that corresponds to the sampling rate of 80%.

The value of the univariate shrinkage is easy to illustrate by the following example. A typical municipality with just under 10 000 residents is represented in the survey by about 1400 subjects, half of them (700) men, and about one-seventh of those (100) in the age group 20–24 (young men). Suppose the employment rate of this group is 80%. Then the standard error of its direct estimator is 4%. The national rate for the young men has municipality-level standard deviation 5.45%, so the national rate is less efficient for estimating the municipality's employment rate than the direct estimator. However, the (univariate) shrinkage estimator has estimated standard error $\sqrt{16 - 16^2/(16 + 5.45^2 + 0.75^2)} \doteq 3.25\%$, a non-trivial improvement over the direct estimator.

The estimates of the national rates of employment are given in Table 10.2. They show that the rates of employment are highest for the middle-aged and are higher for men than for women. The estimated correlation of the municipality-level rates is

Table 10.2. The estimated rates (percentages) of employment of the sex-by-age groups; Norway, 1990. Each cell contains the estimate and estimated standard error (in parentheses).

	Age group				
	T (16–19)	Y (20–24)	M (25–59)	V (60–66)	R (67+)
Men	46.0 (1.1)	80.3 (0.7)	88.6 (0.6)	57.7 (1.4)	9.9 (0.6)
Women	43.7 (1.2)	74.3 (1.0)	76.5 (0.8)	39.8 (1.4)	3.9 (0.3)

Table 10.3. The estimated variances of the municipality-level rates of employment of the sex-by-age groups.

	Age group				
	T (16–19)	Y (20–24)	M (25–59)	V (60–66)	R (67+)
Men	9.31	5.45	3.87	10.30	4.08
Women	9.91	6.57	5.19	9.41	1.92

$$\frac{1}{100}\begin{pmatrix} 100 & 49 & 44 & 55 & 49 & 50 & 48 & 46 & 44 & 50 \\ 49 & 100 & 60 & 56 & 38 & 42 & 46 & 21 & 41 & 28 \\ 44 & 60 & 100 & 77 & 39 & 33 & 41 & 49 & 60 & 40 \\ 55 & 56 & 77 & 100 & 55 & 37 & 39 & 58 & 75 & 61 \\ 49 & 38 & 39 & 55 & 100 & 32 & 24 & 35 & 51 & 53 \\ 50 & 42 & 33 & 37 & 32 & 100 & 56 & 53 & 49 & 45 \\ 48 & 46 & 41 & 39 & 24 & 56 & 100 & 58 & 46 & 40 \\ 46 & 21 & 49 & 58 & 35 & 53 & 58 & 100 & 65 & 49 \\ 44 & 41 & 60 & 75 & 51 & 49 & 46 & 65 & 100 & 62 \\ 50 & 28 & 40 & 61 & 53 & 45 & 40 & 49 & 62 & 100 \end{pmatrix} \begin{bmatrix} \mathrm{Tm} \\ \mathrm{Ym} \\ \mathrm{Mm} \\ \mathrm{Vm} \\ \mathrm{Rm} \\ \mathrm{Tw} \\ \mathrm{Yw} \\ \mathrm{Mw} \\ \mathrm{Vw} \\ \mathrm{Rw} \end{bmatrix}$$

with the submatrices for men and women separated by added space. The estimated variances of the municipality-level rates are given in Table 10.3. The correlation matrices for men and women (the 5×5 submatrices in the top left-hand and bottom right-hand corners) have higher entries than the correlations between the sexes (the off-diagonal blocks of the correlation matrix). In the off-diagonal blocks, the diagonal elements (the correlations between the two sexes in the same age-group) tend to be higher. The neighbouring age categories tend to have higher correlations. But overall, the correlations of the groups are not very high, suggesting that shrinkage estimation is not substantially more efficient than direct estimation.

The result of the analysis is a table of 166×10 estimates and associated standard errors. It is not informative to present them in a tabular form, or indeed, in a set of maps, each for one or two of the sex-by-age groups. The estimates are presented graphically in Figure 10.9, in separate panels for the sexes (columns) and sizes of the municipalities (rows). In each panel, a municipality is represented by the two sets of connected segments, one for the direct (sample) and one for the shrinkage estimates. The estimates of employment rates for the five age groups of each sex are connected by solid lines and the sets of direct (sample) and shrinkage estimates are placed side by side. To reduce the clutter, the estimates are drawn only for random samples of municipalities; for the population range 6000–8000, one in two, and for the population range 10 000–50 000, one in four municipalities are selected at random. For the other two population ranges, all municipalities are represented in the diagrams.

We see that only modest shrinkage takes place, as the 'shrinkage curves' are aligned only slightly more than the 'sample curves' of the estimated rates. However, even the sample curves are quite close to the average (national) trend, drawn by thick dashes, so there is little scope for extensive shrinkage. This is a consequence of the large sample sizes and only moderate correlation among the employment rates of the age groups. Also, the vertical axes of the plots cover the entire range 0–100%, so the variation for each age group is displayed without focus. The curves are similar across the population sizes of the municipalities; that justifies our decision to include the enumerated municipalities in the estimation of the municipality-level variation. The greater dispersion of the estimated employment rates for women, in the group Mw in particular, reflects their greater municipality-level variation. First, the direct estimates are more dispersed (except for the retirement-aged), because the employment rates tend to be closer to 50%, where the binary variance $p(1-p)$ attains its maximum. Second, less shrinkage takes place because there is greater heterogeneity among the municipality-level employment rates of women, except for the elderly.

The gains in precision can be assessed directly, by inspecting the estimated standard errors, but it is more practical to look at the ratios of the estimated standard errors for the two estimators. We define the relative and absolute reductions of the standard error by

$$1 - \sqrt{\frac{\text{eMSE}(\tilde{p}_{k,d})}{\text{var}(\hat{p}_{k,d})}}$$

and

$$\sqrt{\text{var}(\hat{p}_{k,d})} - \sqrt{\text{eMSE}(\tilde{p}_{k,d})}\,,$$

respectively, for category k in municipality d. The naive estimates of these quantities are plotted in Figure 10.10 using a layout similar to that in Figure 10.9. The diagrams show that shrinkage is least effective for the middle-aged. As they cover a range of 35 years, their subsample sizes are much greater than for the other groups, so improvement in estimation for them is less important

Figure 10.9. The direct (sample) and multivariate shrinkage estimates of the sex-by-age municipality-level employment rates in the sampled (not enumerated) Norwegian municipalities. The national estimates are drawn by thick dashes.

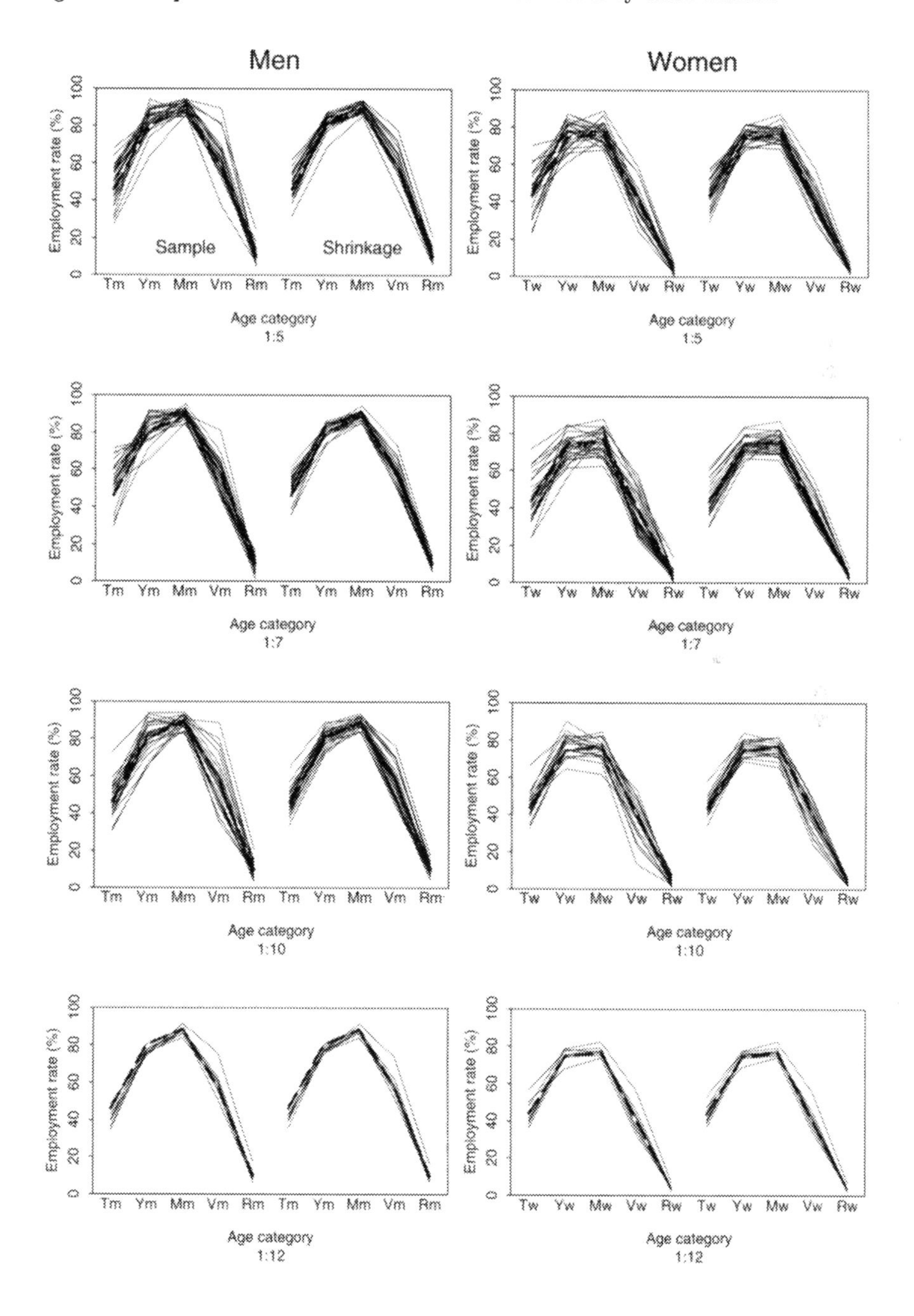

Figure 10.10. The estimated gains in precision of the shrinkage over direct estimators of the sex-by-age municipality-level employment rates in the sampled (not enumerated) Norwegian municipalities.

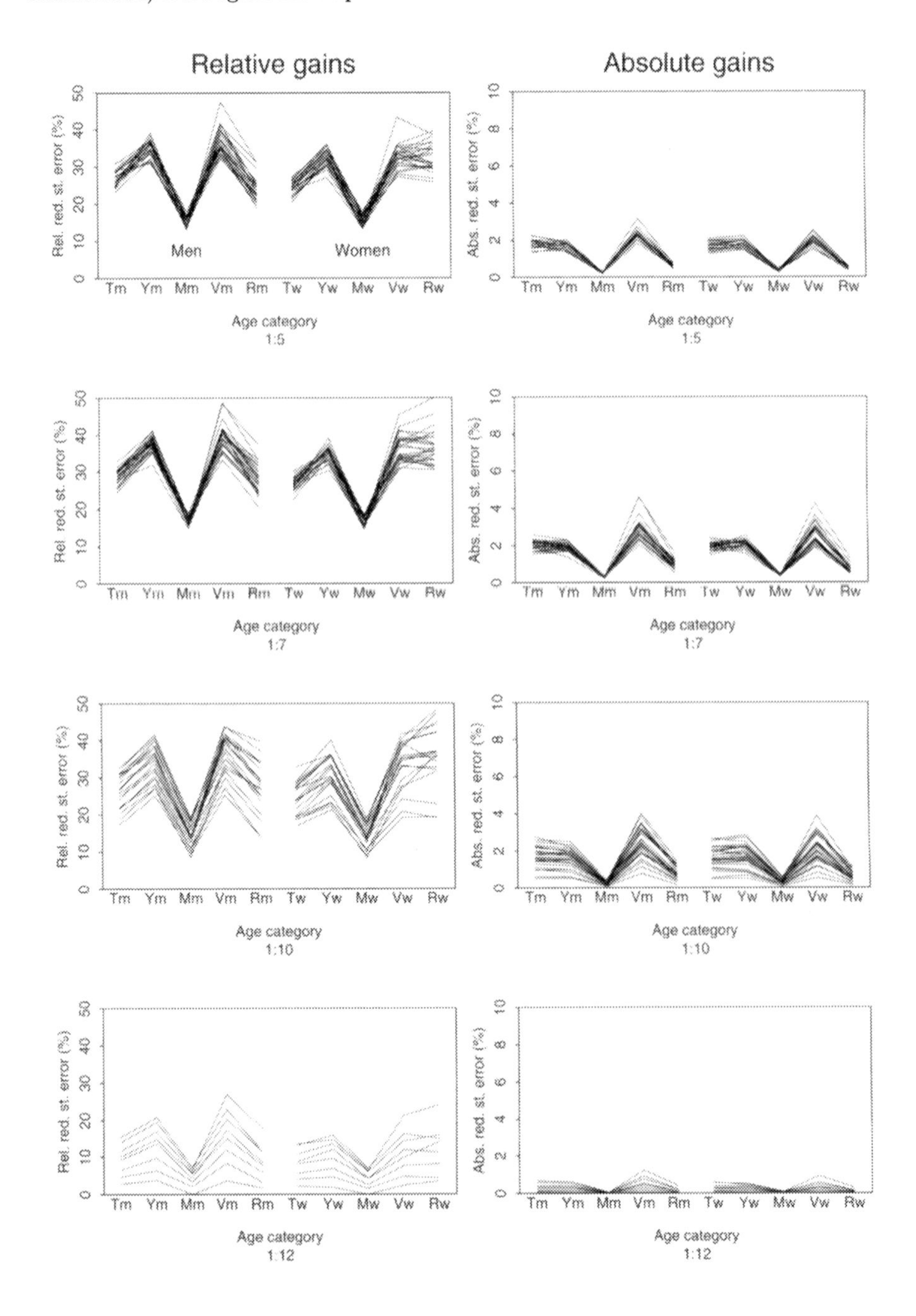

than for the much less numerous groups. The estimated gains differ much less across the sexes, although the differences in the gains are perceptible for the retirement-aged in particular. This is a consequence of the much smaller municipality-level variance for the retirement-aged women than men, see Table 10.3.

The improvement in estimating the municipality-level sex-by-age rates of employment can be summarised by counting the estimated rates that would be reported as being sufficiently precise. With direct estimation, 271 items are not reported (16% of the 10×166 estimated rates), and 326 are reported in parentheses (borderline precision, RSE 0.20–0.30). With shrinkage estimation, only 171 items (10%) would not be reported and 127 (8%) would be reported in parentheses. The most substantial improvement occurs for teenagers. With direct estimation, nine items are not reported and 117 are reported in parentheses, whereas with shrinkage estimation every item would be reported and only 30 of them in parentheses. This comparison of the direct and shrinkage estimators favours shrinkage slightly because the standard error of the direct estimator is estimated with greater precision than its shrinkage counterpart. This is not only due to ignoring the uncertainty about the municipality-level variance matrix, but also because eMSE is used instead of MSE.

10.3.1 Composition of the labour force by industrial sectors

The municipalities require the numbers or percentages of workers in each of the nine industrial sectors listed on page 283. Although the overall sample size for each municipality is quite large, the sample sizes for some of the industrial sectors are quite modest. The sectors AF (agriculture and fisheries), MN (manufacturing) and SP (social and personal services) have widely differing representation in the municipalities, whereas CB (construction) and TC (transport and communications) are distributed much more evenly. This information is presented in Table 10.4, listing the estimated national composition of employment, with the estimated standard errors attached, and the estimated municipality-level standard deviations of the rates. It may appear surprising that the municipality-level variances for MQ (mining and oil production) and EW (utilities) are so small. The rates for these sectors are very small in most municipalities, so the substantial rates in a few municipalities where they are concentrated (cities, locations of power stations, and the like) do not 'raise' the municipality-level variation to the levels for other sectors that employ much greater fractions of the labour force. In other words, comparisons of variances (or standard deviations) of rates are meaningful only when the underlying (national or average) rates are similar.

The distinct skew (non-normality) of the municipality-level rates is not an obstacle to applying multivariate shrinkage, although it would be a problem with estimation based on a model that assumes normality of the municipality-level deviations. In any case, the multivariate shrinkage in not very effective because most of the correlations in $\hat{\mathbf{\Sigma}}_{\mathrm{B}}$ are small. Instead of reproducing the

Table 10.4. The estimated national rates of employment in industrial sectors and the estimated municipality-level standard deviations; Norway, 1990.

	Industrial sector								
	AF	MQ	MN	EW	CB	WR	TC	FB	SP
Estimate	6.09	1.17	15.85	1.07	7.53	18.10	7.75	7.69	34.75
St. error	1.50	0.32	1.04	0.20	0.38	0.75	0.30	0.61	0.87
$\sqrt{\text{diag}(\hat{\Sigma}_B)}$	10.56	2.24	7.31	1.42	2.63	5.27	2.10	4.28	6.06

(9×9) estimated correlation matrix, we discuss only the correlation submatrix for the sectors AF, WR and FB,

$$\frac{1}{100}\begin{pmatrix} 100 & -74 & -76 \\ -74 & 100 & 75 \\ -76 & -74 & 100 \end{pmatrix}.$$

It contains the highest correlations (in absolute value). Next in the order of magnitude are the correlations between CB and FB (-0.51) and of AF with MN (0.50) and SP (0.40). The high correlations can be attributed to the concentration of some sectors in cities and towns (banking, wholesale and retail) and others in rural areas (agriculture and fishing). But the division is not so clear-cut because the correlations for some other sectors are much smaller than might be expected. Commuting to work across municipality boundaries may be one reason for this.

Thus, multivariate shrinkage is only slightly more effective than univariate shrinkage, and the estimated gains in precision are very modest for both, especially for AF and MN which have large municipality-level variances, and for MQ because it is unrelated to any other sector. The estimated gains over direct estimation exceed 10% for CB and TC for the municipalities with the smallest sample sizes (population) in each group of municipalities with the sampling fractions 1:5, 1:7 and 1:10 (population size 6000–50 000), and for WR and FB for fewer municipalities with the sampling fractions 1:5 and 1:7 (population size 6000–10 000). Most of these gains would be realised by univariate shrinkage, and appreciable additional gain (say, more than 1%) is realised by multivariate shrinkage only for AF, WR and FR for a few municipalities.

Since these assessments of the gains may be optimistic, multivariate shrinkage is not advisable. In any case, we would get at most a meagre return for the complex computing involved. Nevertheless, the expenditure on computing, in terms of the analysts' time and cost of equipment, is minute in comparison with the effort required to collect and process the data.

The data on the employment status, involving a mix of enumeration and sampling, provide us with a unique opportunity to assess the properties of the shrinkage estimator empirically. We draw a subsample from the available dataset, apply the direct and shrinkage estimators, and compare the direct and (multivariate) shrinkage estimates for the 282 originally enumerated municipalities with their population rates established in the original survey. The comparison can be based on the count of 'winners' — how many times each estimator is closer to the target, or on the totals of 'discrepancies', such as $\sum_d (\hat{p}_{dk} - p_{dk})^2$ and $\sum_d (\hat{p}^{\mathrm{C}}_{dk} - p_{dk})^2$, or $\sum_d (\hat{p}_{dk} - p_{dk})^2/(p_{dk} + 0.001)$ and $\sum_d (\hat{p}^{\mathrm{C}}_{dk} - p_{dk})^2/(p_{dk} + 0.001)$, for the respective direct and shrinkage estimates of the rates for municipality d and sex-by-age group (or sector) k. The latter pair of summaries impose relatively greater penalty for a given difference when the population rate p_{dk} is small. The totals are calculated over the municipalities that were originally enumerated. The denominator is increased by a token rate of 0.1% to avoid dividing by zero.

These comparisons confirm the superiority of the multivariate shrinkage estimator, for both sex-by-age groups and industrial sectors, although the gains are far from impressive. For example, the multivariate shrinkage estimator of the rates for the sex-by-age groups is superior for between 52.4% and 63.5% of the municipalities. The percentage is smallest for middle-aged men and women and greatest for women over the age of 66. For the industrial sectors, the percentages of municipalities are even smaller, but exceed 50% for all municipalities except one (MN, 49.8%), and that can probably be attributed to chance. The discrepancy statistics favour multivariate shrinkage for every sex-by-age group and industrial sector.

Although the primary purpose of the study, to estimate the rates and composition of employment, may be regarded as a failure because only trivial gains over the direct estimator were achieved, the application of shrinkage is not detrimental to efficiency. An important result is the estimated variance structure of the municipality-level employment rates for the subpopulations, because it informs us about the efficiency of the shrinkage estimator in surveys that might be planned in the future. However, national surveys of employment in Norway have been superseded since the 1990 Census by a comprehensive national register. In fact, one purpose of the survey was to assess the quality of the employment register at the time.

10.4 The Scottish House Condition Survey

The Scottish House Condition Survey (SHCS) collects information about the extent of disrepair of the housing stock in Scotland. This section discusses estimation of the funds required to bring all housing units (dwellings) up to a specified standard, based on the survey conducted in 1996. Since then, the survey was conducted in 2002; the collected information is being processed and analysed at the time of writing.

In 1996, over 18 000 dwellings were included in the survey. The sample comprised 11 000 dwellings drawn by a systematic sampling design from the

Figure 10.11. The subsample sizes of the Scottish unitary authorities in SHCS 1996. Each authority is represented by a vertical bar of height equal to the authority's subsample size, split into segments according to period of construction (age).

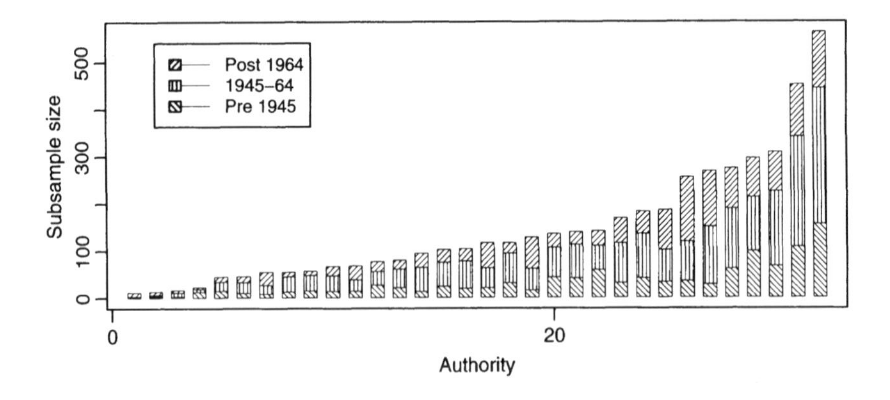

list of all addresses in Scotland (in December 1995), and over 11 000 dwellings from those included in the previous survey in 1991. Some additional samples were drawn to satisfy specific requests of the clients, for example, for more precise information about certain local authorities. We do not deal with the issue of data incompleteness here (refusals, non-availability, unoccupied dwellings, and the like), but point out that the list of addresses may be out of date and contain dwellings that are (temporarily) not occupied or are not residential. The latter cases do not amount to nonresponse; they are more appropriately classified as imperfections of the sampling frame. Nevertheless, as in most large-scale surveys, nonresponse (non-cooperation) is a serious issue.

In the analysis of the survey, the national means of several variables related to the state of the housing stock were estimated; see [249] and [110]. This section describes estimation of the mean repair costs for publicly owned housing in the Scottish unitary authorities. There are 32 such authorities in Scotland. Their population sizes are very disparate: the Cities of Glasgow and Edinburgh contain a substantial fraction of the population of Scotland (over 5 million), whereas the Orkneys, Shetland Islands, Western Isles, but also East Dunbartonshire, East Renfrewshire and Clackmannanshire, have populations of tens of thousands each, and they are represented in the survey by very small subsamples. The authorities' subsample sizes are graphically represented in Figure 10.11 by vertical bars. Each bar is divided to the subsample sizes of three categories of age of the dwelling, defined below.

There are 4640 publicly owned dwellings in the SHCS sample, about 25% of the entire sample. We point out at the outset that information about privately owned dwellings is an obvious auxiliary information for small-area estimation of quantities related to publicly owned housing. However, the relevant data were not made available when the analysis was conducted.

The key outcome variable is the *comprehensive repair cost* (CRC); it is defined for a dwelling as the cost of repairs required to maintain it to a specified standard over the period of ten years from the present on. The cost comprises a large number of *elements*, such as roof, structural integrity, plumbing, decoration of internal walls, driveway, doors and windows, staircases and electrical wiring. In the survey, trained surveyors visit the sampled dwellings assigned to them and assess all the elements that are applicable for the dwelling. For example, assessment of the roof is not applicable for a flat (apartment), and a single-storey house has no staircase. The assessment for most elements, when applicable, is on the ordinal scale 0–10, related to the replacement cost; the surveyor assigns category k when he or she assesses that the element requires repairs that amount to $10k\%$ of its replacement cost. The issue of inconsistency of the surveyors is addressed in Section 5.4. CRC is calculated using extensive tables that take into account the type, size, location and other details of the dwelling and its maintenance regime. A 'discount' is applied in instances when a lot of repairs are required and economies of scale can reasonably be anticipated.

Our targets are the mean CRC for all publicly owned dwellings and their categories defined by age, in each Scottish unitary authority. The sponsor of the surveys, the Scottish Office, has asked the identity of the authorities not to be revealed. On the one hand, the target quantities are *arithmetic* subpopulation means; on the other, working with log(CRC) has several analytical advantages, foremost among them the proximity of their distribution to normality (with a token £1 added to avoid taking the logarithm of zero). Another difficulty with CRC is the strong heteroscedasticity, common to variables in monetary units.

Small-area estimation of authority-level mean CRC by shrinkage requires a reliable estimate of the sampling variance of the direct estimator. The sampling variance is a function of the within-authority variance of CRC. For the least populous authorities, represented in the sample by only a handful of dwellings each (and in some subpopulations in particular), this variance is estimated with very little precision. If the within-authority variances were similar, the pooled estimator would be much more efficient for the authorities with small and moderate population sizes. However, the sample means (direct estimates) and sample standard deviations for the authorities are strongly associated, approximately linearly, suggesting that this association would be removed by the log transformation of CRC. The sample means and standard deviations are plotted in Figure 10.12, on the linear and log scales. The diameter of each circle is proportional to the subsample size of the authority it represents. Note that one of them, with by far the smallest sample mean and standard deviation, would be an influential observation. The fitted regression, drawn by dashes in panel A, is $380.6 + 0.666\widehat{\mathrm{CRC}}$. The pooled (estimated)

Figure 10.12. The direct estimates of the authority-level means and standard deviations of CRC on the original scale (panel A) and log scale (panel B). The diameters of the circles are proportional to the subsample sizes of the authorities.

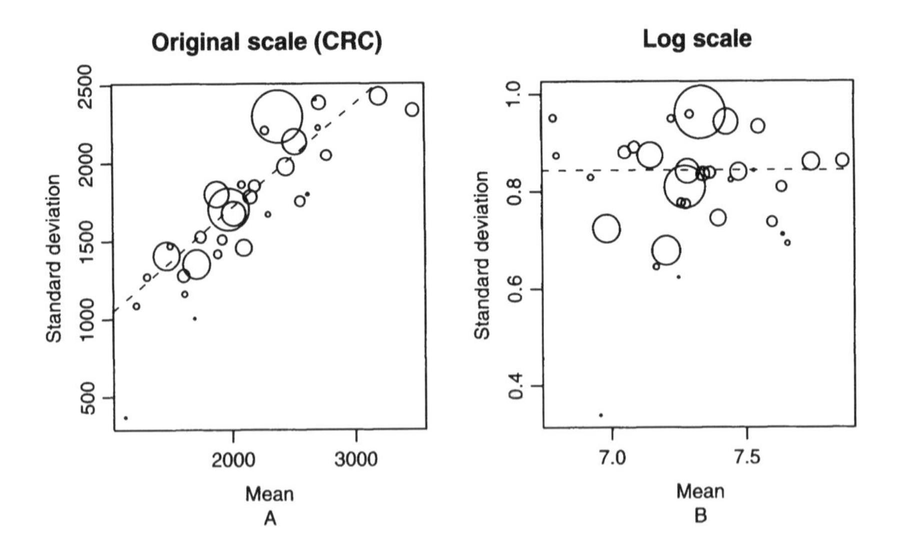

standard deviation on the log scale, equal to 0.844, is drawn by horizontal dashes in panel B.

We apply shrinkage to estimate the within-authority variances on the log scale, where shrinkage to a constant is well motivated. Then we apply the same amount of shrinkage on the linear scale, and estimate the sampling variance of the direct estimator based on this shrinkage variance estimate.

We assume that the estimator of the sampling variance of each authority's sample mean is associated with χ^2 distribution with $n_d - 1$ degrees of freedom. This enables estimation of the authority-level variance of the means (on the log scale) by moment matching. The estimate of the authority-level standard deviation is 0.0805, less than one-tenth of the pooled standard deviation. This indicates that, on the log scale, most of the variation in the estimated sampling variances of the smaller authorities (small n_d) is due to sampling variation. In calculating the shrinkage coefficients, we do not ignore the correlation of the authority and national sample quantities because each of several of the most populous authorities form a sizeable part of the country.

The shrinkage coefficient derived for the log scale is then applied on the original scale, pulling the sample standard deviations toward the fitted linear regression of the standard deviation on the mean. Of course, this is contentious; why should the same extent of shrinkage be suitable on both scales? We can justify this only empirically, arguing that the estimates of the standard

Figure 10.13. Shrinkage estimation of the within-authority standard deviations of CRC. The discs mark the shrinkage estimates and the crosses the direct estimates for the six authorities with the smallest subsample sizes.

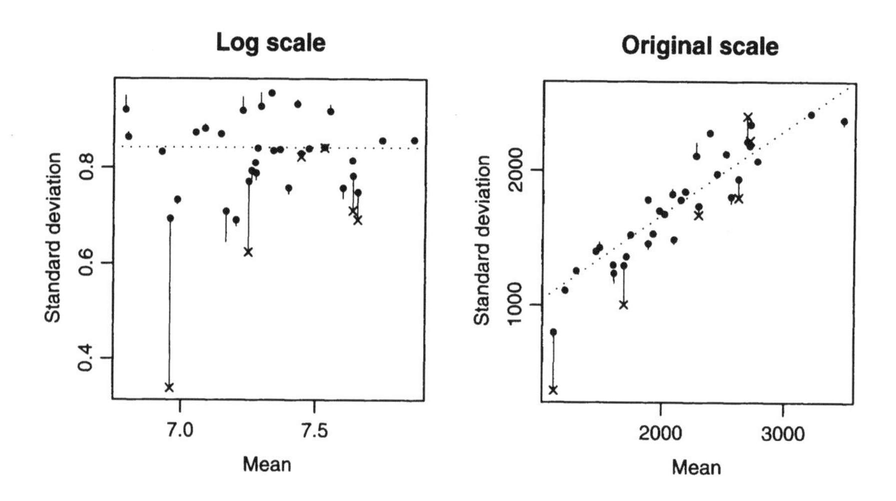

deviations are obviously shrunk in the right direction. In any case, shrinkage brings about substantial changes only for the least populous authorities.

The results of the shrinkage are summarised by the two plots in Figure 10.13. In both panels, the pairs of sample (direct) and shrinkage estimates of the standard deviation are connected by vertical segments. Each shrinkage estimate is marked by a black disc. The sample estimates for the six authorities with the smallest sample sizes are marked by crosses. Shrinkage is substantial only for some of them, because the sample estimate is close to the target of shrinkage in a few instances. The shrinkage coefficient is smaller than 0.1 for seven and exceeds 0.5 for four authorities.

The authority-level means of CRC are estimated by univariate shrinkage. The results are illustrated in Figure 10.14. The vertical segments connecting the sample and shrinkage estimates (the latter marked by black discs) are placed in the ascending order of the sample sizes n_d from left to right. The impression gained at first may be that shrinkage is not particularly useful because the shrinkage estimates differ little from the sample estimates (panel A). However, the changes due to shrinkage should be considered in the context of substantial differences among the authorities, both in the level of CRC and in the sample sizes. The estimate of the authority-level standard deviation is $\hat{\sigma}_{\mathrm{B}} =$ £506.90, almost one quarter of the estimated national mean, £2151.60 (standard error £121.60). Shrinkage *is* redundant for the most populous authorities, but it is very useful for the least populous authorities.

Figure 10.14. Shrinkage estimation of the authority-level mean CRC. The authorities are displayed in the ascending order of their subsample sizes.

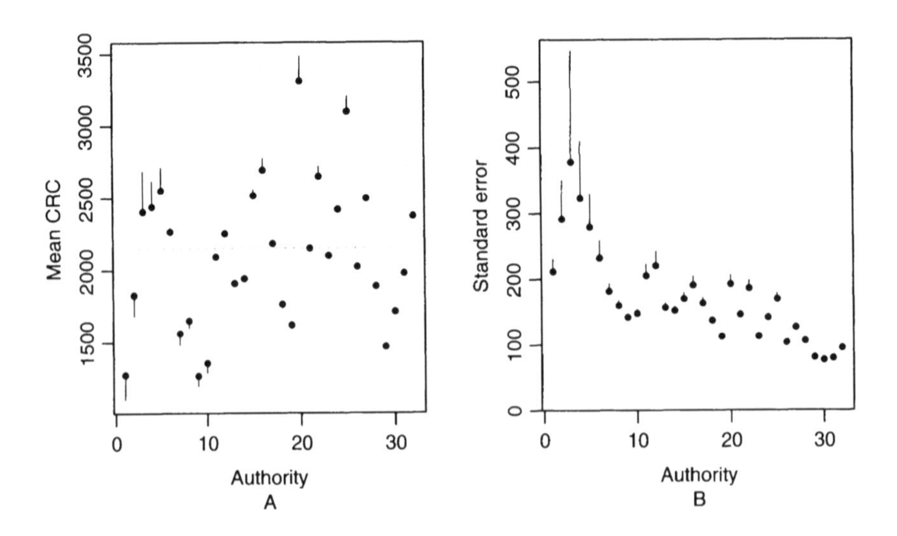

The reduction of the (estimated) standard error (panel B) is strongly associated with the sample size, although the value of the authority's (estimated) mean CRC is also a factor. Thus, the improvement for the authority with the smallest sample size is smaller because so is its sample mean. Despite the considerable shrinkage applied to its within-authority sample variance, the estimated sampling variance of its direct estimator remains smaller than for other authorities of similar size.

10.4.1 Estimation for subpopulations

The age of a residential building is an important correlate of the repair costs, and authorities are interested in the values of mean CRC for dwellings classified by the period of their construction. We consider estimation of the authority-level mean CRC for the subpopulations of dwellings administratively classified in the following categories: pre-1945 (built before 1945), 1945–1964, and post-1964. Their respective national subsample sizes are 1082, 2138 and 1420. The within-authority subsample sizes are indicated in Figure 10.11.

It is essential to estimate these subpopulation quantities simultaneously, by trivariate shrinkage, because the subsample sizes for several age-by-authority combinations are small, and the mean CRCs within the authorities are likely to be correlated. Where more funds are required to repair old buildings, more funds are likely to be needed also for repairing more recently constructed buildings.

The national subsample means of CRC for the respective age-categories pre-1945, 1945–1964 and post-1964 are £2522.80, £2190.00 and £1811.50.

Their estimated standard errors are £214.50, £136.40 and £114.40, respectively. The latter is smaller than the estimated standard error of the national mean CRC. This 'paradox' arises because the values of CRC for post-1964 dwellings tend to be lower and less dispersed than the costs in general. As anticipated, the authority-level means are highly correlated; their estimated correlation matrix is

$$\frac{1}{100}\begin{pmatrix} 100 & 70 & 53 \\ 70 & 100 & 63 \\ 53 & 63 & 100 \end{pmatrix} \qquad \begin{bmatrix} \text{Pre 1945} \\ \text{1945–1964} \\ \text{Post 1964} \end{bmatrix}$$

and the corresponding estimated standard deviations are £817.7, £541.3 and £461.4. Note that higher (national) means are associated with greater authority-level variation.

The results of trivariate shrinkage estimation of the age-specific means of CRC in the authorities are displayed in Figure 10.15. In the top panel, the segments connecting the direct and shrinkage estimates and in the bottom panel their estimated standard errors are plotted. The shrinkage estimates are marked by symbols that distinguish among the three categories of age, with the authorities placed in the order of their (overall) subsample sizes. The national estimates of mean CRC are marked by the three horizontal dashed lines.

Although some extreme shrinkage takes place for 'small' authorities, the extent of shrinkage is not associated with the subsample size very strongly. There are three reasons for this. First, the categories of age are not represented in the authorities' subsamples evenly. Second, small authorities are typically associated with little auxiliary information because the subsample sizes for the other two categories tend to be small. And third, higher means are associated with higher variances of the age-by-authority combinations. As a consequence, more shrinkage takes place in the downward direction; the shrinkage on the log scale would be closer to symmetry.

The standard errors are reduced much more for the means of the pre-1945 dwellings, for which the auxiliary information is relatively richer. Also, in some more populous authorities, only a small fraction of the housing stock remains from before 1945. Estimation of the mean CRC for such stock in the authorities exploits the similarity with the mean CRC for the other two categories that have substantial subsample sizes in the survey.

10.5 Suggested reading

The sections of this chapter are adapted from [164] (Section 10.1), [156] (Section 10.2), [160] (Section 10.3) and [167] (Section 10.4), where further details can be found. `Splus`, [279], and `R`, [41] and [215], were used for all the computing. There is no software package in which these computations could be

Figure 10.15. Trivariate shrinkage estimation of the age-specific mean CRC in the Scottish authorities.

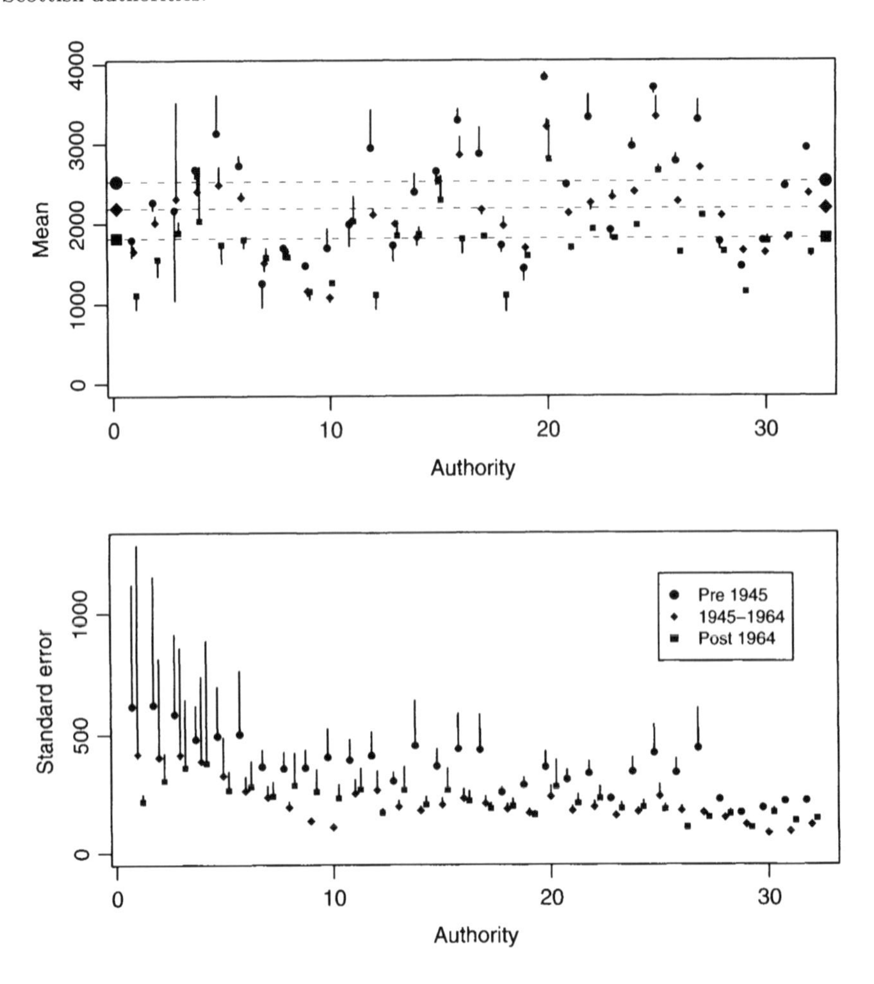

carried out in a modular form. The customisation for each specific problem is essential, but the programming effort required is not extensive.

A range of applications of small-area methods at Statistics Canada is outlined by [74]. Reference [246] is a collection of applications of small-area methods in U.S. Government programmes and [27] is an account of methods used for estimation of the mean income and the rates of poverty in small areas in the U.S.A., with an agenda for future development. The potential of administrative registers as sources of auxiliary information is discussed by [275]. References [62] and [63] are motivated by the practice of small-area estimation in the Italian National Statistics Institute.

Experience with population registers in the Scandinavian countries is discussed by [195], [168] and [276]. See [277] and [7] for accounts from two post-communist countries.

Four papers on several aspects of composite estimation in the Canadian Labour Force Survey, exploiting the similarity over time, appeared in [266]. A model-based approach to small-area estimation for cross-classifications is presented by [287]. An important consideration in their approach is structure preservation — that the estimates should have the same margins as the available population quantities. For motivation of this approach, called SPREE, see [214].

Part III

Combining estimators

11

Model selection

Sir, there is nothing wrong with the shoe.
It's your foot ...

We can motivate the problem of small-area estimation as selecting between two alternative models, A and B. Model A assumes that the population quantities θ_d for districts $d = 1, \ldots, D$ are unrelated, so each θ_d can be estimated only from the subsample of subjects from district d. Model B assumes that these quantities coincide, $\theta_1 = \theta_2 = \ldots = \theta_D$; that is, the country is homogeneous with respect to θ_D. In most established approaches, we choose one of the models, A or B, and proceed by relying on it, assuming that it is appropriate for estimating each θ_d, and possibly other population quantities as well. In Chapter 6, we found this approach poorly suited for small-area estimation. In this chapter, we apply the method found to be suitable for small areas to the standard model-selection problem.

11.1 The problem

The information we would like to have about a population is a description in terms of a set of parameters, such as $\theta_1, \ldots, \theta_D$, and possibly the area-level variance σ_B^2 in a small-area setting. For a general problem, we specify the space of possible values of these parameters, the *parameter space*, denoted by $\boldsymbol{\Theta}$. The parameter values will be estimated by identifying a data-based element of this space. The space $\boldsymbol{\Theta}$ should be delineated generously; if it does not contain the value of the parameter, the estimation process is severely handicapped. By the term *model* we understand a subset of $\boldsymbol{\Theta}$ (or the space itself). For example, model A introduced above corresponds to all configurations of $\theta_1, \ldots, \theta_D$, (the entire parameter space), whereas model B to the subset defined by the constraint that $\theta_1 = \ldots = \theta_D$.

In ordinary regression, models are frequently identified with sets of regression variables. For example,

$$y_i = \beta_0 + x_i\beta_1 + \varepsilon_i\,, \qquad i = 1, \ldots, n\,, \tag{11.1}$$

is a model with parameters $(\beta_0, \beta_1, \sigma^2)$, associated with the covariate x, and

$$y_i = \beta_0 + \varepsilon_i \tag{11.2}$$

is another, with parameters (β_0, σ^2); it is derived from (11.1) by imposing the constraint that $\beta_1 = 0$, that is, by 'excluding' x from the model in (11.1). In both models, we make the usual assumptions of normality, independence of the ε_i and homoscedasticity, and that the values $x_1, \ldots, x_n$ are set a priori. Other models may have different assumptions.

The model in (11.1) is characterised by the class of distributions

$$\mathbf{y} \sim \mathcal{N}(\beta_0 \mathbf{1}_n + \mathbf{x}\beta_1, \sigma^2 \mathbf{I}_n),$$

with arbitrary (real) scalars β_0 and β_1 and non-negative σ^2. We use the matrix notation with $\mathbf{y} = (y_1, \ldots, y_n)^\top$ and $\mathbf{x} = (x_{1,}, \ldots, x_n)^\top$. The model in (11.2) is characterised by

$$\mathbf{y} \sim \mathcal{N}(\beta_0 \mathbf{1}_n, \sigma^2 \mathbf{I}_n).$$

It is a special case of the model in (11.1); it is said to be a *submodel* of (11.1). While we are satisfied that the data behave according to a model, say (11.1), we cannot identify the parameter values (β_0, β_1 and σ^2) according to which the data are generated. Instead of identifying, we estimate them, in the case of (11.1) by ordinary least squares (OLS). Efficient estimation of each parameter β_0, β_1 and σ^2 amounts to making a choice, informed by $\mathbf{y}$, of values of $\hat{\beta}_0$, $\hat{\beta}_1$ and $\hat{\sigma}^2$ in the parameter space, so that their MSEs are as small as possible. The estimation would involve less uncertainty if we could reduce the 'candidate' parameter space — if we could concentrate our search on a narrower range of possible values of β_0, β_1 and σ^2. The submodel in (11.2) can be regarded as such a reduction, defined by $\beta_1 = 0$. It is easy to verify that if indeed $\beta_1 = 0$ estimation of σ^2 is more efficient with (11.2) than with (11.1), where we regard β_1 as unknown. Thus, the incentive to narrow down the parameter values to a smaller set (reduce the model) is obvious, but so are the risks — we should not assume that $\beta_1 = 0$, unless *all* nonzero values of β_1 can be ruled out. Thus, model reduction does not come free, because the decision to rely, or not, on a submodel is usually not correct with certainty. In practice, a submodel is adopted when we fail to find evidence against it that is stronger than an a priori specified threshold. This section concludes that this is a highly questionable practice, and the remainder of the chapter develops an alternative approach.

We consider the following general setting. A mechanism is defined for generating values of a set of variables $\mathbf{Y}$ using a matrix of covariates $\mathbf{X}$. The covariates $\mathbf{X}$ are fixed, that is, in replications of the study their values would be unchanged, although the values of $\mathbf{Y}$ might be different as the mechanism involves some randomness (inconsistency). A regression model for dataset $(\mathbf{X}, \mathbf{Y})$, comprising matrices of outcomes $\mathbf{Y}$ and covariates $\mathbf{X}$, is specified as a class of (joint) conditional distributions $(\mathbf{Y} \mid \mathbf{X})$. A particular model, A, is assumed to be *valid*, that is, $(\mathbf{Y} \mid \mathbf{X})$ belongs to its class of distributions. The distributions are described by their vectors of *parameters* $\boldsymbol{\xi}$ or, more precisely, by the parameter space defined by all the possible values of the vector of parameters $\boldsymbol{\xi}$.

Ideally, we would like to establish the value of a quantity θ that is a function of the underlying distribution or its characterisation by $\boldsymbol{\xi}$; $\theta = \theta(\boldsymbol{\xi})$. An estimator $\hat{\theta}_{\mathrm{A}} = \hat{\theta}_{\mathrm{A}}(\mathbf{Y}; \mathbf{X})$ is available; given that model A is valid it has good properties — no bias and sampling variance smaller than some of its competitors that also assume that model A is valid. If a specified submodel B of A were also valid, θ could be estimated more efficiently, by an unbiased estimator $\hat{\theta}_{\mathrm{B}}$. Other submodels of A, some of them also submodels of B, may be considered, each associated with an estimator of θ that is unbiased *if* the submodel is valid. The analyst has an incentive to search for submodels that are valid, because θ can then be estimated more efficiently. At the extreme, if the parameter space were reduced to a single vector $\boldsymbol{\xi}$, the target θ could be established without any estimation error.

Established approaches define rules for selecting between model A and its submodel B. If model B is selected, it is from then on assumed to be valid, and either the estimator $\hat{\theta}_{\mathrm{B}}$ is applied or further reduction of the parameter space is sought by exploring one or several submodels of B. Such a model selection procedure can be based on hypothesis testing, e.g., based on the likelihood ratio statistic, or on related criteria, such as the Akaike or Bayes information criteria (AIC and BIC), and the like. In hypothesis testing, model B is regarded as the null-hypothesis (special case), and evidence is sought against it, in favour of A or, more precisely, in favour of the complement of B in A (denoted by A\B). If such evidence is found, model B is regarded as not valid; otherwise the reduction to model B is deemed appropriate. More generally, a statistic $u_{\mathrm{A,B}}(\mathbf{Y}, \mathbf{X})$ is evaluated and compared against a critical value $u^*_{\mathrm{A,B}}(\mathbf{Y}, \mathbf{X})$; if $u > u^*$, model B is rejected, and model B is regarded as valid otherwise.

A profound deficiency of such an approach is that the choice (decision) made to reduce the candidate parameter space is usually not correct with certainty. Errors of two kinds can be committed. First, by failing to reduce model A to B we miss out on some variance (MSE) reduction. Second, by reducing model A to B inappropriately we incur bias and we underestimate $\mathrm{MSE}(\hat{\theta}_{\mathrm{B}})$. Hypothesis testing involves a logical inconsistency. Failure to reject the null-hypothesis is inappropriately regarded as its confirmation and action is taken that would be suitable only when the null-hypothesis is correct. In a typical hypothesis test, the size of the test is set, by convention, to 0.05, and the power of the test for a range of alternatives (distributions in A\B) falls short of 1.0. When several hypothesis tests are carried out in the search for a 'small' submodel of A, the probability of ending up with an invalid model, or a valid model that should have been reduced (further), becomes too large and is usually impossible to evaluate or even approximate. However, instead of the probability of identifying the appropriate model we should be concerned with the quality of the inferential statements made under inappropriate assumptions.

The analyst may document the exhaustive attempts at model reduction by showing that each parameter retained in the model is essential (could not be eliminated by constraining it to zero or to another 'special' value). We argue in this section that such an effort is misdirected on several counts. First, the decisions made during model selection are not correct with certainty, but they are regarded as such. Second, the model selection process is subject to uncertainty, that is, a different model may be selected in a replication. The distribution of an estimator chosen a priori differs from the distribution of an estimator obtained by selection, but the inferential statement has no means of reflecting this. By way of an example, suppose model C has been selected and the value of the estimator $\hat{\theta}_{\mathrm{C}}$ is quoted, together with its estimated standard error $\hat{s}_{\mathrm{C}} = \sqrt{\widehat{\mathrm{var}}(\hat{\theta}_{\mathrm{C}})}$. The distribution of the estimator is bound to depend on the details of how the selection was made: which models were compared, in what order, with what criteria and other details, but also on the models that would have been considered had some of the intermediate decisions gone in different ways. In brief, the conditional distribution of an estimator given a model selection process differs from its unconditional distribution.

The third line of argument against model selection is that its ambition is to find the most efficient of the estimators based on the candidate models. We develop a method that has a higher ambition, to outperform each of these models. The ambition is not always fulfilled, but the method does not have the weaknesses of the approaches based on model selection.

We start by introducing some terminology. Suppose the candidate models are indexed by integers 0, 1, ..., and model 0 is regarded as valid a priori. In most practical settings, models $m = 1, 2, \ldots, M$ would be its submodels. For example, in a setting with two candidate models, 1 and 2, suppose neither is a submodel of the other. We could then also consider a model 0 for which both 1 and 2 are submodels. The derivations that follow make no assumptions about the relationship of model 0 to the other models.

Each model m is associated with an estimator $\hat{\theta}_m$ of the same target θ. If model m is valid, $\hat{\theta}_m$ is unbiased and may have some other desirable properties. We refer to $\hat{\theta}_m$, $m = 1, \ldots, M$, as the *single-model based estimators*. The *selection process* is defined as the function that assigns to each conceivable dataset $\mathbf{Y}$ a selected model m. We omit $\mathbf{X}$ from the 'dataset' because it is assumed to be fixed. The aim of the selection process is to identify a *minimal valid model*; this is a model that is valid, but none of its submodels among the models 1, 2, ... , m are. The minimal valid model is in most practical settings unique. Let I_m be the indicator of the selected model (selection indicator); $I_m = 1$ when model m is selected, and $I_m = 0$ otherwise. Finally, let $\mathcal{M}$ be the selected model; that is, $\mathcal{M} = m$ when $I_m = 1$.

The *estimation process* is the collection of all operations applied to the data between compiling the dataset $\mathbf{Y}$ and formulating a statement of the form

$$(\hat{\theta}\,, \hat{s})$$

(estimate, estimated standard error), or similar. We are concerned with estimation processes that comprise two steps: model selection and estimation based on the selected model. The result of such an estimation process is the *selected-model based estimator* defined as

$$\hat{\theta}_{\mathcal{M}} = I_0\hat{\theta}_0 + I_1\hat{\theta}_1 + \cdots + I_M\hat{\theta}_M \,. \tag{11.3}$$

This formulation makes it clear that the distribution of $\hat{\theta}_{\mathcal{M}}$ depends not only on the selected model but on

- *all* the models that have a positive probability of being selected;
- the details of the selection process — the joint distribution of $\mathcal{M}$ and the estimators $\hat{\theta}_m$,

as well as the distribution $(\mathbf{Y}\,|\,\mathbf{X})$. The distribution of $\hat{\theta}_{\mathcal{M}}$ is difficult to establish even in some very simple cases, when the probabilities $p_m = \mathrm{P}(I_m = 1\,|\,\boldsymbol{\xi})$ and the joint distribution of the estimators $\hat{\theta}_m$ are known. The source of the difficulty is that the selection indicators I_m are correlated with the estimators $\hat{\theta}_m$, both within and across models m. The selected-model based estimator $\hat{\theta}_{\mathcal{M}}$ is a *mixture*. The expectation and variance of a mixture are easy to derive only when the mixing indicators (I_m) and the distributions being mixed (of $\hat{\theta}_m$) are mutually independent. When the model selection process is disregarded, as is the common practice, quoting the estimated standard error of a selected-model based estimator corresponds to

$$\hat{s}_{\mathcal{M}} = I_0\hat{s}_0 + I_1\hat{s}_1 + \cdots + I_M\hat{s}_M \,.$$

We will give examples and general derivations showing that $\hat{\theta}_{\mathcal{M}}$ is not unbiased and $\hat{s}^2_{\mathcal{M}}$ grossly underestimates $\mathrm{var}(\hat{\theta}_{\mathcal{M}})$.

We consider the distributions of $\hat{\theta}_m$, $m = 0, 1, \ldots, M$, assuming model 0, being aware that the other models, even if selected, may not be valid. Instead of attempting to reduce the parameter space, while not abandoning validity, we aim to achieve efficiency directly, without relying on models judged to be valid by fallible criteria. The approach can be motivated by an example from small-area estimation. By selecting one of the candidate models, A, that each district has a different population mean, or B, that the districts have identical means, we end up applying for every district d either the direct estimator $\hat{\theta}_d$ or the national estimator $\hat{\theta}$. This approach, discussed in Section 6.2.1, was dismissed soon thereafter.

11.1.1 EM algorithm

In this section, we point out a contradiction of the attempt to find a minimal valid model. Suppose each single-model based estimator is based on maximum likelihood (ML). If we knew that a particular model m^* is the minimal valid model, estimation of θ would entail evaluation of the single-model based estimator $\hat{\theta}_{m^*}$. We can regard m^* as the missing data (item) and apply the EM algorithm. In its estimation step (E), we calculate the conditional probabilities $\hat{p}_m$ that model m is the minimal valid model, given the data and the current values of the model parameter estimates. In the subsequent maximisation step (M), we evaluate $\hat{\theta}_{\mathcal{M}}$ with the selection indicators I_m replaced by the probabilities $\hat{p}_m$, that is,

$$\hat{\theta}_{\mathrm{EM}} = \hat{p}_0\hat{\theta}_0 + \hat{p}_1\hat{\theta}_1 + \cdots + \hat{p}_M\hat{\theta}_M \,. \tag{11.4}$$

Unless all but one of the probabilities $\hat{p}_m$ vanish, the ML estimator is a convex combination of the single-model based estimators. Suppose a model and its submodel m are among the candidate models, and the submodel is defined by restricting one of the model parameters, ξ, from an interval, such as $(-\infty, +\infty)$, to zero. As zero is but one of innumerably many possible values, the submodel would be associated with probability $\hat{p}_m = 0$, unless there is some specific information that supports the hypothesis $\xi = 0$, at the exclusion of all other values of ξ, even those arbitrarily close to zero. This suggests that the iterations of EM algorithm would conclude with $\hat{p}_0 = 1$, that is, at the starting point — model 0.

This example of the EM algorithm leads to a contradiction because validity of the model is regarded as an imperative. An estimator based on an invalid model may be more efficient than its counterpart for a valid model if the departure from validity is only slight, but the invalid model is much simpler.

The conclusion that the most complex model yields the ML estimator may be paradoxical for finite sample sizes. However, in large (infinite) samples any bias implies inefficiency (inconsistency), since the variance inflation due to redundant model terms is infinitesimally small, so long as the number of parameters in the asymptotic consideration increases at a much slower rate than the number of observations. The ML estimator with a valid model is optimal in asymptotics; in finite samples some invalid models may be more efficient.

11.1.2 Example

Figure 11.1 presents the results of a simulation of the selected-model based estimator of the mean for a group in the setting of a balanced one-way random-effect analysis of variance (rANOVA) with $K = 8$ groups, $J = 10$ observations in each group, overall mean $\mu = 0$, within-group variance $\sigma_1^2 = 1$ and between-group variance $\sigma_{\mathrm{B}}^2 = 0.25$. The target of estimation is the mean of group 1, $\mu_1 = 0.35$. Ten thousand values of the estimator $\hat{\mu}_{1,\mathcal{M}}$ are generated, together with the estimates of the nominal sampling variance, $\hat{s}^2_{\mathcal{M}}$, that would be reported conventionally. The hypothesis test of equal group-level means is applied, with 5% significance level and symmetric confidence interval based on the t-statistic.

Panels A and B present the respective histograms of the simulated estimates $\hat{\mu}_{1,\mathcal{M}}$ and estimated sampling variances (MSEs) $\hat{s}^2_{1,\mathcal{M}}$, with the parts

Figure 11.1. Histograms of the simulated values of the selected-model based estimator of the group-level mean μ_1 (panel A) and the associated reported (estimated) sampling variance (panel B). Shading in both panels represents the values generated when the hypothesis of equal means in rANOVA is not rejected.

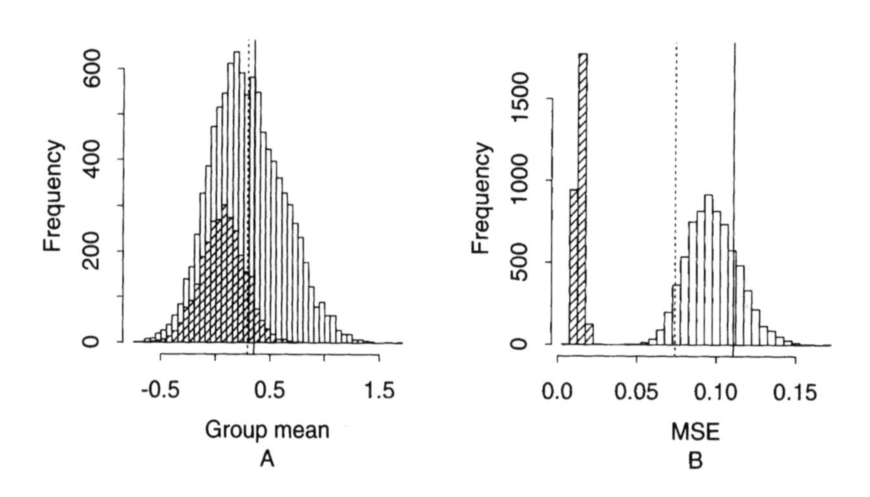

that correspond to failure to reject the null-hypothesis shaded. The target values, $\mu_1 = 0.35$ and $\mathrm{MSE}(\hat{\mu}_{1,\mathcal{M}}) = 0.111$, the latter established by the replications, are marked by vertical solid lines and the means of the replicate values of their respective estimates by vertical dots. Contrary to the conventional claim, the estimator $\hat{\mu}_{1,\mathcal{M}}$ is biased and its distribution deviates from normality. It is arguable whether the bias, -0.061 is substantial or not. However, the bias of $\hat{s}^2_{1,\mathcal{M}}$ in estimating $\mathrm{MSE}(\hat{\mu}_{1,\mathcal{M}})$ is substantial and the distribution of $\hat{s}^2_{1,\mathcal{M}}$ bears no resemblance to a χ^2. Its sets of realised values for the two outcomes of the hypothesis test are prefectly separated. Figure 11.1 illustrates that model selection cannot be ignored and that statements that are conditional on the selected model can be grossly misleading. Model selection is not conducive to efficiency.

Note that the conditional distributions of $\hat{\mu}_{1,\mathcal{M}}$, given the selected model, differ substantially. This property is specific to the model selection applied and the target μ_1. Estimation of the within-group variance σ^2_{W} provides an example of conditional distributions that are much more similar. Figure 11.2 summarises the simulated values of the selected-model based estimator $\hat{\sigma}^2_{\mathrm{W},\mathcal{M}}$ in the same set of replications as in Figure 11.1. The estimator has only a small bias and the two conditional distributions, given the outcome of the hypothesis test, differ only slightly.

Figure 11.2. Histogram of the simulated values of the selected-model based estimator of the within-group variance σ_W^2 in one-way balanced rANOVA. Shading represents the values generated when the hypothesis of equal means is not rejected.

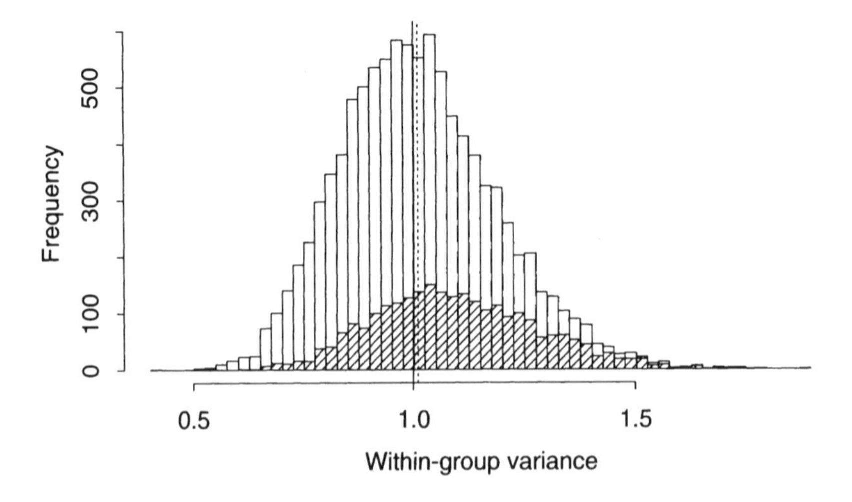

11.2 Why model selection fails

In this section, we show that the two properties pointed out in the previous section, distinctness of the conditional distributions $(\hat{\theta}_{\mathcal{M}} \,|\, \mathcal{M})$, that is, the dependence of $\hat{\theta}_{\mathcal{M}}$ on $\mathcal{M}$, and the negative bias (underestimation) of $\hat{s}^2_{\mathcal{M}}$, are connected. Let $p_0 = \mathrm{P}(\mathcal{M} = 0)$ be the probability that model 0 is selected, and $p_1 = \mathrm{P}(\mathcal{M} = 1)$ its complement. Elementary operations yield the identities

$$\begin{aligned} \mathrm{E}(\hat{\theta}_{\mathcal{M}}) - \theta &= p_0 \mathrm{E}(\hat{\theta}_0 \,|\, \mathcal{M} = 0) + p_1 \mathrm{E}(\hat{\theta}_1 \,|\, \mathcal{M} = 1) - \theta \\ &= p_1 \mathrm{E}(\hat{\theta}_1 - \hat{\theta}_0 \,|\, \mathcal{M} = 1) \end{aligned} \tag{11.5}$$

(as $\hat{\theta}_0$ is unbiased) and

$$\begin{aligned} \mathrm{MSE}(\hat{\theta}_{\mathcal{M}}\,;\,\theta) &= p_0 \mathrm{MSE}(\hat{\theta}_0\,;\,\theta \,|\, \mathcal{M} = 0) + p_1 \mathrm{MSE}(\hat{\theta}_1\,;\,\theta \,|\, \mathcal{M} = 1) \\ &= p_0 \mathrm{var}(\hat{\theta}_0 \,|\, \mathcal{M} = 0) + p_1 \mathrm{var}(\hat{\theta}_1 \,|\, \mathcal{M} = 1) \\ &\quad + p_0 \left\{ \mathrm{E}(\hat{\theta}_0 \,|\, \mathcal{M} = 0) - \theta \right\}^2 + p_1 \left\{ \mathrm{E}(\hat{\theta}_1 \,|\, \mathcal{M} = 1) - \theta \right\}^2 . \end{aligned} \tag{11.6}$$

obtained after substituting $p_0 \mathrm{E}(\hat{\theta}_0 \,|\, \mathcal{M} = 0) + p_1 \mathrm{E}(\hat{\theta}_0 \,|\, \mathcal{M} = 1)$ for θ. (Note that the conditioning is on the model choice, not on the appropriate model.) These identities show when and why the selected-model based estimator is biased and its MSE underestimated. The bias of $\hat{\theta}_{\mathcal{M}}$ arises when the single-model based estimators have different conditional expectations, given the selection of their models, and the probability of selecting the submodel, p_1, is not trivial. Usually $\mathrm{E}(\hat{\theta}_1 \,|\, \mathcal{M} = 1) \doteq \theta$, but $\mathrm{E}(\hat{\theta}_0 \,|\, \mathcal{M} = 0)$ differs from θ substantially when p_0 is smaller than 1.0. The first two terms in the concluding expression in (11.6) are estimated with little or no bias by $\hat{s}^2_{\mathcal{M}}$. However, the sum of the last terms is positive whenever model selection is subject to uncertainty ($p_0 p_1 > 0$) and the conditional means of $\hat{\theta}_0$ and $\hat{\theta}_1$, given the choice of the respective models, differ. That is the case in Figure 11.1. Thus, model-selection based estimation can be dishonest (its sampling variation is underestimated). There are no means of identifying model selection processes that have this deficiency, other than by simulations. The derivations in (11.5) and (11.6) are general, applying to all selection procedures with two alternatives (options). Some procedures may have greater probabilities of leading to the appropriate choice (the minimal valid model), but no improvement will rule out the occasional selection of an inappropriate model. Although reducing the conditional probabilities of choosing an inappropriate model is a natural goal, our analysis suggests that this may not be effective and is insufficient to make the conventional statements based on the selected model $\mathcal{M}$ valid (honest).

11.2.1 Limitations of model selection

The two examples in Section 11.1.2 suggest that model selection should be informed by the purpose to which the selected model is to be applied. In this respect, any solution that concludes with a single choice is very rigid. It may be qualified by an assessment of our confidence in it, but provides no prescription for reflecting this confidence (or its lack) in the applications and inferences that follow. The conclusions of inferences made may state, as a caveat, that they are based on a model that may not be appropriate (valid), but a typical user of such a conclusion (client) would not know how to account for the implied uncertainty. In any case, the uncertainty is difficult to evaluate or describe because it depends on the range of models considered and on the process of model selection that was employed.

Model selection has two serious limitations. First, it contemplates no other choices than the candidate single-model based estimators, even though in the perspective of (11.3), $\hat{\theta}_{\mathcal{M}}$ is an estimator different from either single-model based candidate $\hat{\theta}_m$. The candidate estimator based on a model that is rejected only narrowly is treated in the same way as the estimator based on a model that is rejected outright, with a great deal of confidence. The second limitation is that the same model is selected irrespective of the target of estimation. The possible 'error' committed in model selection leaves its mark on every estimator and predictor based on the selected model.

The first limitation is effectively addressed by *Bayes factors* in [104]. Instead of selecting one of the estimators, their convex combination,

$$\widetilde{\theta} = b_1\hat{\theta}_1 + \cdots + b_K\hat{\theta}_K \,,$$

is used. Note the obvious parallels with the EM solution in (11.4). The coefficients (weights, or Bayes factors) b_k are set so as to reflect the strength of support for the alternative models; they are non-negative and add up to unity. The support is defined as the relative size of the likelihood; see [123] and [104] for details and variations on the general theme. Bayes factors are very appealing because they resolve the coarseness of the conventional model selection, but they have the second limitation: the factors $\mathbf{b} = (b_1, \ldots, b_K)^\top$ apply to *every* target, because the support for a model is defined without any regard for the target of inference. Note that the factors are a random vector $\mathbf{b}$. As they are correlated with $\hat{\boldsymbol{\theta}} = (\hat{\theta}_1, \ldots, \hat{\theta}_K)^\top$, establishing the distribution of the composition $\widetilde{\theta}$ is a non-trivial problem even when the joint distribution of $\hat{\boldsymbol{\theta}}$ is known and is simple.

The model is not a function of the target, and so involving the target in the model selection might appear counterintuitive. However, maximising the chance of selecting the appropriate model is not the right goal because an inappropriate choice, even if made with a small probability, may have a disastrous impact on the distribution of the selected-model based estimator. Parallels can be drawn with multiple imputation (MI, Part I). There we considered two stages of analysis — completing the dataset (imputations for missing values) and analysis of the completed dataset. We concluded that the completion by optimal estimation of each missing item is not conducive to efficient estimation. In estimation with model uncertainty, an optimal way of selecting a model is also not conducive to efficient estimation. A common feature of the two general problems is that the uncertainty in the first stage has to be reflected in the second stage, otherwise the composition of the two stages is inefficient, even if either stage on its own would be for its respective purpose. The main difference between MI and estimation under model uncertainty is that with the latter we step beyond the paradigm that associates valid models with efficient inference.

Suppose a non-trivial model M is known to be the minimal valid model and $\hat{\theta}_{\mathrm{M}}$ is an (approximately) unbiased estimator that would be considered as efficient for target θ. For instance, $\hat{\theta}_{\mathrm{M}}$ may be the ML estimator in a regular and easy-to-solve problem. At first glance, it may seem that $\hat{\theta}_{\mathrm{M}}$ cannot be improved on. However, an estimator of θ based on a submodel of M, although biased, has a smaller sampling variance. Should we reject this estimator altogether because the model it is based on is not valid? Does the incurred bias always outweigh the reduction in variance?

For a given target, the estimator based on a simpler but invalid model may have only a slight bias but its variance is reduced substantially; we should not hesitate to use the invalid model for estimating *this* target. For another target, the estimator based on the invalid submodel may have a substantial bias, overwhelming the variance reduction. The simpler model should not be used for estimating this target.

Examples of these two cases were found in Section 11.1.2. In the next section, we address the problem of model uncertainty by setting aside the issues of model validity and simply search for estimators with minimum MSE.

11.3 Synthetic estimation

The combination in (11.4) motivates the estimator introduced in this section. We pursue the path of efficient estimation directly, without the intermediate step of model selection. Instead of the choice among the single-model based estimators $\hat{\theta}_0, \hat{\theta}_1, \ldots, \hat{\theta}_M$, that is, their mixture $\hat{\theta}_{\mathcal{M}}$, we consider the convex combination

$$\hat{\theta}^{\mathrm{S}} = (1 - b_+)\hat{\theta}_0 + b_1\hat{\theta}_1 + \cdots + b_M\hat{\theta}_M , \tag{11.7}$$

in which $b_1, \ldots, b_M$ are some constants and b_+ is their total. Let $\mathbf{b} = (b_1, \ldots, b_M)^\top$, so that $b_+ = \mathbf{b}^\top\mathbf{1}$, and $\hat{\boldsymbol{\theta}} = (\hat{\theta}_1, \ldots, \hat{\theta}_M)^\top$. Note that b_0 and $\hat{\theta}_0$ are not included in $\mathbf{b}$ and $\hat{\boldsymbol{\theta}}$, respectively; this will make the notation more convenient. Let $\boldsymbol{\Delta} = \mathrm{E}(\hat{\boldsymbol{\theta}}) - \theta\mathbf{1}$ be the vector of biases, $\mathbf{V} = \mathrm{var}(\hat{\boldsymbol{\theta}})$ the variance matrix of the estimators, and $\mathbf{C} = \mathrm{cov}(\hat{\boldsymbol{\theta}}, \hat{\theta}_0)$ the vector of their covariances with the unbiased estimator $\hat{\theta}_0$. The variance (and MSE) of $\hat{\theta}_0$ is denoted by V_0. All the (co-)variances and biases are evaluated under model 0, or another model assumed to be valid a priori. We assume that the estimators $\hat{\theta}_m$ are distinct, that is, none of the differences $\hat{\theta}_m - \hat{\theta}_{m'}$, $m \neq m'$, vanish with probability 1.0. If any pair of such estimators does, one of them can be omitted without any loss.

We call $\hat{\theta}^{\mathrm{S}}$ a *synthetic estimator* because it is composed by synthesis of the candidate models. We can write more compactly

$$\hat{\theta}^{\mathrm{S}}(\mathbf{b}) = (1 - b_+)\hat{\theta}_0 + \mathbf{b}^\top\hat{\boldsymbol{\theta}} . \tag{11.8}$$

The addition of the argument $\mathbf{b}$ to $\hat{\theta}^{\mathrm{S}}$ is essential, because we will consider a range of values of $\mathbf{b}$ and, after identifying an optimum, $\mathbf{b}^*$, estimate it, by $\hat{\mathbf{b}}^*$.

We find the vector $\mathbf{b}$ for which $\hat{\theta}^{\mathrm{S}}$ attains its minimum MSE. Elementary operations yield the identities

$$\begin{aligned}
\mathrm{MSE}\{\hat{\theta}^{\mathrm{S}}(\mathbf{b})\} &= (1 - b_+)^2 V_0 + \mathbf{b}^\top\mathbf{V}\mathbf{b} + 2(1 - b_+)\mathbf{C}^\top\mathbf{b} + (\mathbf{b}^\top\boldsymbol{\Delta})^2 \\
&= V_0 - 2\mathbf{b}^\top(V_0\mathbf{1} - \mathbf{C}) + \mathbf{b}^\top(V_0\mathbf{1}\mathbf{1}^\top - \mathbf{C}\mathbf{1}^\top - \mathbf{1}\mathbf{C}^\top + \mathbf{V} + \boldsymbol{\Delta}\boldsymbol{\Delta}^\top)\mathbf{b} \\
&= V_0 - 2\mathbf{b}^\top\mathbf{P} + \mathbf{b}^\top\mathbf{Q}\mathbf{b} ,
\end{aligned} \tag{11.9}$$

with $\mathbf{P} = \mathrm{cov}(\hat{\theta}_0\mathbf{1} - \hat{\boldsymbol{\theta}}, \hat{\theta}_0)$ and $\mathbf{Q} = \mathrm{E}\left\{(\hat{\theta}_0\mathbf{1} - \hat{\boldsymbol{\theta}})(\hat{\theta}_0\mathbf{1} - \hat{\boldsymbol{\theta}})^\top\right\}$. This MSE is a quadratic function of $\mathbf{b}$. Its (matrix-)quadratic term, $\mathbf{Q}$, is non-negative definite, so the MSE has a minimum. We assume that $\mathbf{Q}$ is non-singular, otherwise one or several estimators would have to be excluded from $\hat{\boldsymbol{\theta}}$, but the purpose of that would be only to obtain a unique minimum, one of those attained also with the original $\mathbf{P}$ and $\mathbf{Q}$. The minimum of $\mathrm{MSE}\{\hat{\theta}^{\mathrm{S}}(\mathbf{b})\}$ is found as the root of its vector of first-order partial differentials:

$$\frac{\partial \mathrm{MSE}(\hat{\theta}^{\mathrm{S}})}{\partial \mathbf{b}} = 2\left(\mathbf{Q}\,\mathbf{b} - \mathbf{P}\right) , \tag{11.10}$$

that is, $\mathbf{b}^* = \mathbf{Q}^{-1}\mathbf{P}$, if $\mathbf{Q}$ is non-singular. The minimum attained is

$$\mathrm{MSE}\left\{\hat{\theta}^{\mathrm{S}}(\mathbf{b}^*)\right\} = V_0 - \mathbf{P}^{\top}\mathbf{Q}^{-1}\mathbf{P}.$$

If the value of $\mathbf{b}^*$ could be established the *ideal synthetic estimator* $\hat{\theta}^{\mathrm{S}}(\mathbf{b}^*)$ would be at least as efficient as either of the candidate estimators $\hat{\theta}_m$, because these estimators are special cases of the convex combination in (11.8), with $\mathbf{b}$ equal to $\mathbf{0}$ (for $\hat{\theta}_0$) or to the appropriate indicator vector (with its components equal to zero, except for the mth element equal to unity for $\hat{\theta}_m$).

In most settings, $\mathbf{b}^*$ depends on unknown parameters, and so has to be estimated. Unlike $\hat{\theta}^{\mathrm{S}}(\mathbf{b}^*)$, the synthetic estimator $\hat{\theta}^{\mathrm{S}}(\hat{\mathbf{b}}^*)$, with $\mathbf{b}$ estimated, is not necessarily more efficient than each candidate estimator $\hat{\theta}_m$. Of course, the efficiency of $\hat{\theta}^{\mathrm{S}}(\hat{\mathbf{b}}^*)$ depends on the estimator $\hat{\mathbf{b}}^*$. The properties of $\hat{\theta}^{\mathrm{S}}(\hat{\mathbf{b}}^*)$ are difficult to explore even in some simple cases, but so are the properties of the selected-model based estimator $\hat{\theta}_{\mathcal{M}}$.

11.3.1 One submodel

The properties of the general synthetic estimator are easier to discuss when there are only two candidate models, that is, $M = 1$, and the alternative model 1 is a submodel of the a priori valid model 0. When $M = 1$, $\mathbf{P}$ and $\mathbf{Q}$ are scalars, and the weight assigned to model 1 in the ideal synthetic estimator is

$$b^* = \frac{V_0 - C}{V_0 + V - 2C + \Delta^2} ,$$

where V, C and Δ are the respective univariate versions of $\mathbf{V}$, $\mathbf{C}$ and $\mathbf{\Delta}$. The synthetic estimator coincides with $\hat{\theta}_0$ only when $V_0 = C$. In this case, as

$$\mathrm{var}\begin{pmatrix} \hat{\theta}_0 \\ \hat{\theta}_1 \end{pmatrix} = \begin{pmatrix} V_0 & C \\ C & V \end{pmatrix} ,$$

necessarily $V > C$; otherwise the 'variance' matrix would have a negative eigenvalue. When $V_0 = C$ and $(\hat{\theta}_0, \hat{\theta}_1)$ has a bivariate normal distribution, $\hat{\theta}_1$ can be expressed as $\hat{\theta}_1 = \hat{\theta}_0 + \delta$ with a random variable $\delta \sim \mathcal{N}(d, V - V_0)$ independent of $\hat{\theta}_0$. Thus, $b^* = 0$ only when the estimator based on model 1 can be formed from the unbiased (model-0 based) estimator by adding 'white noise' to it. In a typical setting, $V < V_0$, so $C < V_0$ and $b^* > 0$. The coefficient b^* exceeds unity when $V - C + \Delta^2 < 0$. In the settings explored in Sections

11.4 and 11.5, $V = C$ and $\Delta > 0$, so $b^* < 1$ and synthetic estimation has a natural interpretation as combining the (constituent) single-model based estimators with positive weights $1 - b^*$ and b^*.

A single-model based estimator with variance greater than an alternative estimator should not be discarded. This conclusion contradicts the aim of model selection. When $\hat{\theta}_0$ and $\hat{\theta}_1$ are independent ($C = 0$) and unbiased ($\Delta = 0$), the synthetic estimator based on them has $b^* = V_0/(V_0 + V)$. It is also unbiased, and its sampling variance, $V_0 V/(V_0 + V)$, is smaller than $\min(V_0, V)$. Whenever $C < V_0$, the biased estimator $\hat{\theta}_1$ contributes to $\hat{\theta}^{\mathrm{S}}$, even when its variance is greater than V_0. Thus, synthesis has a potential to outperform model selection. The principal hurdle in realising this potential is that the coefficient b^* has to be estimated.

Suppose we substitute for b^* a value $b^\dagger \neq b^*$. For example, $b^\dagger$ may be an estimate of b^*. Of interest is the sensitivity of $\hat{\theta}^{\mathrm{S}}(b)$ to b, that is, what extent of the 'error' $b^\dagger - b^*$ (or $b^\dagger/b^*$) can be committed without $\hat{\theta}^{\mathrm{S}}(b^\dagger)$ losing its superiority over the single-model based estimators $\hat{\theta}_0 = \hat{\theta}^{\mathrm{S}}(0)$ and $\hat{\theta}_1 = \hat{\theta}^{\mathrm{S}}(1)$. We have

$$\mathrm{MSE}\left\{\hat{\theta}^{\mathrm{S}}(b^\dagger)\right\} = V_0 - 2b^\dagger(V_0 - C) + {b^\dagger}^2(V_0 + V - 2C + \Delta^2)\,,$$

and this is smaller than both $\mathrm{var}(\hat{\theta}_0) = V_0$ and $\mathrm{MSE}(\hat{\theta}_1) = V + \Delta^2$ when

$$2b^* - 1 < b^\dagger < 2b^*\,. \qquad (11.11)$$

As $0 < b^\dagger < 1$, only one of these inequalities is relevant; the first when $b^* > \frac{1}{2}$, and the second otherwise. Figure 11.3 displays four examples. In each panel, $\mathrm{MSE}(\hat{\theta}^{\mathrm{S}})$ is plotted as a function of b. In panel A, the MSE attains its minimum at $b^* = 0.625$, marked by vertical dashes. The MSE is lower than for both $\hat{\theta}_0$ and $\hat{\theta}_1$ while $0.25 < b < 1.0$, so a considerable 'error' in the guess (or estimation) of b^* is allowed. Panel B presents the mirror-image setting (reflected around $b = 0.5$). Here $b^* = 0.375$ and $\hat{\theta}^{\mathrm{S}}$ is superior to both $\hat{\theta}_0$ and $\hat{\theta}_1$ for $0.0 < b < 0.75$, so the synthetic estimator is quite robust to the setting of b.

Panels C and D present a pair of mirror-ïmage settings in which $\hat{\theta}^{\mathrm{S}}$ is much less robust with respect to the value of b. In panel C, $b^* = 0.125$, and the synthetic estimator is more efficient than for both $\hat{\theta}_0$ and $\hat{\theta}_1$ only when $0.0 < b < 0.25$. However, the MSE is a flat function of b even to the right of $b = 0.25$, so when b moderately exceeds 0.25, $\mathrm{MSE}\{\hat{\theta}^{\mathrm{S}}(b)\}$ exceeds $V_0 = \mathrm{var}(\hat{\theta}_0)$ only slightly.

The MSE of the synthetic estimator with $0 < b^* < 1$ decreases at $b = 0$ and increases at $b = 1$. If we know that $V_0 < V + \Delta^2$, but are not certain about the value of b^*, we need to be concerned only about outperforming $\hat{\theta}_0$. The chances of that are increased by erring on the side of smaller b, because the MSE is more likely to be decreasing at that value of b. However, if too small a value of b is chosen, synthesis is far from optimal; a greater value of

Figure 11.3. The MSE of a synthetic estimator as a function of the coefficient b. Settings with different values of V_0, V, C and Δ.

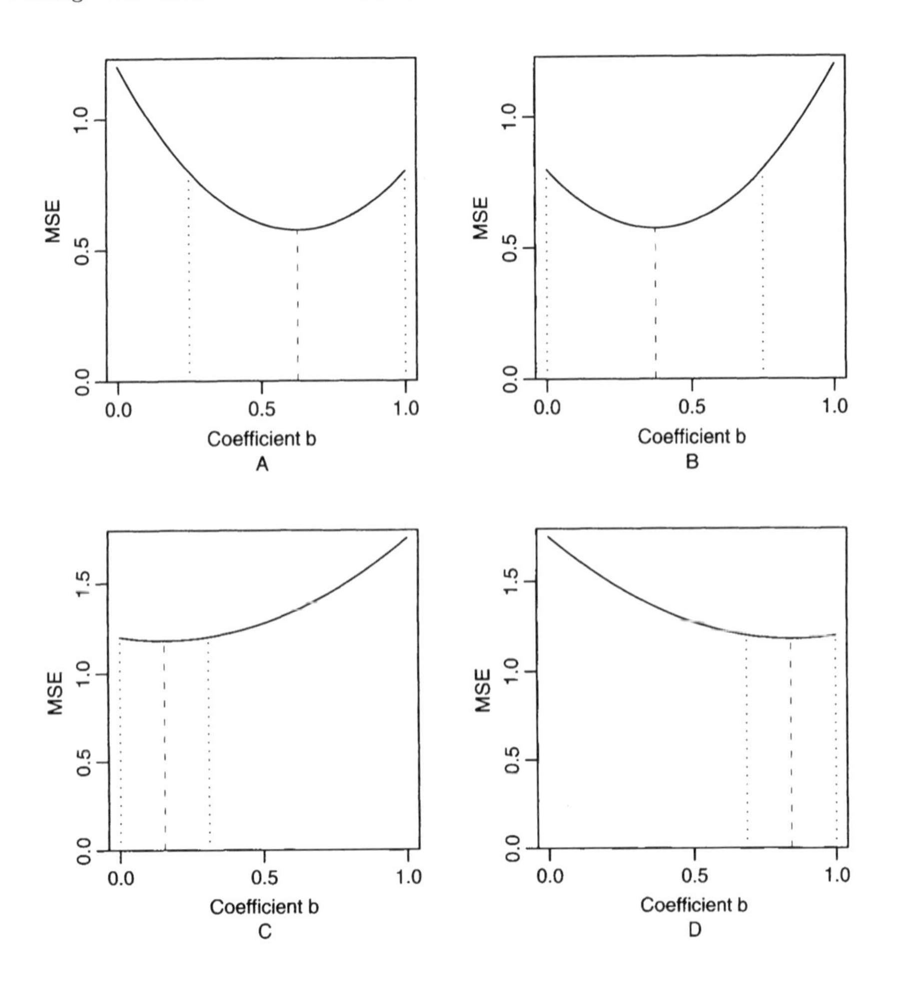

b would yield a much smaller MSE. Note the parallels with the discussion of composite estimation for small areas in Section 6.3.2.

11.4 Analysis of variance

This section discusses applications of synthetic estimation to ANOVA. We consider the one-way model

$$y_{kj} = \mu + \delta_k + \varepsilon_{kj} \,, \qquad (11.12)$$

with an unknown mean μ, group-level deviations δ_k and within-group deviations $\varepsilon_{kj} \sim \mathcal{N}(0, \sigma_W^2)$, and the usual assumptions of mutual independence of the ε's. The deviations δ_k are unknown parameters. For simplicity, we assume a balanced design, with groups $k = 1, \ldots, K$ and J observations in each group ($j = 1, \ldots, J$). The overall sample size is denoted by N; $N = JK$.

We are interested in estimating the mean of a group, say, $\mu_1 = \mu + \delta_1$. The commonly contemplated options are the within-group mean $\hat{\mu}_{1,A} = (y_{11} + y_{12} + \cdots + y_{1J})/J$ and the sample mean $\hat{\mu}_B = (y_{11} + \cdots + y_{1J} + y_{21} + \cdots + y_{KJ})/N$. They are implied by the established test of the hypothesis that the groups have identical means. Presumably, when the hypothesis is rejected μ_1 would be estimated by $\hat{\mu}_{1,A}$, and if not rejected, by $\hat{\mu}_B$.

For the ideal synthetic estimator of μ_1, we require the following quantities:

$$
\begin{aligned}
\operatorname{var}(\hat{\mu}_{1,A}) &= V_0 = \frac{\sigma_W^2}{J} \\
\operatorname{var}(\hat{\mu}_B) &= V = \frac{\sigma_W^2}{N} \\
\operatorname{cov}(\hat{\mu}_{1,A}, \hat{\mu}_B) &= C = \frac{\sigma_W^2}{N} \\
\mathrm{E}(\hat{\mu}_B) - \mu_1 &= \Delta = -\delta_1 .
\end{aligned}
\tag{11.13}
$$

The expression for V holds even when model B applies but, in general, V, C and Δ are evaluated assuming model A. From (11.13), we have

$$
\mathrm{MSE}\left\{\hat{\theta}^{\mathrm{S}}(b)\right\} = \sigma_W^2 \left\{\frac{1}{J} - 2bg + b^2(g + \gamma_1^2)\right\},
$$

where $g = 1/J - 1/N = (K-1)/N$ and $\gamma_1 = \delta_1/\sigma_W$ is the relative deviation of group 1. The optimal coefficient is

$$
b^* = \frac{g}{g + \gamma_1^2},
$$

and the corresponding MSE is

$$
\mathrm{MSE}\left\{\hat{\theta}^{\mathrm{S}}(b^*)\right\} = \sigma_W^2 \left(\frac{1}{J} - \frac{g^2}{g + \gamma_1^2}\right).
\tag{11.14}
$$

This represents a reduction of MSE by $\sigma_W^2 g^2/(g + \gamma_1^2)$ over the variance of $\hat{\mu}_{1,A}$ and by $\sigma_W^2 g \gamma_1^2/(g + \gamma_1^2)$ over the MSE of $\hat{\mu}_B$. But these gains would be realised only if γ_1 were known, and in that case, $\hat{\mu}_B + \gamma_1 \hat{\sigma}_W$ would be a more efficient estimator of μ_1.

If a value $\gamma_\dagger \neq \gamma_1$ is applied, the conditions in (11.11) translate to

$$
\frac{g\gamma_\dagger^2}{2g + \gamma_\dagger^2} < \gamma_1^2 < 2\gamma_\dagger^2 + g .
\tag{11.15}
$$

The inequality on the left-hand side is always satisfied when $\gamma_1^2 > g$ and on the right-hand side when $\gamma_1^2 < g$. The interval in (11.15) is wider than $(\frac{1}{2}\gamma_1^2, 2\gamma_1^2)$. Nevertheless, the interval is quite narrow when γ_1 is small. That happens when $\mu_1 \doteq \mu$, when $\hat{\mu}_{\mathrm{B}}$ is more efficient than $\hat{\mu}_{\mathrm{A}}$. In Section 11.4.1, we consider a class of synthetic estimators that are less efficient than $\hat{\mu}_{\mathrm{B}}$ when μ_1 is in the vicinity of μ, but are much more efficient than $\hat{\mu}_{\mathrm{B}}$ when μ_1 is distant from μ, when $\mathrm{MSE}(\hat{\mu}_{\mathrm{B}})$ is very inefficient.

The coefficient b^* can be interpreted as a *shrinkage* coefficient, pulling the unbiased estimator $\hat{\mu}_{1,\mathrm{A}}$ toward the low-variance (stable) but biased estimator $\hat{\mu}_{\mathrm{B}}$. A parallel can be drawn with the setting of small-area estimation, regarding each group k as a district.

11.4.1 Minimax estimation

Since $\mathrm{MSE}(\hat{\mu}_{\mathrm{B}}\,;\mu_1)$ is an increasing function of γ_1^2, efficient estimation is a greater priority for large values of γ_1^2. Suppose we have a priori information that γ_1^2 does not exceed a given value Γ^2. We apply the synthetic estimator $\hat{\mu}_1^{\mathrm{S}}$ with b^* evaluated at $\gamma_1^2 = \Gamma^2$, and explore the properties of this estimator, denoted by $\hat{\mu}_{1,\Gamma^2}^{\mathrm{S}}$, when in fact $\gamma_1^2 < \Gamma^2$.

The MSE of this estimator is

$$\mathrm{MSE}(\hat{\mu}_{1,\Gamma^2}^{\mathrm{S}}) = \sigma_{\mathrm{W}}^2 \left\{ \frac{1}{J} - \frac{2g^2}{g+\Gamma^2} + \frac{g^2(g+\gamma_1^2)}{(g+\Gamma^2)^2} \right\} .$$

The estimator is more efficient than $\hat{\mu}_{1,\mathrm{A}}$ when

$$\gamma_1^2 < g + 2\Gamma^2 ,$$

and more efficient than $\hat{\mu}_{\mathrm{B}}$ when

$$\gamma_1^2 > \frac{g\Gamma^2}{2g+\Gamma^2} ;$$

the two inequalities are derived similarly to (11.15). So, $\hat{\mu}_{1,\Gamma^2}^{\mathrm{S}}$ is more efficient than $\hat{\mu}_{1,\mathrm{A}}$ for values of γ_1^2 well in excess of Γ^2 and more efficient than $\hat{\mu}_{\mathrm{B}}$ for all but the smallest values of γ_1^2 for which $\hat{\mu}_{\mathrm{B}}$ has a very small MSE. The threshold $g\Gamma^2/(2g+\Gamma^2)$ is smaller than both g and $\Gamma^2/2$. The MSE of $\hat{\mu}_{1,\Gamma^2}^{\mathrm{S}}$ is a linear increasing function of γ_1^2, but its slope on γ_1^2, equal to $\sigma_{\mathrm{W}}^2 g^2/(g+\Gamma^2)^2$, is not as steep as for $\mathrm{MSE}(\hat{\mu}_{\mathrm{B}})$.

The MSEs of the estimators $\hat{\mu}_{1,\mathrm{A}}$, $\hat{\mu}_{\mathrm{B}}$ and $\hat{\mu}_{1,\Gamma^2}^{\mathrm{S}}$, as functions of the relative deviation γ_1, are compared in Figure 11.4 for the following setting: $K = 8$ groups, $J = 10$ observations within groups, $\sigma_{\mathrm{W}}^2 = 1$, and assuming $\Gamma^2 = 0.4$ and $\Gamma^2 = 0.25$. All the MSE's considered are symmetric functions of γ_1, so it suffices to discuss their behaviour for $\gamma_1 > 0$. The synthetic estimator $\hat{\mu}_{1,0.4}^{\mathrm{S}}$ provides an effective protection against the large bias of $\hat{\mu}_{\mathrm{B}}$, while being uniformly more efficient than $\hat{\mu}_{1,\mathrm{A}}$. As $\hat{\mu}_{1,0.4}^{\mathrm{S}}$ is efficient when $\gamma_1^2 = \Gamma^2 = 0.4$,

Figure 11.4. The single-model based (A — $\hat{\mu}_{1,\text{A}}$ and B — $\hat{\mu}_{\text{B}}$) and minimax synthetic estimators (0.25 — $\hat{\mu}^{\text{S}}_{1,0.25}$ and 0.4 — $\hat{\mu}^{\text{S}}_{1,0.40}$) of the mean of a group in ANOVA. The vertical dashes mark the upper limits $\Gamma = 0.5$ and $\Gamma = \sqrt{0.4}$.

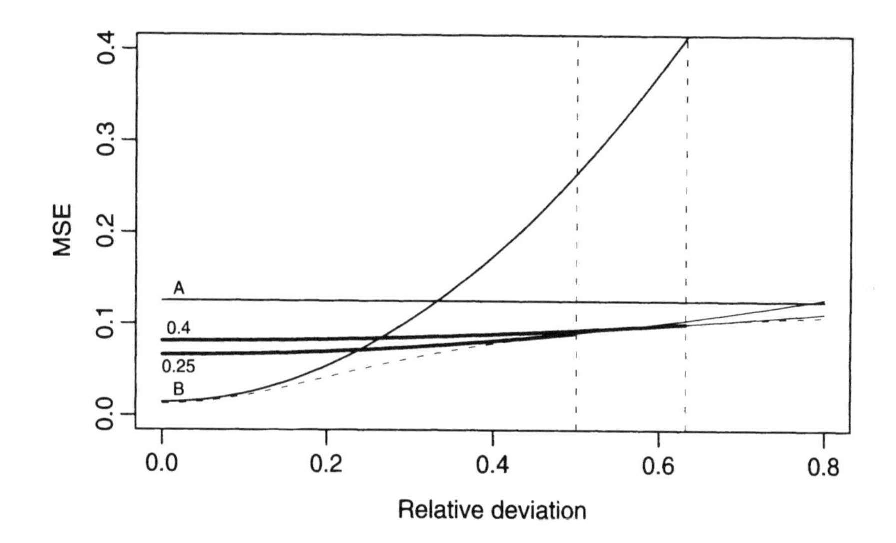

and attains the highest MSE at that value, $\hat{\mu}^{\text{S}}_{1,0.4}$ is the minimax estimator of μ_1 ; it is superior in the worst plausible scenario for all the synthetic estimators $\hat{\mu}^{\text{S}}_1(b)$.

When Γ^2 can be set to a smaller value, say, $\Gamma^2 = 0.25$, $\hat{\mu}^{\text{S}}_{1,0.25}$ is more efficient than $\hat{\mu}^{\text{S}}_{1,0.4}$ for all values of γ_1^2 up to 0.25 and slightly beyond. Thus, 'tighter' information about γ_1 is rewarded by (uniformly) more efficient estimation. There is some leeway — the penalty for basing $\hat{\mu}^{\text{S}}_{1,\Gamma^2}$ on too small a value of Γ^2 becomes harsh only when γ_1^2 exceeds Γ^2 by a wide margin. The curve drawn in Figure 11.4 by short dashes is the MSE of the ideal synthetic estimator, based on the actual value of γ_1. It represents a lower bound for the MSE; $\hat{\mu}_{\text{B}}$ attains it for $\gamma_1 = 0$, $\hat{\mu}^{\text{S}}_{1,\Gamma^2}$ for $\gamma_1 = \Gamma$, and the MSE approaches $\text{var}(\hat{\mu}_{1,\text{A}})$, very slowly, as γ_1 diverges to $+\infty$.

11.4.2 Estimating σ^2_{W}

In this section, we derive the synthetic estimator of the within-group variance σ^2_{W}. We show that synthetic estimators of μ_1 and σ^2_{W} have different ideal coefficients b^*. The need for such flexibility in estimation was anticipated in Section 11.2.

For the single-model based estimators

$$\hat{\sigma}^2_{\mathrm{W,A}} = \frac{1}{N-K} \sum_{k=1}^{K} \sum_{j=1}^{J} (y_{jk} - \hat{\mu}_{k,\mathrm{A}})^2$$

$$\hat{\sigma}^2_{\mathrm{W,B}} = \frac{1}{N-1} \sum_{k=1}^{K} \sum_{j=1}^{J} (y_{jk} - \hat{\mu}_{\mathrm{B}})^2 \,,$$

based on the $N-K$ and $N-1$ degrees of freedom, respectively, we have

$$\begin{aligned}
\mathrm{var}(\hat{\sigma}^2_{\mathrm{W,A}}) &= V_0 = \frac{2\sigma^4_{\mathrm{W}}}{N-K} \\
\mathrm{MSE}(\hat{\sigma}^2_{\mathrm{W,B}}) &= V = \frac{2\sigma^4_{\mathrm{W}}}{N-1} + \frac{4\sigma^2_{\mathrm{W}}}{(N-1)^2} \sum_{k=1}^{K} \delta_i^2 \\
\mathrm{cov}(\hat{\sigma}^2_{\mathrm{W,A}}\,, \hat{\sigma}^2_{\mathrm{W,B}}) &= C = \frac{2\sigma^4_{\mathrm{W}}}{N-1} \\
\mathrm{E}(\hat{\sigma}^2_{\mathrm{W,B}}) - \sigma^2_{\mathrm{W}} &= \Delta = \frac{J}{N-1} \sum_{k=1}^{K} \delta_k^2 \,.
\end{aligned} \tag{11.16}$$

Hence the ideal coefficient for estimating σ^2_{W} is

$$\begin{aligned}
b^* &= \frac{2q\sigma^4_{\mathrm{W}}}{2q\sigma^4_{\mathrm{W}} + 4\sigma^2_{\mathrm{W}} \sum_k \delta_k^2 + J^2 \left(\sum_k \delta_k^2\right)^2} \\
&= \frac{2q}{2q + 4\sum_k \gamma_k^2 + J^2 \left(\sum_k \gamma_k^2\right)^2} \,,
\end{aligned} \tag{11.17}$$

where $q = (K-1)(N-1)/(N-K)$. The ideal coefficient $b^* = b^*_{\sigma^2_{\mathrm{W}}}$ differs from its counterpart $b^*_{\mu_1}$; it depends on the relative deviations γ_k exchangeably, through their sum of squares, whereas $b^*_{\mu_1}$ depends only on γ_1.

The minimax synthetic estimator of σ^2_{W} can be derived in analogy with its counterpart for μ_1, although the algebra is somewhat more involved. However, in most settings, $\hat{\sigma}^2_{\mathrm{W,B}}$ is not worth considering, and b^* or its estimator is quite small. This can be motivated by considering the degrees of freedom of the two candidate estimators. In the setting considered earlier, $\hat{\sigma}^2_{\mathrm{W,A}}$ is associated with $N-K = 72$ degrees of freedom. With $\hat{\sigma}^2_{\mathrm{W,B}}$ we gain an additional $K-1 = 7$ degrees of freedom. The increase by about 10%, at the risk of incurring bias, is hardly worth it. In contrast, the alternatives available for estimating μ_1 are based on either $J = 10$ on $N = 80$ observations; the threat of bias should be assessed differently, in view of an overwhelming reduction of the sampling variance.

The naive estimation of $\sum_k \delta_k^2$ is very inefficient, unless the within-group sample size J is substantial. We may estimate this sum of squares from the finite-sample variance $\sigma^2_{\mathrm{B}} = \mathrm{var}_{\mathcal{K}}(\delta_{\mathcal{K}})$. The subscript $\mathcal{K}$ is used to indicate expectation or variance over the groups k, similarly to $\mathcal{D}$ for districts in small-area estimation. Simple moment matching yields the estimator

$$\hat{\sigma}_{\mathrm{B}}^2 = \sum_{k=1}^{K} (\hat{\mu}_{k,\mathrm{A}} - \hat{\mu}_{\mathrm{B}})^2 - \frac{K}{J} \hat{\sigma}_{\mathrm{W}}^2 .$$

Some advantage is derived by erring on the side of smaller b. This can be achieved by overestimating σ_{B}^2, that is, making the groups to appear more dispersed.

11.4.3 Estimated coefficient $\hat{b}^*$

In this section we return to the problem of estimating μ_1 in one-way balanced ANOVA. In practice, b^* has to be estimated, and $\hat{\mu}^{\mathrm{S}}(\hat{b}^*)$ need not be more efficient than both candidates $\hat{\mu}_{1,\mathrm{A}}$ and $\hat{\mu}_{\mathrm{B}}$. We can ensure that the synthetic estimator is more efficient than the unbiased estimator $\hat{\mu}_{1,\mathrm{A}}$ by reducing $\hat{b}^*$ so much that it is very likely smaller than b^*. However, by 'shrinking' $\hat{b}^*$ too much we may forego much of the advantage of synthetic estimation.

To assess the loss of efficiency due to not knowing b^*, we express the MSE of $\hat{\mu}_1^{\mathrm{S}}$ by conditioning on $\hat{b}^*$:

$$\begin{aligned}
\mathrm{MSE}\left(\hat{\mu}_1^{\mathrm{S}}; \mu_1\right) &= \mathrm{E}\left\{\mathrm{var}(\hat{\mu}_1^{\mathrm{S}} \,|\, \hat{b}^*)\right\} + \mathrm{var}\left\{\mathrm{E}(\hat{\mu}_1^{\mathrm{S}} \,|\, \hat{b}^*)\right\} + \left[\mathrm{E}\left\{\mathrm{E}(\hat{\mu}_1^{\mathrm{S}} \,|\, \hat{b}^*)\right\} - \mu_1\right]^2 \\
&= \left\{1 - \mathrm{E}(\hat{b}^*)\right\}^2 \frac{\sigma_{\mathrm{W}}^2}{J} + \left\{\mathrm{E}(\hat{b}^*)\right\}^2 \frac{\sigma_{\mathrm{W}}^2}{N} + 2\mathrm{E}(\hat{b}^*)\left\{1 - \mathrm{E}(\hat{b}^*)\right\} \frac{\sigma_{\mathrm{W}}^2}{N} \\
&\quad + g\sigma_{\mathrm{W}}^2 \,\mathrm{var}(\hat{b}^*) + \delta_1^2 \,\mathrm{var}(\hat{b}^*) + \delta_1^2 \left\{\mathrm{E}(\hat{b}^*)\right\}^2 \\
&= \sigma_{\mathrm{W}}^2 \left[\frac{1}{J} - 2g\mathrm{E}(\hat{b}^*) + (g + \gamma_1^2)\left\{\mathrm{E}(\hat{b}^*)\right\}^2 + (g + \gamma_1^2)\,\mathrm{var}(\hat{b}^*)\right] ;
\end{aligned}$$

in the first line, the inner expectation or variance are over the distribution of $\hat{\mu}_1^{\mathrm{S}}$ and the outer over $\hat{b}^*$. When b^* is estimated with little or no bias, $\mathrm{E}(\hat{b}^*) \doteq b^*$,

$$\mathrm{MSE}\left\{\hat{\mu}_1(\hat{b}^*);\, \mu_1\right\} \doteq \mathrm{MSE}\left\{\hat{\mu}_1^{\mathrm{S}}(b^*);\, \mu_1\right\} + \sigma_{\mathrm{W}}^2 (g + 2\gamma_1^2)\,\mathrm{var}(\hat{b}^*) .$$

Hence, the inflation of $\mathrm{MSE}(\hat{\mu}_1^{\mathrm{S}} \,|\, \mu_1)$ owing to (unbiased) estimation of b^* is approximately $\sigma_{\mathrm{W}}^2(g + 2\gamma_1^2)\,\mathrm{var}(\hat{b}^*)$. This can be compared directly with the gains of the ideal synthetic estimator over the single-model based estimators.

The coefficient b^* can be estimated naively, by $(\hat{\mu}_{1,\mathrm{A}} - \hat{\mu}_{\mathrm{B}})^2/\hat{\sigma}_{\mathrm{W,A}}^2$. The numerator and denominator are independent and the ratio has a scaled non-central F-distribution with one and $N - K$ degrees of freedom. The bias of the numerator can be adjusted for, but the adjustment is itself estimated and may result in a negative value of the numerator. In any case, the ratio $\hat{T}/\hat{U}$ of unbiased estimators of some quantities T and U is not an unbiased estimator of T/U; see Section 9.1.1. With a χ^2-distributed denominator (subject to a scale factor), the bias can be corrected. However, the objective is not to estimate b^* without bias, but to estimate μ_1 as efficiently as possible. The pursuit of unbiasedness of the estimators of some intermediate quantities is not conducive to this goal.

11.4.4 Simulations

Apart from introducing synthetic estimators, we want to illustrate the deceitful nature of selected-model based estimators, reinforcing the message of Section 11.1.2. Synthetic estimation also involves dishonesty if we estimate b (or $\mathbf{b}$), and regard the estimate as the ideal coefficient b. Since the distribution of neither $\hat{\mu}_1^{\mathrm{S}}(\hat{b}^*)$ nor $\hat{\mu}_{1,\mathcal{M}}$ is available in any analytical form, we compare them by simulations. For $\hat{\mu}_{1,\mathcal{M}}$, we use the standard hypothesis testing process with 5% significance level, using the obvious F-test statistic. The statistic depends on all the data, so we have to set the (population) means of all $K = 8$ groups. The results are described for the vector of means $\boldsymbol{\mu} = (\delta, \delta, -\delta, -\delta, 0, 0, 0, 0)^\top$. We set $\mu = 0$ and $\sigma_{\mathrm{W}}^2 = 1$; the value of σ_{W}^2 is immaterial for estimating the relative deviation γ_1. The actual outcomes y_{kj} are not required in the simulations, as it suffices to generate $\hat{\delta}_1 \sim \mathcal{N}(\delta, g)$ and, independently, $(N-K)\hat{\sigma}_{\mathrm{W}}^2 \sim \chi^2_{N-K}$.

The empirical MSEs of the two single-model based, the ideal and estimated-shrinkage synthetic, and the selected-model based estimators are compared in Figure 11.5. Panel A shows that the selected-model based estimator $\hat{\mu}_{1,\mathcal{M}}$ (nearly) coincides with the sample mean $\hat{\mu}_{\mathrm{B}}$ in the range $|\gamma_1| < 1.3$, and they are both efficient only for very small values of γ_1, $|\gamma_1| < 0.2$. The synthetic estimator with b^* estimated is less efficient than $\hat{\mu}_{1,\mathcal{M}}$ for small values of γ_1, slightly less efficient than $\hat{\mu}_{1,\mathrm{A}}$ for $\gamma_1 \in (0.5, 1.0)$, and for $|\gamma_1| > 1$ its performance is indistinguishable from $\hat{\mu}_{1,\mathrm{A}}$. Panel B zooms in on the comparison of the synthetic estimator and the within-group mean $\hat{\mu}_{1,\mathrm{A}}$. Unlike the ideal synthetic estimator (drawn by dots), $\hat{\mu}_1^{\mathrm{S}}(\hat{b}^*)$ is not uniformly more efficient than $\hat{\mu}_{1,\mathrm{A}}$, but it is less efficient only slightly and in a narrow range.

In conclusion, the selected-model based estimator is a very poor choice, but the synthetic estimator does not deliver on the promise of outperforming both single-model based estimators. Against $\hat{\mu}_{\mathrm{B}}$ it 'fails' for small $|\gamma_1|$, when $\mathrm{MSE}(\hat{\mu}_{\mathrm{B}}; \mu_1)$ is small, so this cannot be regarded as a serious deficiency. Against $\hat{\mu}_{1,\mathrm{A}}$ it fails for intermediate values of $|\gamma_1|$, so that should be regarded as a more serious drawback.

We suggested earlier that erring on the side of lower coefficient b is preferable. The impact of using $r\hat{b}^* = rg/(g + \hat{\gamma}_1^2)$ instead of $\hat{b}^*$ is studied in Figure 11.6 for factors $r = 0.5, 0.6, \ldots, 1$. The diagram shows that a reduction of $\hat{b}^*$ improves the efficiency of $\hat{\mu}_1^{\mathrm{S}}$ in the range where it is least efficient, $(0.5, 1.0)$.

Figure 11.5. The root-MSEs of estimators of μ_1 as functions of the relative deviation δ_1.

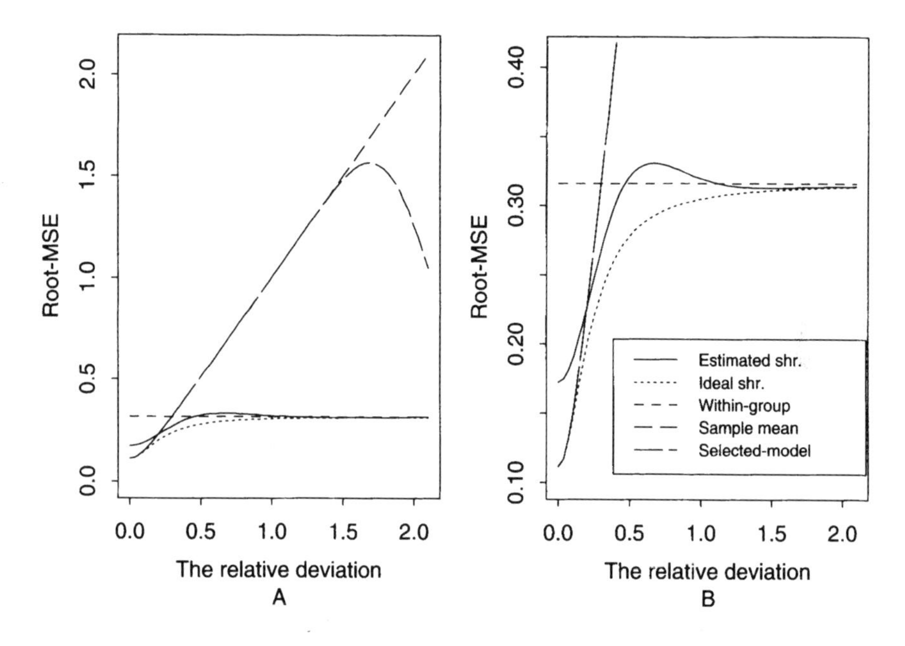

For 1.28-fold reduction of $\hat{b}^*$, $r = 0.78$, $\hat{\mu}_1^{\mathrm{S}}(r\hat{b}^*)$ is uniformly more efficient than $\hat{\mu}_{1,\mathrm{A}}$. This improvement comes at the expense of reduced efficiency for the smallest values of γ_1. Such a trade-off is advantageous if we prefer avoiding any circumstances in which μ_1 is estimated with large MSE to retaining a chance that μ_1 may be estimated with high precision.

11.4.5 ANOVA with random effects

In the random-effect version of (11.12), the group-level deviations δ_k are assumed to be a random sample from $\mathcal{N}(0, \sigma_{\mathrm{B}}^2)$. As μ_1 is a random variable in this model, its estimation is meaningful only by a reference to replications in which it is held fixed. Therefore, all the items required for (ideal) synthetic estimation are derived *conditionally* on μ_1:

$$\begin{aligned}
\operatorname{var}(\hat{\mu}_{1,\mathrm{A}} \,|\, \mu_1) &= V_0 = \frac{\sigma_{\mathrm{W}}^2}{J} \\
\operatorname{MSE}(\hat{\mu}_{\mathrm{B}}\,;\, \mu_1 \,|\, \mu_1) &= V = \frac{\sigma_{\mathrm{W}}^2}{N} + \frac{(K-1)\sigma_{\mathrm{B}}^2}{K^2} \\
\operatorname{cov}(\hat{\mu}_{1,\mathrm{A}}\,,\, \hat{\mu}_{\mathrm{B}} \,|\, \mu_1) &= C = \frac{\sigma_{\mathrm{W}}^2}{N}
\end{aligned}$$

Figure 11.6. The root-MSEs of synthetic estimators of μ_1 with underestimated coefficient $\hat{b}^*$.

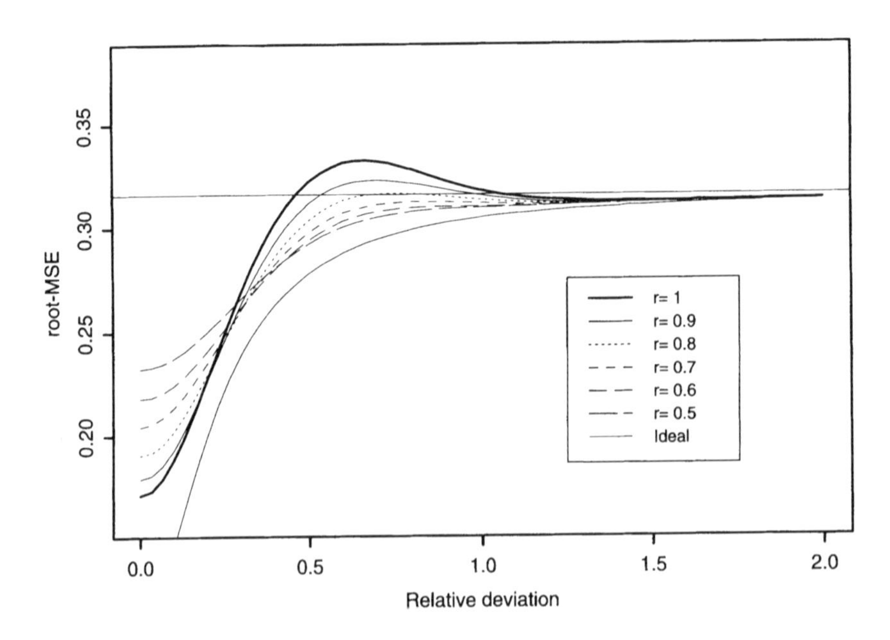

$$\mathrm{E}(\hat{\mu}_{\mathrm{B}} \mid \mu_1) - \mu_1 = \quad \Delta = -\delta_1 \frac{K-1}{K} . \tag{11.18}$$

For example, without conditioning, $V_0 = \sigma_{\mathrm{B}}^2 + \sigma_{\mathrm{W}}^2/J$. Note that in the expression for V, we indicate μ_1 as both the target and the condition, because μ_1 is regarded as fixed, unlike the means of the other groups. The ideal coefficient is

$$b^* = \frac{g}{g + \{\omega + \gamma_1^2(K-1)\}(K-1)/K^2} ,$$

where $\omega = \sigma_{\mathrm{B}}^2/\sigma_{\mathrm{W}}^2$ is the variance ratio. Estimation of b^* is simplified by replacing γ_1^2 with its expectation over the groups, equal to ω. As in Section 11.4.4, conservatism corresponds to underestimating b^*, or overestimating γ_1^2 or ω. To affect this, γ_1^2 can be replaced by a multiple of ω, such as 2ω.

The ideal synthetic estimator $\hat{\mu}_1^{\mathrm{S}}(b^*)$ has MSE (conditional on μ_1)

$$\sigma_{\mathrm{W}}^2 \left\{ \frac{1}{J} - \frac{g^2}{g + \omega(K-1)/K^2 + \gamma_1^2(K-1)^2/K^2} \right\} .$$

It is smaller than its counterpart for fixed effects, (11.14), when

$$\gamma_1^2 < \omega \frac{K(K-1)}{2K-1} .$$

Thus, the assumption of randomness of the deviations δ_k leads to more precise estimation of the within-group mean for groups with smaller absolute deviations $|\,\delta_k\,|$. It is more useful when a greater number of groups K is observed and when the variance ratio ω is greater. These comparisons are slightly unfair to the fixed-effect ANOVA because in the rANOVA, $\hat{b}^*$ requires estimation of ω in addition to γ_1^2. The advantages of random-effect ANOVA cannot be attributed to borrowing strength (as in [194]), because a form of borrowing strength takes place in synthetic estimation even for fixed effects, although this is not exploited in ML estimation.

11.5 Ordinary regression

This section develops synthetic estimation first for simple regression, then extends it to multiple regression, and concludes with an outline of further generalisations.

We consider the problem of predicting the outcome y^* in response to a stimulus x^* given that the stimulus and outcome are related by the simple regression model

$$y = \beta_0 + \beta_1 x + \varepsilon \tag{11.19}$$

with the usual assumptions of homoscedasticity, independence and normality of ε. The values of the parameters β_0, β_1 and $\sigma^2 = \mathrm{var}(\varepsilon)$ are not known and all the information about them is contained in a random sample $\mathbf{y} = (y_1, \ldots, y_n)^\top$ of outcomes generated in response to a vector of stimuli $\mathbf{x} = (x_1, \ldots, x_n)^\top$. To avoid the problem becoming trivial, assume that x^* differs from the sample mean $\overline{x} = (x_1 + \cdots + x_n)/n$ and that the values of x are not all identical. No generality is lost by assuming that $\overline{x} = 0$ because a change in the origin of x can be compensated by a change in the intercept β_0. Denote by $S_x = x_1^2 + \cdots + x_n^2$ the sum of squares of the x's.

Predicting y^* can be regarded as a problem of estimating $\beta_0 + \beta_1 x^*$, although the meaning of β_0 and β_1 has to be connected with the assumed model. Alternatively, y^* can be regarded as $\mathrm{E}(y \,|\, x = x^*)$. The obvious predictor of y^* is $\hat{\beta}_0 + \hat{\beta}_1 x^*$, where $(\hat{\beta}_0, \hat{\beta}_1)$ is the ordinary least squares estimator of (β_0, β_1). It may be worth considering the submodel

$$y = \mu + \varepsilon$$

that does not involve x, because the degree of freedom saved may outweigh the bias that is due to lack of validity of the model. The predictor based on this model is the sample mean $\overline{y} = (y_1 + \cdots + y_n)/n$.

The expressions required for synthetic estimation are

$$\mathrm{var}(\hat{y}^*) = \quad V = \sigma^2 \left(\frac{1}{n} + \frac{x^{*2}}{S_x} \right)$$

$$\begin{aligned}
\mathrm{var}(\overline{y}) &= V_1 = \frac{\sigma^2}{n} \\
\mathrm{cov}(\hat{y}^*, \overline{y}) &= C = \frac{\sigma^2}{n} \\
\mathrm{E}(\overline{y}) - y^* &= \Delta = -\beta_1 x^* ,
\end{aligned}$$

evaluated assuming the model in (11.19). Hence

$$b^* = \frac{\sigma^2 x^{*2}/S_x}{\sigma^2 x^{*2}/S_x + \beta_1^2 x^{*2}} = \frac{1}{1+\gamma^2 S_x} ,$$

where $\gamma^2 = \beta_1^2/\sigma^2$ is the squared relative slope. The corresponding MSE is

$$\mathrm{MSE}\left\{\hat{y}^{\mathrm{S}}(b^*)\,|\,x^*\right\} = \sigma^2\left(\frac{1}{n} + \frac{x^{*2}\gamma^2}{1+\gamma^2 S_x}\right) .$$

As γ^2 is not known, and depends on the slope β_1, we seem not to have resolved much. The form of b^* suggests that, if we were wedded to the choice between $\hat{y}^*$ and $\overline{y}$, an approach superior to model selection might be based on whether or not γ^2, or $\hat{\gamma}^2$, exceeds $1/S_x$. However, the convex combination of the candidate estimators widens the horizon considerably. In particular, b^* never vanishes and equals to unity only when the submodel is valid ($\gamma = 0$). In the latter case, $\hat{y}^*$ would be genuinely burdened by the degree of freedom used up for estimating the slope $\beta_1 = 0$. The optimal coefficient b^* does not depend on x^*.

ANOVA can be regarded as a special case of ordinary regression, and so some of the discussion of the synthetic estimators in Section 11.4 carries over to simple regression with only minimum changes. Thus, if an incorrect value $\gamma_\dagger^2$ of γ^2 is used the synthetic predictor $\hat{y}^{\mathrm{S}\dagger}$ is more efficient than both $\hat{y}^*$ and $\overline{y}$, so long as

$$\frac{\gamma_\dagger^2}{2+\gamma_\dagger^2/S_x} < \gamma^2 < 2\gamma_\dagger^2 + \frac{1}{S_x} . \tag{11.20}$$

The squared relative slope γ^2 can be estimated naively, although the bias of its numerator $\hat{\beta}^2$ can be adjusted straightforwardly using the identity $\mathrm{E}\{(\hat{\beta}_1)^2\} = \mathrm{E}(\hat{\beta}_1^2) - \mathrm{var}(\hat{\beta}_1)$. The drawback of such an adjustment is that it may result in a negative estimate of $\hat{\beta}_1^2$. The bias of $1/\hat{\sigma}^2$ can be adjusted for similarly. Apart from reducing the bias of the elements contributing to $\hat{b}^*$, it may be more constructive to weigh the consequences of under- and overestimating b^*. As in ANOVA, it is preferable to err on the side of smaller b^*, and this can be arranged by overestimating γ^2. The impact of such (or further) reduction of b^* can be explored by simulations.

11.5.1 Estimating σ^2

The fact that synthetic prediction of y^* combines the candidate estimators with the same coefficient b^* for every value of x^* is quite unusual. A different coefficient is obtained for estimating the residual variance σ^2. The single-model based estimators are the mean residual square, $\hat{\sigma}_0^2 = \hat{\mathbf{e}}^\top\hat{\mathbf{e}}/(n-2)$, where $\hat{\mathbf{e}} = \mathbf{y} - \hat{\beta}_0 - \hat{\beta}_1\mathbf{x}$, and $\hat{\sigma}_1^2 = \hat{\mathbf{e}}_0^\top\hat{\mathbf{e}}_0/(n-1)$, where $\hat{\mathbf{e}}_0 = \mathbf{y} - \overline{y}\mathbf{1}$. It can reasonably be expected that for moderate to large n the regression-based $\hat{\sigma}_0^2$ will be preferred because it is hardly worth sacrificing unbiasedness for only one additional degree of freedom. The ideal synthetic estimator of σ^2 is based on the following identities:

$$\begin{aligned}
\operatorname{var}(\hat{\sigma}_0^2) &= V_0 = \frac{2\sigma^4}{n-2} \\
\operatorname{var}(\hat{\sigma}_1^2) &= V = \frac{2\sigma^4}{n-1} \\
\operatorname{cov}(\hat{\sigma}_0^2, \hat{\sigma}_0^2) &= C = \frac{2\sigma^4}{n-2} \\
\mathrm{E}(\hat{\sigma}_1^2) - \sigma^2 &= \Delta = \frac{\beta_1^2 S_x}{n-1} .
\end{aligned}$$

Hence the optimal coefficient is

$$b^* = \frac{2}{2 + \gamma^4 S_x^2 (n-2)/(n-1)} . \tag{11.21}$$

For all but very small n, the fraction $(n-2)/(n-1)$ can be ignored. Then b^* has the same form as for predicting y^*, with $\gamma^2 S_x$ replaced by $(\gamma^2 S_x)^2/2$. Thus, the optimal coefficients for predicting y^* and estimating σ^2 differ substantially. Figure 11.7 shows this graphically for sample size $n = 20$. The horizontal axis is for $u = \gamma^2 S_x$. The vertical axis is cut off at $b = 0.5$, to improve the resolution of the plot. The coefficient b^* for y^* exceeds its counterpart for σ^2 for $u > 2$. The two functions, $b^*_{y^*}(u)$ and $b^*_{\sigma^2}(u)$ cross at $u = 2$, that is, when $\beta_1^2 = 2\sigma^2/S_x$. So, when the slope β_1 is very shallow the submodel is preferred more for estimating σ^2 than for prediction of y^*. However, the weight given to the submodel for estimating σ^2 drops precipitously toward zero with increasing u, so that, for instance, it is about 0.005, ten times smaller than its counterpart for y^*, when $u = 20$.

11.5.2 Several covariates

Suppose first that only two models, A (valid) and its submodel B are considered, with respective vectors of covariates $\mathbf{x}_\mathrm{A}$ and $\mathbf{x}_\mathrm{B}$, so that $\mathbf{x}_\mathrm{B}$ is formed by deleting one or several variables in $\mathbf{x}_\mathrm{A}$. The respective regression-design matrices are denoted by $\mathbf{X}_\mathrm{A}$ and $\mathbf{X}_\mathrm{B}$, and their cross-products by $\mathbf{S}_\mathrm{AB} = \mathbf{X}_\mathrm{A}^\top\mathbf{X}_\mathrm{B}$, $\mathbf{S}_\mathrm{A} = \mathbf{X}_\mathrm{A}^\top\mathbf{X}_\mathrm{A}$, and the like. Denote by $\mathbf{x}_\mathrm{D}$ the vector of variables included in model A, but not in B. No generality is lost by assuming that $\mathbf{x}_\mathrm{D}$ comprises the right-most components of $\mathbf{x}_\mathrm{A}$, so that $\mathbf{x}_\mathrm{A} = (\mathbf{x}_\mathrm{B}, \mathbf{x}_\mathrm{D})$, and that $\mathbf{x}_\mathrm{B}$ and

Figure 11.7. The optimal shrinkage coefficients b^* for predicting y^* and for estimating σ^2 in simple regression. The curve drawn by dots approximates b^* in (11.21) by replacing $(n-2)/(n-1)$ with 1.0.

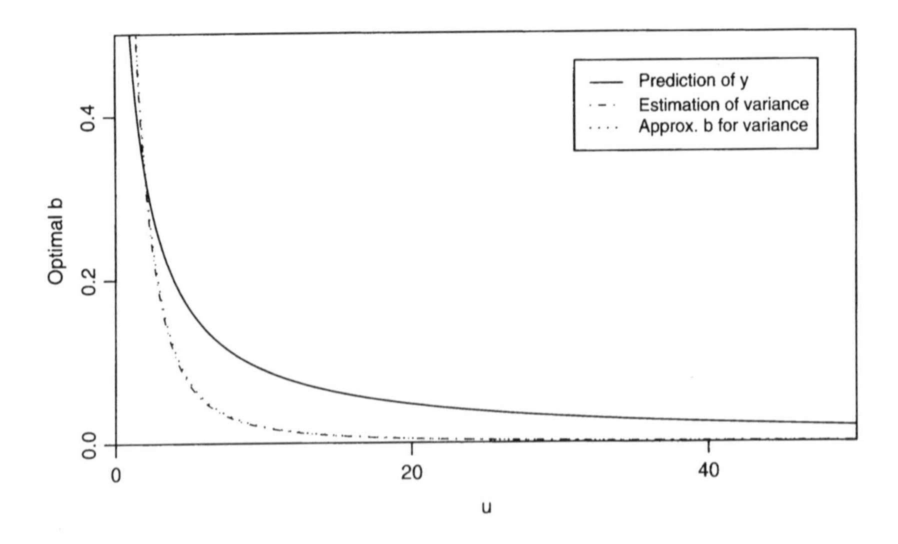

$\mathbf{x}_\mathrm{D}$ are orthogonal, $\mathbf{S}_\mathrm{BD} = \mathbf{0}$. Further, we assume that $\mathbf{x}_\mathrm{A}$ are centred; that is, $\mathbf{X}_\mathrm{A}^\top \mathbf{1}_n = (n, \mathbf{0})^\top$, where n is the sample size.

Let $\hat{y}_\mathrm{A}$ be the linear predictor of y for a vector of covariates $\mathbf{x}_\mathrm{A}^* = (\mathbf{x}_\mathrm{B}^*, \mathbf{x}_\mathrm{D}^*)$, based on the (valid) model A, and let $\hat{y}_\mathrm{B}$ be its counterpart based on model B; $\hat{y}_\mathrm{A} = \mathbf{x}_\mathrm{A}^* \hat{\boldsymbol{\beta}}_\mathrm{A}$ and $\hat{y}_\mathrm{B} = \mathbf{x}_\mathrm{B}^* \hat{\boldsymbol{\beta}}_\mathrm{B}$. To avoid trivial cases, we assume that $\mathbf{X}_\mathrm{A}$ is of full rank and $\mathbf{x}_\mathrm{D}^* \neq \mathbf{0}$.

The elements required for synthetic estimation are

$$
\begin{aligned}
V &= \sigma^2 \mathbf{x}_\mathrm{A}^* \mathbf{S}_\mathrm{A}^{-1} \mathbf{x}_\mathrm{A}^{*\top} \\
V_1 &= \sigma^2 \mathbf{x}_\mathrm{B}^* \mathbf{S}_\mathrm{B}^{-1} \mathbf{x}_\mathrm{B}^{*\top} \\
C &= \sigma^2 \mathbf{x}_\mathrm{B}^* \mathbf{S}_\mathrm{B}^{-1} \mathbf{x}_\mathrm{B}^{*\top} \\
D &= -\mathbf{x}_\mathrm{D}^* \boldsymbol{\beta}_\mathrm{D} \,,
\end{aligned}
$$

derived directly from the expressions $\hat{\boldsymbol{\beta}}_\mathrm{A} = \mathbf{S}_\mathrm{A}^{-1} \mathbf{X}_\mathrm{A}^\top \mathbf{y}$ and $\hat{\boldsymbol{\beta}}_\mathrm{B} = \mathbf{S}_\mathrm{B}^{-1} \mathbf{X}_\mathrm{B}^\top \mathbf{y}$, its equivalent for model B, and realising that $\mathbf{S}_\mathrm{BD} = \mathbf{X}_\mathrm{B}^\top \mathbf{X}_\mathrm{D} = \mathbf{0}$.

The optimal coefficient is

$$
b^* = \left\{ 1 + \frac{(\mathbf{x}_\mathrm{D}^* \boldsymbol{\beta}_\mathrm{D})^2}{\sigma^2 \mathbf{x}_\mathrm{D}^* \mathbf{S}_\mathrm{D}^{-1} \mathbf{x}_\mathrm{D}^{*\top}} \right\}^{-1} .
$$

Unlike in the univariate case, b^* depends on the value of $\mathbf{x}^*$. However, it depends on $\mathbf{x}^*$ only through the direction of its subvector $\mathbf{x}^*_{\mathrm{D}}$, as $\mathbf{x}^*_{\mathrm{D}}$ and $c\mathbf{x}^*_{\mathrm{D}}$ are associated with the same coefficient b^* for any $c \neq 0$.

For problems with several candidate models, no conceptual difficulties arise, as the vector $\mathbf{P}$ and matrix $\mathbf{Q}$ defined in (11.9) require variances, covariances and biases, all of them assuming the validity of the 'super'-model 0, similar to the case of two candidate models. The vector $\mathbf{P}$ and matrix $\mathbf{Q}$ have to be estimated but, apart from σ^2, the only uncertainty is about the biases, linear functions of $\boldsymbol{\beta}$, whose squares and cross-products contribute to $\mathbf{Q}$. The analysis of the synthetic estimator with two candidate models suggests that overestimation of the variances and underestimation of the covariances in $\mathbf{Q}$ contribute to efficiency, but it is difficult to formulate a general rule about the extent of such an adjustment that is useful.

In problems with many alternative models, the matrix $\mathbf{Q}$ is likely to be ill-conditioned. This can be interpreted that there are numerous competing compositions of the single-model based estimators that are close to the ideal synthetic estimator. As $\mathbf{Q}$ is estimated, and the inverse of the estimate used, the naive (or probably any other) estimator of $\hat{\mathbf{b}}^*$ is not very efficient, the advantage of the wide space of compositions is not converted to efficient estimation. The handicap of a narrower space of compositions may be overcome by more efficient estimation of the elements of $\mathbf{Q}^{-1}$ when $\mathbf{Q}$ has smaller dimensions.

The balance between casting our 'modelling net' too wide and focussing on too small a set of models is difficult to find and insights by other means than from simulations are hard to come by. Making sure that *the* 'good' model is not omitted is essential, but it does not guarantee efficient estimation. In model selection approaches, this model or its close competitor has to be identified. In synthetic estimation submodels of the minimal valid model may contribute to more efficient estimation, but do not necessarily outweigh the influence of some of its submodels.

11.6 Discussion

An obvious limitation of the synthetic estimator is that a large system of linear equations, $\hat{\mathbf{b}}^* = \hat{\mathbf{Q}}^{-1}\hat{\mathbf{P}}$, has to be solved, with each quantity involved in $\mathbf{P}$ and $\mathbf{Q}$ estimated. Thus, ill-conditioning and non-linear transformation of an estimator may conspire to erode the efficiency of the synthetic estimator. In contrast, model selection does not encounter such problems because the selection can be conducted in stages. However, each of these stages is problematic, and the deficiencies are likely to compound over the stages. Synthetic estimation can also be conducted in stages. The candidate models are divided into groups and synthesis is first applied in each group separately. Synthesis is then applied 'across' the groups, by combining the within-group synthetic estimators. Some efficiency is lost in the process but synthesis becomes computationally manageable. If the synthesis within a group is still not manageable, the models in the group can be sub-divided and synthesis carried out in another stage. While conventional model selection works, in effect, on the same principle, with choice made between pairs of models, multi-stage synthesis is more flexible because elementary synthesis can be applied to several models at a time, limited only by the concerns about robustness and stability of $\hat{\mathbf{Q}}^{-1}$. In other words, multi-stage model selection can be improved by replacing each model selection step by synthesis, and further improvement is achieved by reducing the number of stages. The term 'improvement' has to be qualified carefully. Synthesis is not uniformly more efficient than model selection but, in ordinary regression, it protects inferences from excessive deficiencies. The estimated conditional sampling variance $\hat{s}^2_{\mathcal{M}}$ underestimates the unconditional MSE of the selected-model based estimator, and the cause of such dishonesty is not only the unacknowledged bias of $\hat{\theta}_{\mathcal{M}}$.

The synthetic estimator is also biased, and there is no unbiased estimator of its MSE. The naively estimated MSE of the ideal synthetic estimator underestimates the MSE of the estimator $\hat{\theta}^{\mathrm{S}}(\hat{b}^*)$, but the underestimation is not as blatant as with model selection.

Identifying a dataset, together with its context, with a single (minimal valid) model is an attractive proposition, but it is a poor practice to disregard models that come in a close second in a contest in which the judging is imperfect. Using an estimator or any other form of inference based on the model that won the contest, even if correctly selected, is not as efficient as generally perceived because the estimator based on an invalid submodel may be more efficient. And the combination of the two estimators may be more efficient still. This suggests that the generally adopted standard of ML estimation with the appropriate model should be raised to the *optimal combination* of the ML estimators for such a model and for (some of) its submodels. The ML estimator with a valid model is efficient only asymptotically; for finite samples, submodels can contribute to the efficiency. Reference [163] presents an example in which a patently inappropriate model, which describes the modelled setting very poorly, is assigned a weight close to unity for estimating a quantity of interest. Of course, for another quantity, a different combination of the single-model based estimators is used.

One purpose of model selection is to eliminate unimportant covariates. Synthetic estimation provides an alternative to hypothesis testing, although it may appear as rather relunctant to discard any covariates. With synthesis, it is appropriate to discard a covariate if the coefficient associated with any model that involves it is very small for the range of inferences (targets) considered. This requires specifying the range of targets as well as the threshold b° for which any model with coefficient $|\,\hat{b}^*\,| < b^\circ$ would be regarded as redundant. (In principle, the coefficient b^* may be negative.) A more rigorous criterion may be that, if all models that involve the covariate in question are discarded, the MSE of the synthetic estimator is increased by not more than a given threshold for every target. Of course, it is not advisable to propose a threshold that would be suitable as a convention, similar to the 5% level of significance in hypothesis testing.

Nuisance parameters are quantities that are not involved in the target of estimation, but the estimator of the target and its distribution depend on their values. Handling nuisance parameters is an issue related to model selection. Should the target be estimated using the estimated values of the nuisance parameters, or should a default value, such as $\mathbf{0}$, be assumed for them? The latter option is attractive because the reduced model it implies is associated with greater efficiency *if* the reduction is appropriate. Synthetic estimation arbitrates between these two extreme positions, and moves the problem from the dichotomy to a continuum, searching for the best combination of the alternative single-model based estimators.

11.7 Other applications of synthesis

Synthesis is applicable generally, whenever there is a set of alternative estimators of a target. Simply, instead of choosing one of them, aiming to match the efficiency of the most efficient of them, the estimators are combined; the combination may be more efficient than either of the candidate estimators.

11.7.1 Meta-analysis

In *meta-analysis*, studies $k = 1, \ldots, K$ are conducted, each yielding an unbiased estimator $\hat{\theta}_k$, and its associated estimated sampling variance $\hat{s}_k^2$. The studies aim to estimate the same quantity θ, such as a treatment effect that applies universally to all the (human) subjects suffering from a particular condition. As a consequence of the study-specific settings, conventions, measurement and assessment instruments, and the like, the estimators $\hat{\theta}_k$ are not unbiased for θ, although they are unbiased for the context specific to study k. For example, the studies may be conducted in different countries, different years, recruiting subjects through different agents or channels, and using slightly different protocols. The estimators based on most studies have sampling variances that are too large for a particular purpose, so pooling information across the studies is necessary. Also, it would be a waste not to take advantage of all the studies, since they relate to the same set of treatments and the biases for settings different from any specific study are at most moderate.

Standard approaches to meta-analysis estimate θ assuming that the study-specific parameters are a random sample from a distribution centred around θ. An alternative viewpoint accepts that there is no universal treatment effect θ and defines a target θ^* that applies for a specific setting used by one of the studies, k^*, so that it is estimated without bias by $\hat{\theta}_{k^*}$. The other studies estimate this target with bias, but they can nevertheless contribute to estimating θ_{k^*}. No estimates of the biases are available, but they are known not to be very large. In fact, the between-study variance of θ_k, $k = 1, \ldots, K$, can be estimated, in analogy with small-area estimation. A conservative application of synthesis bases coefficients $\hat{\mathbf{b}}$ in the synthetic estimator $\hat{\theta}^{\mathrm{S}}_{k^*} = (1 - b_+)\hat{\theta}_{k^*} + \hat{\mathbf{b}}\hat{\boldsymbol{\theta}}_{-k^*}$ on an overestimate of the (squared) bias for each study. The squared bias can be replaced by the estimated study-level variance, or by its suitable overestimate. The resulting estimator combines the unbiased estimator with 'full' weight, reflecting its (estimated) sampling variance, and the other estimators with reduced weights, corresponding to their sampling variances inflated by a factor. Extensions of this approach impose a structure on the studies; some are closer to the context of the target, so the inflation factor for them is smaller than for studies with a more distant context. Such an approach can incorporate expert judgement; as it is subjective, it is essential to accompany it with a sensitivity analysis exploring some deviations from the adopted way of setting the coefficients $\mathbf{b}$.

11.7.2 Multiple sources and prior information

A typical setting with several estimators of the same quantity arises when several, say $K + 1$, studies are conducted independently, so that their estimators $\hat{\theta}_k$, $k = 0, \ldots, K$, of the same target θ are mutually independent. Meta-analysis can be regarded as their special case. Suppose the estimator for the study that is assigned index 0 has no bias. One of the estimators $\hat{\theta}_k$ has to be unbiased, or have a known bias, otherwise the problem of estimating θ is ill-posed. When all the estimators are unbiased, synthesis yields the estimator that combines the single-study estimators with coefficients that reflect their relative precisions. To show this, we evaluate the vector of ideal coefficients $\mathbf{b}^*$, given that the vector of covariances $\mathbf{C}$ vanishes:

$$\mathbf{b}^* = \left(\mathbf{V} + V_0\mathbf{1}\mathbf{1}^\top\right)^{-1}\mathbf{1}V_0 ,$$

where $\mathbf{V}$ is the (diagonal) sampling variance matrix of the estimators $\hat{\boldsymbol{\theta}} = (\hat{\theta}_1, \ldots, \hat{\theta}_K)^\top$. The inverse of the matrix can be expressed as

$$\left(\mathbf{V} + V_0\mathbf{1}\mathbf{1}^\top\right)^{-1} = \mathbf{V}^{-1} - \mathbf{V}^{-1}\frac{V_0}{1 + \mathbf{1}^\top\mathbf{V}^{-1}\mathbf{1}V_0}\mathbf{1}\mathbf{1}^\top\mathbf{V}^{-1} ,$$

and hence

$$\begin{aligned}
\mathbf{b}^* &= \left(\mathbf{I} - \mathbf{V}^{-1}\frac{V_0}{1 + \mathbf{1}^\top\mathbf{V}^{-1}\mathbf{1}V_0}\mathbf{1}\mathbf{1}^\top\right)\mathbf{V}^{-1}\mathbf{1}V_0 \\
&= \frac{1}{1/V_0 + \mathbf{1}^\top\mathbf{V}^{-1}\mathbf{1}}\mathbf{V}^{-1}\mathbf{1} .
\end{aligned}$$

The result now follows by realising that $\mathbf{V}^{-1}\mathbf{1}$ is the vector of the precisions (reciprocals of the variances) of the single-study estimators (with study 0 omitted), and $\mathbf{1}^\top \mathbf{V}^{-1}\mathbf{1}$ is their total. If another study is completed and its data becomes available, the synthesis need not be conducted for the $K+2$ studies because the combination is identical to the synthesis of the estimator based on studies $0, \ldots, K$ combined with the new study $K+1$. Such an updating would be suboptimal if the estimators were correlated.

The task of incorporating prior information in Bayesian analysis is a special case of such an updating. The prior information about θ is expressed in the form of a *prior distribution* θ_0 and data from a study (source) is used to update it and obtain the *posterior distribution* of θ. Without the Bayesian perspective and computational machinery, this task can be regarded as synthesis of the prior (old-data) and new (current-study) estimators of θ. With synthesis, we operate only with the first two moments (means and variances) of the estimators, so all evaluations are much simpler and require no input about the shapes and types of the distributions involved. In contrast, Bayes methods are much more involved, but their outcome is the posterior distribution of θ, a much more detailed and complete inferential statement, although the detail is sometimes difficult digest and interpret.

11.7.3 Secondary outcomes and auxiliary information

Studies designed to estimate a target θ, based on a variable y, often record several other variables $\mathbf{x}$ that are intended for other analyses, or to support the evidence obtained about the value of θ. They are referred to as *secondary* variables (or outcomes), and y as primary. Usually, the estimator based on y is treated formally and the estimators based on the secondary variables informally, leaving the interpretation largely to the client. The roles of the variables in $\mathbf{x}$ can be formalised by agreeing on the largest plausible bias associated with each variable and combining the single-variable based estimators, assuming these biases. The impact of the assumptions about the biases can be explored by sensitivity analysis.

This problem can be formulated also as estimating one component of the vector $\boldsymbol{\theta}$, say $\mathbf{w}^\top \boldsymbol{\theta}$, where $\mathbf{w} = (1, 0, \ldots, 0)^\top$. Apart from the obvious, estimating $\mathbf{w}^\top \boldsymbol{\theta}$ by $\mathbf{w}^\top \hat{\boldsymbol{\theta}}$, other convex combinations $\mathbf{u}^\top \hat{\boldsymbol{\theta}}$ may be considered. This may be useful when the components of $\hat{\boldsymbol{\theta}}$ are highly correlated. For example, $\hat{\theta}_2$ may contribute to estimating θ_1 when $\mathrm{var}(\hat{\theta}_2)$ is much smaller than $\mathrm{var}(\hat{\theta}_1)$, the two estimators are highly correlated, and the underlying quantities θ_1 and θ_2 differ insubstantially. In practice, a single realisation of $\hat{\boldsymbol{\theta}}$ cannot inform us about this, and so synthesis is not useful. When some external information is available, the auxiliary estimators in $\hat{\boldsymbol{\theta}}$ can be exploited, although the covariances and biases required for the synthesis are only estimated. Drawing parallels with multivariate shrinkage estimation for small areas is left as an exercise.

11.8 Suggested reading

The deficiency of ignoring model uncertainty is highlighted by [26] and [50]. However lucid and eloquent they may have been, much of the current statistical practice is firmly wedded to the idea of selecting one model — to find *the best* model, [137] and [122]. ANOVA is the most elementary example of this, familiar to most of us from university lectures and textbooks. The likelihood ratio is probably the most popular criterion used for model selection. The Akaike information criterion (AIC), the Bayes information criterion (BIC), [283], and Mallows' C_p, [176], are attempts to 'correct' some of its deficiencies. Reference [288], among others, shows that they come way short.

Although model selection is a quintessentially small-scale data problem (asymptotically, any model-related question is resolved correctly with high probability), there is scope for studying asymptotic properties of model selection procedures, [265] and [255].

Bayes factors is the subject of [123], [216] and [104] in the (original) Bayesian perspective and [103] formulate Bayes factors for the frequentist. The method described in this chapter was originally proposed by [163], expressing the 'heretical' view that bad (poorly fitting) models may be useful for estimation or prediction, and documenting it on an example.

The term and subject of meta-analysis were greatly promoted by [98]. It is the methodological staple of the systematic reviews, [280]. Publication bias is a term for the poor representation of the studies reported in the literature among all the conducted studies; [35] describes a sensitivity analysis that protects the inferences from this problem. A Bayesian method for pooling information across two samples is described in [54]. An open and unaddressed problem is how to deal with the fact that the collection of studies in a meta-analysis does not have a sampling design (even if every study did have one), and so the population of contexts may not be represented well among them.

11.9 Exercises

1. Generate a set of about $n = 50$ outcomes from a simple regression model (11.1) with the (non-constant) values of x specified in some simple way, such as $c, 2c, \ldots, nc$, and residual variance $\sigma^2 = 1$. Apply your favourite criterion for selecting between the models in (11.1) and (11.2). Replicate this exercise (with the same set of values of x) 1000 times and count the number of times each model is selected. Conduct a similar exercise with an (automatic) diagnostic procedure. Find, by trial and error, a regression slope β_1 for which either model is selected about the same number of times. Comment on the fallibility of both of these procedures.
2. Relate the mean and variance of the mixture $\hat{\theta}_{\mathcal{M}}$ in (11.3) to the means and variances of the single-model based estimators $\hat{\theta}_0, \ldots, \hat{\theta}_M$ when the selection $\mathcal{M}$ is independent of these estimators.

Hint: Express the moments of $\hat{\theta}_{\mathcal{M}}$ in terms of the conditional moments of $\hat{\theta}_{\mathcal{M}}$ given $\mathcal{M}$.

3. Describe and implement the EM algorithm for fitting a mixture of two (univariate or multivariate) normal distributions. For help, consult [44] or [184].
4. Review the theoretical results about the efficiency of the ML estimators (see, e.g., [37]) and relate them to how they are used (by yourself and others) in practice.
5. Replicate the example described in Section 11.1.2, not necessarily with the same values of the parameters and sample sizes. Use your favourite model selection criterion.
6. Prove the rules for matrix differentiation of a quadratic form, used in (11.10). Consult [173] if necessary.
7. Discuss the traditional way of using the (one-way) ANOVA table for a severely unbalanced design and assess the drawbacks of estimating the means of groups represented by the largest and smallest samples. Generalise the results about the ideal synthetic estimator for the ANOVA setting in Section 11.4 to unbalanced designs. Derive the corresponding minimax estimator (Section 11.4.1).
8. Compare the ideal shrinkage coefficients b_{μ_1} and b_{σ^2}, either graphically for a range of settings, or analytically as far as it is possible.
9. Prove the inequalities in (11.20) and discuss them in the context of a simple regression problem (real or simulated) of your choice. Explore the MSE of prediction, for a given value of x, as a function of an incorrect value of ω.
10. Derive the ideal synthetic estimator that minimises a criterion for efficiency different from the MSE. For example, if efficiency is defined by small $\mathrm{var}(\hat{\theta}) + r\{\mathrm{E}(\hat{\theta} - \theta)^2\}$, greater emphasis is placed on bias reduction when $r > 1$. Show that the coefficient b associated with a biased estimator is a decreasing function of r. Consider the limit $r \rightarrow +\infty$, and compare the limiting synthetic estimator with the preference for estimators based on valid models.
11. Consider the setting with $K + 1$ studies yielding mutually independent estimators $\hat{\theta}_k$, $k = 0, 1, \ldots, K$, of the same target θ. Let their sampling variances be v_k and suppose $\hat{\theta}_0$ is unbiased. Suppose further that the bias of each $\hat{\theta}_k$ does not exceed a positive value Δ_k. Show that the MSE of the synthetic estimator, that is based on the assumption that the biases are equal to Δ_k, is an increasing function of the bias of each estimator $\hat{\theta}_k$, and derive the loss of efficiency due to not knowing the biases.

    Hint: Define the ratios r_k of the bias of $\hat{\theta}_k$ and the largest plausible bias Δ_k.

References

1. Agresti, A.: *Categorical Data Analysis*. Wiley, New York (1990)
2. Aitkin, M.: A general maximum likelihood analysis of variance components in generalized linear models. *Biometrics* **55**, 117–128 (1999)
3. Aitkin, M., and Wilson, G. T.: Mixture models, outliers, and the EM algorithm. *Technometrics* **22**, 325–331 (1980)
4. Anderson, D., and Aitkin, M.: Variance component models with binary response: Interviewer variability. *Journal of the Royal Statistical Society* Ser. B **47**, 203–210 (1985)
5. Arora, V., and Lahiri, P.: On the superiority of the Bayesian method over the BLUP in small area estimation problems. *Statistica Sinica* **7**, 1053–1063 (1997)
6. Baker, S. G., Freedman, L. S., and Parmar, M. K. B.: Using replicate observations in observer agreement studies with binary assessments. *Biometrics* **47**, 1327–1338 (1991)
7. Balicki, A., and Szreder, M.: Usefulness of official registers in sample surveys in Poland. *Statistics in Transition* **3**, 315–328 (1997)
8. Barnard, J., and Meng, X.-L.: Applications of multiple imputation in medical studies: From AIDS to NHANES. *Statistical Methods in Medical Research* **8**, 17–36 (1999)
9. Barnard, J., and Rubin, D. B.: Small-sample degrees of freedom with multiple imputation. *Biometrika* **86**, 948–955 (1999)
10. Battese, G. E., Harter, R. M., and Fuller, W. A.: An error components model for prediction of county crop areas using survey and satellite data. *Journal of the American Statistical Association* **83**, 28–36 (1988)
11. Beale, E. M. L., and Little, R. J. A.: Missing values in multivariate analysis. *Journal of the Royal Statistical Society* Ser. B **37**, 129–146 (1975)
12. Becker, M. P., Yang, I., and Lange, K.: EM algorithms without missing data. *Statistical Methods in Medical Research* **6**, 38–54 (1997)
13. Becker, N. G.: Uses of the EM algorithm in the analysis of data on HIV/AIDS and other infectious diseases. *Statistics in Medical Research* **6**, 24–37 (1997)
14. Becker, R. A., Chambers, J. M., and Wilks, A. R.: *The New S Language. A Programming Environment for Data Analysis and Graphics*. Wadsworth & Brooks/Cole, Pacific Grove, CA (1988)

15. Belin, T. R., Diffendal, G., Mack, S., Rubin, D. B., Schafer, J. L., and Zaslavsky, A.: Hierarchical logistic regression models for imputation of unresolved enumeration status in undercount estimation. *Journal of the American Statistical Association* **88**, 1149–1159 (1993)
16. Belin, T. R., and Rubin, D. B.: A method for calibrating false match rates in record linkage. *Journal of the American Statistical Association* **90**, 694–707 (1995)
17. Berry, C. C., Flatt, S. W., and Pierce, J. P.: Correcting unit nonresponse via response modeling and raking in the California Tobacco Survey. *Journal of Official Statistics* **12**, 349–363 (1996)
18. Binder, D. A., and Théberge, A.: Estimation of the variance of raking-ratio estimators. *Canadian Journal of Statistics* **16** Suppl. 47–55 (1988)
19. Booth, J. G., and Hobert, J. P.: Standard errors of prediction in generalized linear mixed models. *Journal of the American Statistical Association* **83**, 262–272 (1998)
20. Booth, J. G., and Hobert, J. P. M.: Maximizing generalized linear mixed model likelihoods with an automated Monte Carlo EM algorithm. *Journal of the Royal Statistical Society* Ser. B **61**, 265–285 (1999)
21. Brackstone, G. J., and Rao, J. N. K.: An investigation of raking ratio estimation. *Sankhyā* Ser. C **41**, 97–114 (1979)
22. Breslow, N. E., and Clayton, D.: Approximate inference in generalised linear mixed models. *Journal of the American Statistical Association* **88**, 9–25 (1993)
23. van Buuren, S., Boshuizen, H. C., and Knook, D. L.: Multiple imputation of missing blood pressure covariates in survival analysis. *Statistics in Medicine* **18**, 681–694 (1999)
24. Carlin, B. P., and Louis, T. A.: *Bayes and Empirical Bayes Methods for Data Analysis.* Chapman and Hall, London (1996)
25. Carroll, R. J., Ruppert, D., and Stefanski, L. A.: *Measurement Error in Nonlinear Models.* Chapman and Hall, London (1995)
26. Chatfield, C.: Model uncertainty, data mining and statistical inference. *Journal of the Royal Statistical Society* Ser. A **158**, 419–466 (1995)
27. Citro, C. F., and Kalton, G. (eds): *Small-Area Income and Poverty Estimates. Priorities for 2000 and Beyond.* National Academy Press, Washington, DC (2000)
28. Clayton, D., and Rasbash, J.: Estimation in large crossed random-effect models by data augmentation. *Journal of the Royal Statistical Society* Ser. A **162**, 425–436 (1999)
29. Clogg, C. C., Rubin, D. B., Schenker, N., Schultz, B., and Weidman, L.: Multiple imputation of industry and occupation codes in census public-use samples using Bayesian logistic regression. *Journal of the American Statistical Association* **86**, 68–78 (1991)
30. Cochran, W. G.: *Sampling Techniques.* 3rd ed. Wiley, New York (1977)
31. Coles, S. G., and Dixon, M. J.: Likelihood-based inference for extreme value models. *Extremes* **2**, 5–23 (1999)
32. Cook, J., and Stefanski, L. A.: A simulation-extrapolation method for parametric measurement error models. *Journal of the American Statistical Association* **89**, 1314–1328 (1994)

33. Copas, A. J., and Farewell, V. T.: Dealing with non-ignorable non-response by using an 'enthusiasm-to-respond' variable. *Journal of the Royal Statistical Society* Ser. A **161**, 385–396 (1998)
34. Copas, J. B., and Li, H. G.: Inference for non-random samples. *Journal of the Royal Statistical Society* Ser. B **59**, 55–95 (1997)
35. Copas, J. B., and Shi, J. Q.: A sensitivity analysis for publication bias in systematic reviews. *Statistics in Medicine* **20**, 251–265 (2001)
36. Cox, D. R.: Regression models and life tables. *Journal of the Royal Statistical Society* Ser. B **34**, 187–220 (1972)
37. Cox, D. R., and Hinkley, D. V.: *Theoretical Statistics.* Chapman and Hall, London (1974)
38. Cox, D. R., and Oakes, D.: *Analysis of Survival Data.* Chapman and Hall, London (1984)
39. Czajka, J. L., Hirabayashi, S. M., Little, R. J. A., and Rubin, D. B.: Projecting from advance data using propensity modeling: An application to income and tax statistics. *Journal of Business and Economic Statistics* **10**, 117–131 (1992)
40. d'Agostino, R. B.: Propensity score methods for bias reduction in the comparison of a treatment to a non-randomized control group. *Statistics in Medicine* **17**, 2265–2281 (1998)
41. Dalgaard, P.: *Introductory Statistics with R.* Springer, New York (2002)
42. Datta, G. S., Day, B., and Basawa, I.: Empirical best linear unbiased and empirical Bayes prediction in multivariate small area estimation. *Journal of Statistical Planning and Inference* **75**, 269–279 (1999)
43. Deeley, J. J., and Smith, A. F. M.: Quantitative refinements for comparisons of institutional performance. *Journal of the Royal Statistical Society* Ser. B **161**, 5–12 (1998)
44. Dempster, A. P., Laird, N. M., and Rubin, D. B.: Maximum likelihood for incomplete data via the EM algorithm. *Journal of the Royal Statistical Society* Ser. B **39**, 1–38 (1977)
45. Dempster, A. P., Rubin, D. B., and Tsutakawa, R. K.: Estimation in covariance component models. *Journal of the American Statistical Association* **76**, 341–353 (1981)
46. Deville, J.-C., and Särndal, C.-E.: Calibration estimators in survey sampling. *Journal of the American Statistical Association* **87**, 376–382 (1992)
47. Deville, J.-C., Särndal, C.-E., and Sautory, O.: Generalized raking procedures in survey sampling. *Journal of the American Statistical Association* **88**, 1013–1020 (1993)
48. Diggle, P., and Kenward, M. G.: Informative drop-out in longitudinal data analysis. *Applied Statistics* **43**, 49–93 (1994)
49. Drake, C.: Effects of misspecification of the propensity score on estimators of treatment effect. *Biometrics* **49**, 1231–1236 (1993)
50. Draper, D.: Assessment and propagation of model uncertainty. *Journal of the Royal Statistical Society* Ser. B **57**, 45–97 (1995)
51. Draper, N. R., and Smith, H.: *Applied Regression Analysis.* 2nd ed. Wiley, New York (1981)
52. Drew, J. D., Singh, M. P., and Choudry, G. H.: Evaluation of small area estimation techniques for the Canadian Labour Force Survey. *Survey Methodology* **8**, 17–46 (1982)

53. Duncan, T. E., Duncan, S. C., and Li, F.: A comparison of model- and multiple imputation-based approaches to longitudinal analyses with partial missingness. *Structural Equation Modelling* **5**, 1–21 (1998)
54. van Eeden, C., and Zidek, J. V.: Combining the data from two normal populations to estimate the mean of one when their means difference is bounded. *Journal of Multivariate Analysis* **88**, 19–46 (2004)
55. Efron, B., and Morris, C.: Limiting the risk of Bayes and empirical Bayes estimators — Part I: The Bayes case. *Journal of the American Statistical Association* **66**, 807–815 (1971)
56. Efron, B., and Morris, C.: Limiting the risk of Bayes and empirical Bayes estimators — Part II: The empirical Bayes case. *Journal of the American Statistical Association* **67**, 130–139 (1972)
57. Efron, B., and Morris, C.: Stein's estimation rule and its competitors — an empirical Bayes approach. *Journal of the American Statistical Association* **68**, 117–130 (1973)
58. Efron, B., and Morris, C.: Data analysis using Stein's estimator and its generalizations. *Journal of the American Statistical Association* **70**, 311–319 (1975)
59. Ericksen, E.: A method of combining sample survey data and symptomatic indicators to obtain population estimates for local areas. *Demography* **10**, 147–160 (1973)
60. Ericksen, E.: A regression method for estimating population changes of local areas. *Journal of the American Statistical Association* **69**, 867–875 (1974)
61. Ewing, J. A.: Detecting alcoholism: The CAGE questionnaire. *Journal of the American Medical Association* **252**, 1905–1907 (1984)
62. Falorsi, P. D., Falorsi, S., and Russo, A.: Empirical comparison of small area estimation methods for the Italian Labour Force Survey. *Survey Methodology* **20**, 171–178 (1994)
63. Falorsi, P. D., and Russo, A.: A conditional analysis of some small area estimators in two stage sampling. *Journal of Official Statistics* **15**, 537–550 (1999)
64. Faucett, C. L., Schenker, N., and Taylor, J. M. G.: Survival analysis using auxiliary variables via multiple imputation, with application to AIDS clinical trial data. *Biometrics* **58**, 37–47 (2002)
65. Fay, R. E.: Application of multivariate regression to small domain estimation. In: Platek, R., Rao, J. N. K., Särndal, C.-E., and Singh, M. P. (eds), *Small Area Statistics. An International Symposium,* pp. 91–102. Wiley, New York (1987)
66. Fay, R. E.: Alternative paradigms for the analysis of imputed survey data. *Journal of the American Statistical Association* **91**, 490–498 (1996)
67. Fay, R. E., and Herriot, R. A.: Estimates of income for small places: an application of James-Stein procedures to census data. *Journal of the American Statistical Association* **74**, 269–277 (1979)
68. Fitzmaurice, G. M., Heath, A. F., and Clifford, P.: Logistic regression models for binary panel data with attrition. *Journal of the Royal Statistical Society* Ser. A **159**, 249–263 (1996)
69. Fitzmaurice, G. M., and Laird, N. M.: Regression models for mixed discrete and continuous responses with potentially missing values. *Biometrics* **53**, 110–122 (1997)

70. Fitzmaurice, G. M., Laird, N. M., and Lipsitz, S., R.: Analysing incomplete longitudinal binary responses: A likelihood-based approach. *Biometrics* **50**, 601–612 (1994)
71. Fitzmaurice, G. M., Laird, N. M., and Zahner, G. E. P.: Multivariate logistic models for incomplete binary responses. *Journal of the American Statistical Association* **91**, 99–108 (1996)
72. Friedl, H., and Kauermann, G.: Standard errors for EM estimates in generalized linear models with random effects. *Biometrics* **56**, 761–767 (2000)
73. Fuller, W. A.: *Measurement Error Models.* Wiley, New York (1987)
74. Gambino, J., and Dick, P.: Small area estimation practice at Statistics Canada. *Statistics in Transition* **4**, 597–610 (2000)
75. Gelfand, A. E., and Smith, A. F. M.: Sampling-based approaches to calculating marginal densities. *Journal of the American Statistical Association* **85**, 398–409 (1990)
76. Gelfand, A. E., Hills, S. E., Racine-Poon, A., and Smith, A. F. M.: Illustration of Bayesian inference in normal data models using Gibbs sampling. *Journal of the American Statistical Association* **85**, 972–985 (1990)
77. Gelman, A., Carlin, J. B., Stern, H. S., and Rubin, D. B.: *Bayesian Data Analysis.* Chapman and Hall, London (1995)
78. Gelman, A., King, G., and Liu, C.: Not asked and not answered: Multiple imputation for multiple surveys. *Journal of the American Statistical Association* **93**, 846–857 (1998)
79. Gelman, A., and Price, P. N.: All maps of parameter estimates are misleading. *Statistics in Medicine* **18**, 3221–3234 (1999)
80. Ghosh, M., and Lahiri, P.: A hierarchical Bayes approach to small area estimation with auxiliary information. In: Goel, P. K., and Iyengar, N. S. (eds), *Bayesian Analysis in Statistics and Econometrics*, pp. 107–125. Springer, New York (1992)
81. Ghosh, M., Nangia, N., and Kim, D. H.: Estimation of median income of four-person families: A Bayesian time series approach. *Journal of the American Statistical Association* **91**, 1423–1431 (1996)
82. Ghosh, M., Natarajan, K., Stroud, T. W. F., and Carlin, B.: Generalized linear models for small-area estimation. *Journal of the American Statistical Association* **93**, 273–282 (1998)
83. Ghosh, M., and Rao, J. N. K.: Small area estimation. An appraisal. *Statistical Science* **9**, 55–93 (1994)
84. Gilks, W. R., Richardson, S., and Spiegelhalter, D. J.: *Markov Chain Monte Carlo Methods in Practice.* Chapman and Hall, London (1996)
85. Goldstein, H.: *Multilevel Statistical Models.* 2nd ed. Edward Arnold, London (1995)
86. Goldstein, H., and Rasbash, J.: Improved approximations for multilevel models with binary responses. *Journal of the Royal Statistical Society* Ser. A **159**, 505–513 (1996)
87. Goldstein, H., and Spiegelhalter, D.: League tables and their limitations: Statistical issues in comparisons of institutional performance. *Journal of the Royal Statistical Society* Ser. A **159**, 385–443 (1996)
88. Gonzalez, M. E., and Hoza, C.: Small-area estimation with application to unemployment and housing estimates. *Journal of the American Statistical Association* **73**, 7–15 (1978)

89. Green, E. J., and Strawderman, W. E.: A James-Stein type estimator for combining unbiased and possibly biased estimators. *Journal of the American Statistical Association* **86**, 1001–1006 (1991)
90. Green, P. J.: On the use of the EM algorithm for penalized likelihood estimation. *Journal of the Royal Statistical Society* Ser. B **52**, 443–452 (1990)
91. Hartley, H. O.: Maximum likelihood estimation from incomplete data. *Biometrics* **14**, 783–823 (1958)
92. Hartley, H. O., and Hocking, R. R.: The analysis of incomplete data. *Biometrics* **27**, 783–808 (1971)
93. Hartley, H. O., and Rao, J. N. K.: Maximum likelihood estimation for the mixed analysis of variance model. *Biometrika* **54**, 93–108 (1967)
94. Harville, D. A.: Bayesian inference for variance components using only error contrasts. *Biometrika* **61**, 383–385 (1974)
95. Harville, D. A.: Maximum likelihood approaches to variance component estimation and to related problems. *Journal of the American Statistical Association* **72**, 320–340 (1977)
96. Harville, D. A.: *Matrix Algebra from a Statistician's Perspective.* Springer, New York (1985)
97. Healy, M. J., and Westmacott, M.: Missing values in experiments analyzed on automatic computers. *Applied Statistics* **5**, 203–206 (1956)
98. Hedges, L. V., and Olkin, I.: *Statistical Methods for Meta-analysis.* Academic Press, New York (1985)
99. Heitjan, D. F., and Little, R. J. A.: Multiple imputation for the Fatal Accident Reporting System. *Applied Statistics* **40**, 13–29 (1991)
100. Heitjan, D. F., and Rubin, D. B.: Inference from coarse data via multiple imputation with application to age heaping. *Journal of the American Statistical Association* **85**, 304–314 (1990)
101. Hemmerle, W. J., and Hartley, H. O.: Computing maximum likelihood estimates for the mixed A.O.V. model using the W transformation. *Technometrics* **15**, 819–831 (1973)
102. Henderson, C. R.: Estimation of variance and covariance components. *Biometrics* **9**, 226–252 (1953)
103. Hjort, N. L., and Claeskens, G.: Frequentist model average estimators. *Journal of the American Statistical Association* **98**, 879–899 (2003)
104. Hoeting, J., Madigan, D., Raftery, A. E., and Volinsky, C. T.: Bayesian model averaging: A tutorial. *Statistical Science* **14**, 381–417 (1998)
105. Holt, D., and Holmes, D. J.: Small domain estimation for unequal probability survey designs. *Survey Methodology* **20**, 23–31 (1994)
106. Holt, D., and Smith, T. M. F.: Post stratification. *Journal of the Royal Statistical Society* Ser. A **142**, 33–46 (1979)
107. Holt, D., Smith, T. M. F., and Tomberlin, T. J.: A model-based approach to estimation for small subgroups of a population. *Journal of the American Statistical Association* **74**, 405–410 (1979)
108. Hopke, P. K., Liu, C., and Rubin, D. B.: Multiple imputation for multivariate data with missing and below-threshold measurements: Time-series concentrations of pollutants in the Arctic. *Biometrics* **57**, 22–33 (2001)
109. Horton, N. J., and Lipsitz, S. R.: Multiple imputation in practice: Comparison of software packages for regression models with missing variables *American Statistician* **55**, 244–254 (2001)

110. House Condition Survey Team, Communities Scotland: Scottish House Condition Survey 2002. Communities Scotland, Edinburgh (2002)
111. Ibrahim, J. G., and Lipsitz, S. R.: Parameter estimation from incomplete data in binomial regression when the missing data mechanism is nonignorable. *Biometrics* **52**, 1071–1078 (1996)
112. Ibrahim, J. G., Lipsitz, S. R., and Chen, M.-H.: Missing covariates in generalized linear models when the missing data mechanism is non-ignorable. *Journal of the Royal Statistical Society* Ser. B **61**, 173–190 (1999)
113. Ibrahim, J. G., and Weisberg, S.: Incomplete data in generalized linear models with continuous covariates. *Australian Journal of Statistics* **34**, 461–470 (1992)
114. Ihaka, R., and Gentleman, R.: R: A language for data analysis and graphics. *Journal of Computational and Graphical Statistics* **5**, 299–314 (1996)
115. James, W., and Stein, C.: Estimation with quadratic loss. In: *Proceedings of the 4th Berkeley Symposium on Mathematical Statistics and Probability*, Vol. 1., pp. 361–379. University of California Press, Berkeley, CA. (1961)
116. Jamshidian, M., and Jennrich, R. I.: Conjugate gradient acceleration of the EM algorithm. *Journal of the American Statistical Association* **88**, 221–228 (1993)
117. Jamshidian, M., and Jennrich, R. I.: Acceleration of the EM algorithm by using quasi-Newton methods. *Journal of the Royal Statistical Society* Ser. B **59**, 569–587 (1997)
118. Jansen, R. C.: Maximum likelihood in a generalized linear finite mixture model by using the EM algorithm. *Biometrics* **49**, 227–231 (1993)
119. Jennrich, R. I., and Sampson, P. F.: Newton-Raphson and related algorithms for maximum likelihood variance component estimation. *Technometrics* **18**, 11–17 (1976)
120. Johnson, E. G., Mazzeo, J., and Kline, D. L.: NAEP Technical Report of the NAEP 1992 Trial State Assessment Program in Mathematics. National Center for Educational Statistics, Washington, DC (1993)
121. Judge, G. G., and Mittelhammer, R. C.: A semiparametric basis for combining estimation problems under quadratic loss. *Journal of the American Statistical Association* **99**, 479–287 (2004)
122. Kadane, J. B., and Lazar, N. A.: Methods and criteria for model selection. *Journal of the American Statistical Association* **99**, 279–290 (2004)
123. Kass, R. E., and Raftery, A. E.: Bayes factors. *Journal of the American Statistical Association* **90**, 773–795 (1995)
124. Kish, L.: *Survey Sampling.* Wiley, New York (1965)
125. Lahiri, P., and Rao, J. N. K.: Robust estimation of the mean square error of small area predictors. *Journal of the American Statistical Association* **90**, 758–766 (1995)
126. Laird, N. M., and Louis, T. A.: Empirical Bayes ranking methods. *Journal of Educational Statistics* **14**, 29–46 (1989)
127. Lange, K.: A quasi Newton acceleration of the EM algorithm. *Statistica Sinica* **5**, 1–18 (1995)
128. Lange, K.: *Numerical Analysis for Statisticians.* Springer, New York (1999)
129. Lange, N., and Ryan, L.: Assessing normality in random effects models. *Annals of Statistics* **17**, 624–643 (1989)
130. Langford, I. H., and Lewis, T.: Outliers in multivariate data. *Journal of the Royal Statistical Society* Ser. A **161**, 121–160 (1998)

131. Lee, Y. and Nelder, J. A.: Hierarchical generalized linear models. *Journal of the Royal Statistical Society* Ser. B **58**, 619–678 (1996)
132. Lee, Y. and Nelder, J. A.: Hierarchical generalized linear models: a synthesis of generalised linear models, random effect models and structured dispersions. *Biometrika* **88**, 987–1006 (2001)
133. Lehtonen, R., and Djerf, K. (eds): Lecture notes on estimation for population domains and small areas. (M. Ghosh: Model-dependent small area estimation — Theory and practice; C.-E. Särndal: Design-based methodologies for domain estimation) Proceedings of the Symposium on Advances in Domain Estimation. *Reviews* 2001/5. Statistics Finland, Helsinki (2001)
134. Lesaffre, E., and Spiessens, B.: On the effect of the number of quadrature points in logistic random-effects model: An example. *Applied Statistics* **50**, 325–335 (2001)
135. Li, K. H., Meng, X.-L., Raghunathan, T. E., and Rubin, D. B.: Significance levels from repeated p values with multiply-imputed data. *Statistica Sinica* **1**, 65–92 (1991)
136. Li, K. H., Raghunathan, T. E., and Rubin, D. B.: Large-sample significance levels from multiply imputed data using moment-based statistics and an F distribution. *Journal of the American Statistical Association* **86**, 1065–1073 (1991)
137. Lindley, D. V.: The choice of variables in multiple regression. *Journal of the Royal Statistical Society* Ser. B **30**, 31–66 (1968)
138. Lindstrom, M. J., and Bates, D. M.: Newton-Raphson and EM algorithms for linear mixed-effects models for repeated measures data. *Journal of the American Statistical Association* **83**, 1014–1022 (1988)
139. Lipsitz, S. R., and Ibrahim, J. G.: A conditional model for incomplete covariates in parametric regression models. *Biometrika* **83**, 916–922 (1996)
140. Lipsitz, S. R., Ibrahim, J. G., and Fitzmaurice, G. M.: Likelihood methods for incomplete longitudinal binary responses with incomplete categorical covariates. *Biometrics* **55**, 214–223 (1999)
141. Lipsitz, S. R., Zhao, L. P., and Molenberghs, G.: A semiparametric method of multiple imputation. *Journal of the Royal Statistical Society* Ser. B **60**, 127–144 (1998)
142. Little, R. J. A.: Survey nonresponse adjustments for estimates of means. *International Statistical Review* **54**, 139–157 (1986)
143. Little, R. J. A.: Regression with missing X's: A review. *Journal of the American Statistical Association* **87**, 1227–1237 (1992)
144. Little, R. J. A.: Pattern-mixture models for multivariate incomplete data. *Journal of the American Statistical Association* **88**, 125–134 (1993)
145. Little, R. J. A.: Modelling the drop-out mechanism in repeated-measures studies. *Journal of the American Statistical Association* **90**, 1112–1121 (1995)
146. Little, R. J. A., and Rubin, D. B.: *Statistical Analysis with Missing Data.* 2nd ed. Wiley, New York (2002)
147. Little, R. J. A., and Schluchter, M. D.: Maximum likelihood for mixed continuous and categorical data. *Biometrika* **72**, 497–512 (1985)
148. Little, R. J. A., and Wang, Y.: Pattern-mixture models for multivariate incomplete data with covariates. *Biometrics* **52**, 98–111 (1996)

149. Longford, N. T.: A fast scoring algorithm for maximum likelihood estimation in unbalanced mixed models with nested random effects. *Biometrika* **74**, 817–827 (1987)
150. Longford, N. T.: *Random Coefficient Models.* Oxford University Press, Oxford (1993)
151. Longford, N. T.: Logistic regression with random coefficients. *Computational Statistics and Data Analysis* **17**, 1–15 (1994)
152. Longford, N. T.: *Models for Uncertainty in Educational Testing.* Springer, New York (1995)
153. Longford, N. T.: Small-area estimation using adjustment by covariates. *Qüestió* **20**, 187–212 (1996)
154. Longford, N. T.: Shrinkage estimation of linear combinations of true scores. *Psychometrika* **62**, 237–244 (1997)
155. Longford, N. T.: An experiment in primary health care provision. *Journal of the Royal Statistical Society* Ser. A **162**, 291–302 (1999)
156. Longford, N. T.: Multivariate shrinkage estimation of small-area means and proportions. *Journal of the Royal Statistical Society* Ser. A **162**, 227–245 (1999)
157. Longford, N. T.: Multiple imputation in an international database of social science surveys. *ZA-Information,* **46**, 72–95 (2000)
158. Longford, N. T.: On estimating the standard errors in multilevel analysis. *The Statistician* **49**, 389–398 (2000)
159. Longford, N. T.: Attitudes to immigration in an international social survey. *Statistics in Transition* **5**, 267–280 (2001)
160. Longford, N. T.: Estimation of the rates and composition of employment in Norwegian municipalities. *Journal of Official Statistics* **17**, 391–406 (2001)
161. Longford, N. T.: Simulation-based diagnostics in random-coefficient models. *Journal of the Royal Statistical Society* Ser. A **164**, 259–273 (2001)
162. Synthetic estimators with moderating influence: the carry-over in cross-over trials revisited. *Statistics in Medicine* **20**, 3189–3203 (2001)
163. Longford, N. T.: An alternative to model selection in ordinary regression. *Statistics and Computing* **13**, 67–80 (2003)
164. Longford, N. T.: Missing data and small-area estimation in the UK Labour Force Survey. *Journal of the Royal Statistical Society* Ser. A **167**, 341–373 (2004)
165. Longford, N. T.: On selection and composition in small area and mapping problems. *Statistical Methods in Medical Research* **14**, 3–16 (2005)
166. Longford, N. T., Ely, M., Hardy, R., and Wadsworth, M. E. J.: Handling missing data in diaries of alcohol consumption. *Journal of the Royal Statistical Society* Ser. A **163**, 381–402 (2000)
167. Longford, N. T., and Macintyre, C.: Mean repair costs of dwellings in Scottish unitary authorities: An application of shrinkage. In: R. Banks et al. (eds), *Leading Survey and Statistical Computing into the New Millenium.* Proceedings of the Third International Conference, pp. 347–354. Association for Survey Computing, Chesham, Bucks (1999)
168. Longva, S., Thomsen, I., and Severeide, P. I.: Reducing costs of censuses in Norway through use of administrative registers. *International Statistical Review* **66**, 223–234 (1998)

169. Louis, T. A.: Finding the observed information matrix when using the EM algorithm. *Journal of the Royal Statistical Society* Ser. B **44**, 226–233 (1982)
170. Lui, K.-J., and Cumberland, W. G.: A model-based approach: composite estimators for small area estimation. *Journal of Official Statistics* **7**, 69–76 (1991)
171. Madow, W. G., Olkin, I., Nisselson, H., and Rubin, D. B. (eds): *Incomplete Data in Sample Surveys.* (Three volumes) Academic Press. New York (1983)
172. Magee, L.: Improving survey-weighted least squares regression. *Journal of the Royal Statistical Society* Ser. B **60**, 115–126 (1998)
173. Magnus, J. R., and Neudecker, H.: *Matrix Differential Calculus with Applications in Statistics and Econometrics.* Wiley, New York (1988)
174. Malec, D., Davis, W. W., and Cao, X.: Model-based small area estimates of overweight prevalence using sample selection adjustment. *Statistics in Medicine* **18**, 3189–3200 (1999)
175. Malec, D., Sedransk, J., Moriarity, C. L., and LeClere, F. B.: Small area inference for binary variables in the National Health Interview Survey. *Journal of the American Statistical Association* **92**, 815–826 (1997)
176. Mallows, C.: Some comments on C_p. *Technometrics* **15**, 661–675 (1973)
177. Mardia, K. V., Kent, J. T., and Bibby, J. M.: *Multivariate Analysis.* Academic Press, London (1979)
178. Marker, D. A.: Organization of small area estimators using a generalized linear regression framework. *Journal of Official Statistics* **15**, 1–24 (1999)
179. Marker, D. A., and Waksberg, J.: Small area estimation for the U. S. National Health Interview Survey. *Statistics in Transition* **1**, 747–768 (1994)
180. McCullagh, P., and Nelder, J. A.: *Generalized Linear Models.* 2nd ed. Chapman and Hall, London (1989)
181. McCulloch, C. E.: Maximum likelihood variance components estimation for binary data. *Journal of the American Statistical Association* **89**, 330–335 (1994)
182. McGibbon, B., and Tomberlin, T. J.: Small area estimates of proportions via empirical Bayes techniques. *Survey Methodology* **15**, 237–252 (1989)
183. McLachlan, G. J., and Krishnan, T.: *The EM Algorithm and Extensions.* Wiley, New York (1997)
184. McLachlan, G., and Peel, D.: *Finite Mixture Models.* Wiley, New York (2000)
185. McLaren, C. E., Wagstaff, M., Brittenham, G. M., and Jacobs, A.: Detection of two-component mixtures of log-normal distributions in grouped, doubly truncated data: Analysis of red blood cell volume distributions. *Biometrics* **47**, 607–622 (1991)
186. Meijlijson, I.: A fast improvement to the EM algorithm on its own terms. *Journal of the Royal Statistical Society* Ser. B **51**, 127–138 (1989)
187. Meng, X.-L.: Multiple imputation with uncongenial sources of input. *Statistical Science* **9**, 538–574 (1994)
188. Meng, X.-L., and van Dyk, D.: The EM algorithm — an old folk-song sung to a fast new tune. *Journal of the Royal Statistical Society* Ser. B **59**, 511–567 (1997)

189. Meng, X.-L., and van Dyk, D.: Fast EM-type implementations for mixed effects models. *Journal of the Royal Statistical Society* Ser. B **60**, 559–578 (1998)
190. Meng, X.-L., and Rubin, D. B.: Using EM to obtain asymptotic variance-covariance matrices: The SEM algorithm. *Journal of the American Statistical Association* **86**, 899–909 (1991)
191. Meng, X.-L., and Rubin, D. B.: Performing likelihood ratio tests with multiply-imputed data sets. *Biometrika* **79**, 103–111 (1992)
192. Molenberghs, G., and Goetghebeur, E.: Simple fitting algorithms for incomplete categorical data. *Journal of the Royal Statistical Society* Ser. B **59**, 401–414 (1997)
193. Molenberghs, G., Kenward, M. G., and Lesaffre, E.: The analysis of longitudinal ordinal data with nonrandom drop-out. *Biometrika* **84**, 33–44 (1997)
194. Morris, C.: Parametric empirical Bayes inference. *Journal of the American Statistical Association* **78**, 47–65 (1983)
195. Myrskylä, P.: Census by questionnaire — Census by registers and administrative records: The experience of Finland. *Journal of Official Statistics* **7**, 457–474 (1991)
196. Navidi, W.: A graphical illustration of the EM algorithm. *American Statistician* **51**, 29–31 (1997)
197. Nelder, J. A., and Pregibon, D.: An extended quasi-likelihood function. *Biometrika* **74**, 221–232 (1987)
198. Nettleton, D.: Convergence properties of the EM algorithm in constrained parameter spaces. *Canadian Journal of Statistics* **27**, 639–648 (1999)
199. Oakes, D.: Direct calculation of the information matrix via the EM algorithm. *Journal of the Royal Statistical Society* Ser. B **61**, 479–482 (1999)
200. Oja, H., Koiranen, M., and Rantakallio, P.: Fitting mixture models to birth weight data: A case study. *Biometrics* **47**, 883–897 (1991)
201. Orchard, T., and Woodbury, M. A.: A missing information principle: Theory and applications. In: *Proceedings of the 6th Berkeley Symposium on Mathematical Statistics and Probability*, Vol. 1., pp. 697–715. University of California, Berkeley, CA. (1972)
202. Pan, W., and Kooperberg, C.: Linear regression for bivariate censored data via multiple imputation. *Statistics in Medicine* **18**, 3111–3121 (1999)
203. Park, T., and Brown, M. B.: Models for categorical data with nonignorable nonresponse. *Journal of the American Statistical Association* **89**, 44–52 (1994)
204. Patterson, H. D., and Thompson, R.: Recovery of inter-block information when block sizes are unequal. *Biometrika* **58**, 545–554 (1971)
205. Pfeffermann, D., and Barnard, C. H.: Some new estimators for small-area means with application to the assessment of farmland values. *Journal of Business and Economic Statistics* **9**, 73–84 (1991)
206. Pfeffermann, D., and Bleuer, S. R.: Robust joint modelling of labour force series of small areas. *Survey Methodology* **19**, 149–163 (1993)
207. Pfeffermann, D., and Burck, L.: Robust small area estimation combining time series and cross-sectional data. *Survey Methodology* **16**, 217–237 (1990)

208. Pfeffermann, D., Feder, M., and Signorelli, D.: Estimation of autocorrelations of survey errors with application to trend estimation in small areas. *Journal of Business and Economic Statistics* **16**, 339–348 (1998)
209. Pinheiro, J. C., and Bates, D. M.: *Mixed-effects Models in S and S-plus.* Springer, New York (2000)
210. Platek, R., Rao, J. N. K., Särndal, C.-E., and Singh, M. P. (eds): *Small Area Statistics. An International Symposium.* Wiley, New York (1987)
211. Potthoff, R. F., Woodbury, M. A., and Manton, K. G.: "Equivalent sample size" and "equivalent degrees of freedom" refinements for inference using survey weights under superpopulation models. *Journal of the American Statistical Association* **87**, 383–396 (1992)
212. Prasad, N. G. N., and Rao, J. N. K.: The estimation of the mean squared error of small-area estimators. *Journal of the American Statistical Association* **85**, 163–171 (1990)
213. Purcell, N. J., and Kish, L.: Estimation for small domains. *Biometrics* **35**, 365–384 (1979)
214. Purcell, N. J., and Kish, L.: Postcensal estimates for local areas (or domains). *International Statistical Review* **48**, 3–18 (1980)
215. R Development Core Team: R: A language and environment for statistical computing. R Foundation for Statistical Computing, Vienna, Austria (2004)
216. Raftery, A. E., Madigan, D., and Hoeting, J. A.: Bayesian model averaging for linear regression models. *Journal of the American Statistical Association* **92**, 179–191 (1997)
217. Raghunathan, T., E.: A quasi-empirical Bayes method for small area estimation. *Journal of the American Statistical Association* **88**, 1444–1448 (1993)
218. Raghunathan, T., E., Lepkowski, J., van Hoewyk, J., and Solenberger, P. W.: A multivariate technique for multiply imputing missing values using a sequence of regression models. *Survey Methodology* **27**, 85–95 (2001)
219. Rai, S. N., and Matthews, D. E.: Improving the EM algorithm. *Biometrics* **49**, 587–591 (1993)
220. Ramsay, J. O., and Silverman, B. W.: *Functional Data Analysis.* Springer, New York (1997)
221. Rao, J. N. K.: On variance estimation with imputed survey data. *Journal of the American Statistical Association* **91**, 499–506 (1996)
222. Rao, J. N. K.: Some recent advances in model-based small area estimation. *Survey Methodology* **25**, 175–186 (1999)
223. Rao, J. N. K.: *Small Area Estimation.* Wiley, New York (2003)
224. Redfern, P.: An alternative view of the 2001 census and future census taking. *Journal of the Royal Statistical Society* Ser. A **167**, 209–228 (2004)
225. Reilly, M.: Data analysis using hot-deck multiple imputation. *The Statistician* **42**, 307–313 (1993)
226. Robinson, G. K.: That BLUP is a good thing: The estimation of random effects. *Statistical Science* **6**, 15–32 (1991)
227. Rodríguez, G., and Goldman, N.: An assessment of estimation procedures for multilevel models with binary responses. *Journal of the Royal Statistical Society* Ser. A **158**, 73–89 (1995)
228. Rosenbaum, P. R.: *Observational Studies.* Springer, New York (1995)
229. Rubin, D. B.: Inference and missing data. *Biometrika* **63**, 581–592 (1976)

230. Rubin, D. B.: Formalizing subjective notions about the effect of nonrespondents in sample surveys. *Journal of the American Statistical Association* **72**, 538–543 (1977)
231. Rubin, D. B.: Using empirical Bayes techniques in the law school validity studies. *Journal of the American Statistical Association* **75**, 801–827 (1980)
232. Rubin, D. B.: Bayesianly justifiable and relevant frequency calculations for the applied statistician. *Annals of Statistics* **12**, 1151–1172 (1984)
233. Rubin, D. B.: *Multiple Imputation for Nonresponse in Surveys.* Wiley, New York (1987)
234. Rubin, D. B.: EM and beyond. *Psychomctrika* **56**, 241–254 (1991)
235. Rubin, D. B.: Computational aspects of analysing random effects/longitudinal models. *Statistics in Medicine* **11**, 1809–1821 (1992)
236. Rubin, D. B.: Satisfying confidentiality constraints through the use of synthetic multiply-imputed micro-data. *Journal of Official Statistics* **9**, 461–468 (1993)
237. Rubin, D. B.: Multiple imputation after 18+ years. *Journal of the American Statistical Association* **91**, 473–489 (1996)
238. Rubin, D. B., and Schenker, N.: Multiple imputation in health-care databases: an overview and some applications. *Statistics in Medicine* **10**, 585–598 (1991)
239. Rubin, D. B., Stern, H., and Vehovar, V.: Handling "Don't know" survey responses: The case of Slovenian plebiscite. *Journal of the American Statistical Association* **90**, 822–828 (1995)
240. Rubin, D. B., and Thomas, N.: Matching using estimated propensity scores: Relating theory to practice. *Biometrics* **52**, 249–264 (1996)
241. Särndal, C.-E.: Design-consistent versus model-dependent estimation for small domains. *Journal of the American Statistical Association* **80**, 624–631 (1984)
242. Särndal, C.-E., Swensson, B., and Wretman, J.: *Model Assisted Survey Sampling.* Springer, New York (1992)
243. Schafer, J. L.: *Analysis of Incomplete Multivariate Data.* Chapman and Hall, London (1996)
244. Schafer, J. L.: Multiple imputation: A primer. *Statistical Methods in Medical Research* **8**, 3–15 (1999)
245. Schafer, J. L., and Olsen, M. K.: Multiple imputation for multivariate missing-data problems: A data analyst's perspective. *Multivariate Behavioral Research* **33**, 545–571 (1998)
246. Schaible, W. L. (ed.): *Indirect Estimators in U. S. Federal Programs.* Lecture Notes in Statistics. Springer, New York (1995)
247. Schenker, N., Treiman, D. J., and Weidmann, L.: Analyses of Public Use Decennial Census Data with multiply imputed industry and occupation codes. *Applied Statistics* **42**, 545–556 (1990)
248. Schirm, L. A., and Preston, S. H.: Census undercount adjustment and the quality of geographic population data. *Journal of the American Statistical Association* **82**, 965–978 (1987)
249. Scottish Homes: *Scottish House Condition Survey. Main Report 1996.* Scottish Homes, Edinburgh (1997)
250. Searle, S. R.: *Matrix Algebra Useful for Statistics.* Wiley, New York (1982)
251. Searle, S. R.: *Linear Models for Unbalanced Data.* Wiley, New York (1987)

252. Searle, S. R., and Henderson, H. V.: Dispersion matrices for variance component models. *Journal of the American Statistical Association* **74**, 465–470 (1979)
253. Seber, G. A. F.: *Linear Regression Analysis.* Wiley, New York (1977)
254. Segal, M. R., Bacchetti, P., and Jewell, N. P.: Variances for maximum penalized likelihood estimates obtained via the EM algorithm. *Journal of the Royal Statistical Society* Ser. B **56** 345–352 (1994)
255. Shao, J.: An asymptotic theory for linear model selection. *Statistica Sinica* **7**, 221–264 (1997)
256. Shen, W., and Louis, T. A.: Triple-goal estimates in two-stage hierarchical models. *Journal of the Royal Statistical Society* Ser. B **60**, 455–471 (1998)
257. Simpson, S., Diamond, I., Tonkin, P., and Tye, R.: Updating small area population estimates in England and Wales. *Journal of the Royal Statistical Society* Ser. A **159**, 235–247 (1996)
258. Singh, A. C., Stukel, D. M., and Pfeffermann, D.: Bayesian *versus* frequentist measures of error in small area estimation. *Journal of the Royal Statistical Society* Ser. B **60**, 377–396 (1998)
259. Singh, M. P., Gambino, J., and Mantel, H. J.: Issues and strategies for small area data. *Survey Methodology* **20**, 3–22 (1994)
260. Spiegelhalter, D., J., Aylin, P., Best, N. G., Evans, S. J. W., and Murray, G. D.: Commissioned analysis of surgical performance using routine data: Lessons from the Bristol inquiry. *Journal of the Royal Statistical Society* Ser. A **165**, 191–231 (2002)
261. Spiess, M., and Keller, F.: A mixed approach and a distribution-free multiple imputation technique for the estimation of a multivariate probit model with missing values. *British Journal of Mathematical and Statistical Psychology* **52**, 1–17 (1999)
262. Stasny, E. A.: Hierarchical models for the probabilities of a survey classification and nonresponse: An example from the National Crime Survey. *Journal of the American Statistical Association* **86**, 296–303 (1991)
263. Statistica Sinica: Special issue on the EM algorithm. *Statistica Sinica* **5**, 1–107 (1995)
264. Stein, C.: Inadmissibility of the usual estimator for the mean of a multivariate normal distribution. In: *Proceedings of the 3rd Berkeley Symposium on Mathematical Statistics and Probability*, Vol. 1, pp. 197–202. University of California Press, Berkeley, CA. (1955)
265. Stone, M.: An asymptotic equivalence of choice of model by cross-validation and Akaike's criterion. *Journal of the Royal Statistical Society* Ser. B **39**, 44–47 (1997)
266. *Survey Methodology*: Volume 1, pp. 1–74 (2001)
267. Swensen, A. R.: Estimating change in a proportion by combining measurements from a true and a fallible classifier. *Scandinavian Journal of Statistics* **15**, 139–145 (1988)
268. Tanner, M. A.: *Tools for Statistical Inference. Methods for the Exploration of Posterior Distributions and Likelihood Functions.* 2nd ed. Springer, New York (1993)
269. Tanner, M. A., and Wong, W. H.: The calculation of posterior distribution by data augmentation. *Journal of the American Statistical Association* **82**, 528–550 (1987)

270. Thisted, R. A.: *Elements of Statistical Computing*. Chapman and Hall, London (1988)
271. Thomas, N., Longford, N. T., and Rolph, J. E.: Empirical Bayes methods for estimating hospital specific mortality rates. *Statistics in Medicine* **13**, 889–903 (1994)
272. Thompson, E. J.: The 1991 census of population in England and Wales. *Journal of the Royal Statistical Society* Ser. A **158**, 203–240 (1995)
273. Thompson, J. R.: Some shrinkage techniques for estimating the mean. *Journal of the American Statistical Association* **63**, 113–122 (1968)
274. Thompson, M. E.: *Theory of Sample Surveys*. Chapman and Hall, London (1997)
275. Thomsen, I., and Holmøy, A. M. K.: Combining data from surveys and administrative record systems. The Norwegian experience. *International Statistical Review* **66**, 201–221 (1998)
276. Thomsen, I., and Zhang, L.-C.: The effects of using administrative registers in economic short term statistics: The Norwegian Labour Force Survey as a case study. *Journal of Official Statistics* **17**, 285–294 (2001)
277. Tršinar, I.: The central register of population of the Republic of Slovenia *Journal of Official Statistics* **11**, 221–223 (1995)
278. Tsutakawa, R. K.: Mixed model for analyzing geographic variability in mortality rates. *Journal of the American Statistical Association* **83**, 37–42 (1988)
279. Venables, W. N., and Ripley, B. D.: *Modern Applied Statistics with S-Plus*. 4th ed. Springer, New York (2002)
280. Villar, J., Mackey, M. E., Carroli, G., Donner, A.: Meta-analyses in systematic reviews of randomized controlled trials in perinatal medicine: comparison of fixed and random effects models. *Statistics in Medicine* **20**, 3635–3647 (2001)
281. Walker, S.: An EM algorithm for nonlinear random effects models. *Biometrics* **52**, 934–944 (1996)
282. Wang, N., and Robins, J.: Large-sample theory for parametric multiple imputation procedures. *Biometrika* **85**, 935–948 (1998)
283. Wasserman, L.: Bayesian model selection and model averaging. *Journal of Mathematical Psychology* **44**, 92–107 (2000)
284. Wei, G. C. G., and Tanner, M. A.: A Monte Carlo implementation of the EM algorithm and the poor man's data augmentation algorithms. *Journal of the American Statistical Association* **85**, 699–704 (1990)
285. Wolter, K. M.: *Introduction to Variance Estimation*. Springer, New York (1985)
286. Wolter, K. M., and Causey, B. D.: Evaluation of procedures for improving population estimates for small areas. *Journal of the American Statistical Association* **86**, 278–284 (1991)
287. Zhang, L.-C., and Chambers, R. (2004) Small area estimates for cross-classifications. *Journal of the Royal Statistical Society* Ser. B **66**, 479–496 (2004)
288. Zhang, P.: Inference after variable selection in linear regression models. *Biometrika* **79**, 741–746 (1992)

Index

BUGS, 139
Gauss, 16
IVEware, 139
MICE, 139
MLwin, 205
R, 15, 139
SAS, 139
SPSS, 139
Solas, 139
Splus, 15, 139
matlab, 16

Akaike information criterion (AIC), 149, 305, 334
ANCOVA (analysis of covariance), 176
ANOVA (analysis of variance), 149, 173, 205, 316
apportionment method, 210
asymptotic, 239
auxiliary
  data, 207
  information, 176, 207, 221, 292, 333
  variable, 33, 181, 207, 221

Bayes
  factor, 311, 334
  information criterion (BIC), 305, 334
  prior, 86
  theorem, 12, 81, 134
bootstrap, 267

censoring, 85
census, 224, 276, 283, 291
  undercount, 170
chained equations, 71
choice
  tailored, 150
  uniform, 149
Cholesky decomposition, 191
coarse data, 84
complete data, 22, 52
  analysis, 37, 54
  estimator, 51, 59, 64
  information, 55
  likelihood, 54
  model, 61
  statistic, 59
  variance, 64
complete information, 52
completed data, 38, 64
  analysis, 64
composite estimator, 151, 212, 240
  ideal, 159, 217
composition, 151, 211, 223, 246
  bivariate, 218
  ideal, 171
  multivariate, 215
  univariate, 217
confidence
  interval, 8, 117
  limit, 8
coverage rate, 8

data
  completion, 40
  editing, 48, 60, 90
  reduction, 37, 39
density

joint, 54
direct
estimator, 147
information, 207
discrepancy statistic, 291
distribution
χ^2, 171, 193, 252, 294, 309
F-, 321
t-, 8
asymptotic, 193
beta, 206
binomial, 127, 202
gamma, 171, 206
log-normal, 114
multinomial, 68, 102, 223
Poisson, 164, 171, 202
posterior, 333
prior, 333
Wishart, 67, 186
district-level
model, 180, 197, 204
variance, 160
donor, 42, 75
pool, 43, 75, 103

E-step (EM algorithm), 54
efficiency, 8
asymptotic, 182
EM algorithm, 53, 114, 269, 307
empirical density, 268
eMSE (expected mean squared error), 154
enumeration, 11
error contrasts, 186
estimate, 4
estimation process, 5
estimator, 4
class, 11
complete-data, 51
minimax, 318
national, 147
selected-model based, 307
single-model based, 306
type, 10
compatible, 10
exponential family, 201

feature, 197, 245
multi-, 197
random, 173
systematic, 173
Fisher scoring algorithm, 54, 186, 202
fraction of the information lost, 55, 66, 116
functional data analysis, 270

Gibbs sampler, 71
GLM (generalised linear models), 47, 200
GMLM (generalised mixed linear models), 235

Hessian matrix, 184, 203
hot deck, 43, 75, 101, 103
multivariate, 76
hypothesis test, 149, 192, 305

ignorable
mechanism, 62
nonresponse, 78
imputation, 27, 37
by experts, 47
deterministic, 40
horizontal, 42
mean, 40
multi-stage, 69, 110
multiple (MI), 51, 59
nearest-neighbour, 42, 75
proper, 66, 103, 114
regression, 45
single, 37, 48, 52
stochastic, 40, 103
vertical, 42
incomplete
data, 19, 22, 52, 292
information, 15, 29
information
complete, 52
complete-data, 55
incomplete, 15, 29
matrix, 204
expected, 184
observed, 184
missing, 55
fraction of, 55, 66, 116
ISSP (International Social Survey Programme), 119
iteratively reweighted least squares, 202

jackknife, 155

kernel density estimation, 268

Labour Force Survey (LFS), 41, 97, 257
latent variable, 11
likelihood
  h-, 235
  complete-data, 54
  ratio, 192
link
  canonical, 202
  function, 201
  identity, 202
  log, 202
  logit, 202
listwise deletion, 127
LOCF (last observation carried forward), 41, 100
log-likelihood, 54

M-step (EM algorithm), 54
Mallows' C_p, 334
manifest variable, 11, 29
  parallel, 17
MAR (missing at random), 30, 52, 62, 111, 124
  direction of departure from, 78
  extent of departure from, 78
match, 43
matching variable, 103
MCAR (missing completely at random), 30, 52
MCMC (Markov chain Monte Carlo) method, 139
measurement process, 80
messy data, 15
meta-analysis, 331
MI (multiple imputation), 51, 59, 240, 270
MI estimator, 64
minimax
  estimator, 318
  property, 225
misclassification, 83, 130
  process, 83
missing
  data, 13
    extent of, 21
    pattern of, 21
  information, 55
    fraction of, 55, 66, 116
  values
    extent of, 19
    pattern of, 19
mixture (distribution), 114, 307
ML (maximum likelihood), 54, 182
MSE (mean squared error), 5, 148, 155
multi-feature, 197

national estimator, 147
Newton method, 231
Newton-Raphson algorithm, 54, 184, 235
NMAR (not missing at random), 31, 52, 62, 72, 78, 107, 121, 127
  extreme, 127
non-informative process, 245
nonresponse, 20
  item, 23
  mechanism, 30, 114
  model, 61
  process, 19, 22, 28, 52
  rate, 21
  unit, 23
NSHD (National Survey of Health and Development), 110
nuisance parameter, 331
numerical quadrature, 203

ordering, 241

parallel regressions, 177, 194
pattern-mixture model, 61
personalisation, 245
plausible
  category, 67
  cost, 138
  distribution, 66, 103
  map, 271
  model, 62
  parameter, 63
  probability, 77
  score, 133, 137
  value, 12, 63, 103
  variance matrix, 67
  vector, 240
population quantity, 3, 22
poststratification, 44

prior
  distribution, 333
  information, 332
priority exponent, 230
process
  assessment, 29
  data collection, 80, 173
  data generating, 28
  data inspection, 244
  estimation, 5, 303
  imputation, 52
  measurement, 80
  misclassification, 17, 83
  model selection, 306
  non-informative, 245
  nonresponse, 19, 22, 28, 52
  nuisance, 52
  sampling, 5, 22, 28, 52, 144
  stochastic, 28
profile likelihood, 194
propensity
  interval, 77
  score, 77
proper imputation, 66, 103, 114

raking, 45
rANCOVA (ANCOVA with random effects), 177
random coefficient model, 177, 197
random-effect model, 91
random-intercept model, 177
ranking, 240, 241, 254
rANOVA (ANOVA with random effects), 174, 205, 308, 323
recipient, 42, 75
record
  complete, 23
  empty, 23
  incomplete, 23
  partial, 23
register, 224, 258, 282
regression part, 179
relative
  precision, 253
  slope, 326
REML (restricted maximum likelihood), 186, 199, 203
residual
  district-level, 196
  subject-level, 196
response
  indicator, 24, 61
  pattern, 24, 121, 124
    group-monotone, 71
    model for, 61
    monotone, 26, 70, 114
  probability of, 31
rMSE (root-MSE), 6
RSE (relative standard error), 284

sample
  quantity, 4, 22
  realised, 4
  representative, 20
  size, planned, 22
sample-completion design, 90
Samples of Anonymised Records (SAR), 276
sampling
  design
    clustered, 98
    planned, 20
    realised, 20
    rotating panel, 97
    systematic, 291
  frame, 16
  mechanism, 3
  process, 5, 22, 28, 52
    quantity, 7, 22
score pattern, 76
score vector, 184, 190
Scottish House Condition Survey (SHCS), 130, 291
selection
  bias, 90
  indicator, 306
  model, 61
sensitivity analysis, 78, 117, 127, 260, 266, 334
separated parameters, 62, 69
shrinkage, 155, 214, 291
  coefficient, 153, 247
    plausible, 241
  estimator, 82, 152, 247
    ideal, 247
    univariate, 221
  matrix, 217
  multivariate, 221, 262

similarity, 144
small area, 143
stratification, 30, 90
  more detailed, 30
subject-level model, 180
sufficient statistics, 53
  minimal, 53
superpopulation, 268
synthetic estimator, 208, 313
  ideal, 314

target, 4
  variable, 181
Taylor expansion, 135, 253
transition probability, 83
two-level
  GLM, 202
  model, 177, 180, 195, 203, 208

UK Labour Force Survey (LFS), 41, 97, 257
UK Women's Cohort Survey, 39

valid model, 304
  minimal, 306
variance
  between-imputation, 64, 138
  district-level, 147
  function, 202
  matrix
    scaled, 181, 198, 213
  ratio, 175, 198, 324
  within-district, 150
variation
  associated with, 179
  part, 179